Prosthetics and Orthotics for Physical Therapists

Prosthetics and Orthotics for Physical Therapists provides physical therapy students, physical therapists, and other allied health clinicians with foundational knowledge in prosthetic and orthotic (P&O) topics. The text and its resources are efficient, impactful, and affordable, including an overview of the history of amputation, artificial limb, prosthetic, and orthotic concepts followed by a review of professional and education concepts related to P&O.

Prosthetics and Orthotics for Physical Therapists is divided into two section: first, Prosthetics and second, Orthotics. The Prosthetics section includes chapters on amputation epidemiology, related surgical concepts, componentry, gait, therapy, outcomes, dermatologic considerations as well as lower and upper extremity amputation principles and concepts. In the Orthotics section, there is an overview of pathology, and chapters on orthotic principles primarily by body region including below and above the knee, spinal and chest, cranial and upper extremity.

Key features and benefits of the book include the concise but clinically focused topics which are supported by evidence when available, and the covering of historic concepts through to the latest topics such as osseointegration and microprocessor-controlled devices. The organization by prosthetic and orthotic divisions, the anatomic and regional body section divisions, and the special topics (i.e. history, epidemiology, education, others) allows discrete compartmentalization of vast content.

This cutting-edge new textbook is ideal for entry level clinicians in training such as physical therapists, occupational therapists, physicians, prosthetists/orthotists or others in physical rehabilitative disciplines. Additionally, the book may serve well as a desk reference for clinicians who may not be specialized in P&O care but manage patients who utilize P&O devices.

M. Jason Highsmith is a dual-licensed physical therapist and prosthetist. He is also a medical scientist with a concentration in clinical trials and patient-oriented translational research. He served in a few positions with the U.S. Department of Veterans Affairs including service as a research physical therapist, the Deputy Chief of Research for the congressionally mandated dual agency VA-DoD Extremity Trauma & Amputation Center of Excellence (EACE) and he currently serves as National Director of the Orthotic, Prosthetic & Pedorthic Clinical Services Program Office.

Prosthetics and Orthotics for Physical Therapists

Edited by M. Jason Highsmith

Routledge
Taylor & Francis Group

NEW YORK AND LONDON

Designed cover image: Tinhouse Design

First published 2025
by Routledge
605 Third Avenue, New York, NY 10158

and by Routledge
4 Park Square, Milton Park, Abingdon, Oxon, OX14 4RN

Routledge is an imprint of the Taylor & Francis Group, an informa business

ISBN: 9781630912512 (hbk)
ISBN: 9781041024279 (pbk)
ISBN: 9781003526025 (ebk)

DOI: 10.4324/9781003526025

Typeset in Minion Pro
by codeMantra

Access the Support Material: www.routledge.com/9781041024279

To my wife Kimberlee—none of this would have been possible without your unwavering support. To my three sons, Lance, Toby, and Miles—you too have sacrificed during this time. I hope one day, you too will become critical thinkers and hard workers and use your talents to help others.

CONTENTS

FIGURES

TABLES

ABOUT THE EDITOR

M. Jason Highsmith is a dual-licensed physical therapist and prosthetist. He is also a medical scientist with a concentration in clinical trials and patient-oriented translational research. He served in a few positions with the U.S. Department of Veterans Affairs including service as a research physical therapist, the Deputy Chief of Research for the congressionally mandated dual agency VA-DoD Extremity Trauma & Amputation Center of Excellence (EACE) and he currently serves as National Director of the Orthotic, Prosthetic & Pedorthic Clinical Services Program Office. Dr. Highsmith began his career in academia at the University of South Florida's (USF) School of Physical Therapy & Rehabilitation Sciences (SPTRS) which is housed within the Morsani College of Medicine in Tampa, FL. He currently maintains a joint appointment there as a Research Professor. Dr. Highsmith serves in the U.S. Army Reserves as a physical therapist, currently at the rank of Major and has held multiple positions in his military career including serving as a clinical physical therapist, Executive Officer and Commander of the 319th Minimal Care Detachment. He has served the profession of orthotics and prosthetics as a research council chair, board member, executive board member and is a past-president of the American Academy of Orthotists & Prosthetists (AAOP). Dr. Highsmith has earned many awards including the American Physical Therapy's Margaret L. Moore Award for Outstanding New Academic Faculty, the USF SPTRS Student Choice Award, the AAOP Research Award and the Force for Good Award from the University of St. Augustine. Militarily, he has received an Army Commendation Medal, multiple Army Achievement Medals and the Army Reserve Component Achievement Medal.

Dr. Highsmith has contributed to and led the development of numerous Clinical Practice Guidelines, Clinical Practice Recommendations, Systematic Reviews, Meta Analyses, and patient facing periodicals. Dr. Highsmith holds two U.S. Patents on artificial limb component designs in partnership with USF. In his personal life, he is married with three sons who all play baseball. He has enjoyed coaching and contributing to the development of his sons and their teammates, many of whom have gone on to play at the high school and collegiate levels.

FOREWORD

We are greatly honored to introduce this essential, groundbreaking work, *Prosthetics and Orthotics for Physical Therapists*, edited by Dr. M. Jason Highsmith, PhD, PT, DPT, CP, FAAOP, a renowned expert whose dedication to advancing the scholarship and clinical practice of prosthetics, orthotics, and physical therapy has shaped the lives of countless individuals, especially those who have served our country. In this first edition, Dr. Highsmith brings together a wealth of knowledge and expertise that will undoubtedly serve as a key resource for practitioners dedicated to improving the care of individuals with limb loss and disabilities.

As physical therapists, we have the privilege and responsibility of not only restoring function but also enhancing the quality of life for our patients. Whether working with those who have undergone amputation or those who live with musculoskeletal and/or neurological pathologies that require orthotic intervention, the role of the physical therapist is critical in achieving optimal outcomes. This text meticulously explores the dynamic interplay between prosthetics, orthotics, and the biomechanics of the movement systems, making it a comprehensive resource for those who wish to deepen their understanding and refine their clinical skills.

The trajectory of Dr. Highsmith's impressive career has spanned both clinical practice and cutting-edge research, making him an unparalleled authority in the intersection of physical therapy and prosthetics/orthotics. As a dual-licensed physical therapist and prosthetist, he brings a unique perspective to the professions—one informed by both hands-on clinical experience and scientific research. His remarkable journey began as a Journeyman Ironworker in Local 397 (Tampa, FL), applying mechanical acumen, cutting, welding, and fitting steel beams and girders to build, repair, and maintain structures, often while safely rappelling. As a Journeyman, Dr. Highsmith laid the foundation to apply this skill set, for his later passion for rehabilitation sciences and patient care through biomechanical analyses of movement. However, it is his extensive work advancing care for Warriors and Veterans, particularly during the 20-year War in Afghanistan (2001–21), Operation Enduring Freedom, that truly sets him apart.

Throughout his career, Dr. Highsmith has been deeply committed to improving the lives of Veterans who have experienced traumatic injuries, including amputations, as a result of their service. His contributions to the U.S. Department of Veterans Affairs (VA) have been profound. Dr. Highsmith's service in key roles, including as a research physical therapist, the Deputy Chief of Research for the VA-Department of Defense, Extremity Trauma & Amputation Center of Excellence (EACE), and currently as the National Director of the Orthotic, Prosthetic & Pedorthic Clinical Services Program Office, VA (Central Office). Through these positions, Dr. Highsmith has had a direct hand in shaping the rehabilitation and care of Veterans, ensuring they receive the best possible treatments and outcomes following their injuries.

Dr. Highsmith's dedication to advancing care for Veterans is reflected in his military service as well. As a U.S. Army Reserve Physical Therapist, he has served in multiple positions, including Clinical Physical Therapist, Executive Officer, and Commander of the 319th Minimal Care Detachment. His leadership in these roles has been instrumental in providing care to military personnel who have sustained injuries during deployment, many of which require complex prosthetic and orthotic interventions.

Beyond his work with Veterans, Dr. Highsmith has made significant contributions to the academic and research communities. He began his academic career at the University of South Florida's School of Physical Therapy & Rehabilitation Sciences (SPTRS) and currently holds a joint appointment there as a Research Professor with the Morsani School of Medicine, Department of Neurology. His research, funded by agencies such as the Department of Defense, the Department of Veterans Affairs, and the National Institutes of Health, has led to over $6 million in extramural funding and has contributed to the development of numerous clinical practice guidelines, recommendations, and systematic reviews that shape modern rehabilitation practices.

As a result of his work, Dr. Highsmith has received numerous accolades, including the prestigious American Physical Therapy's Margaret L. Moore Award for Outstanding New Academic Faculty (2012), the American Academy of Orthotists & Prosthetists (AAOP) Research Award (2016), and multiple military honors, including the Army Commendation Medal. His contributions to evidence-based practice for the health professions, are reflected in over 75 peer-reviewed manuscripts, contributions to key reference texts, and two U.S. patents related to highly innovative artificial limb component designs while mentoring with Dr. Derek James Lura, PhD, ME, Florida Gulf Coast University and in partnership with Dr. Murray Maitland, PT, PhD, FAPTA, University of Washington, Department of Rehabilitation Medicine, Division of Physical Therapy.

This book reflects Dr. Highsmith's deep commitment to improving the lives of those living with amputation and disability, especially those who have served in the military. It presents both a comprehensive guide for the applications of prosthetics and orthotics for enhanced movement and function, along with a heartfelt dedication to the people who have sacrificed for their country. In *Prosthetics and Orthotics for Physical Therapists*, Dr. Highsmith not only shares his wealth of knowledge, and prolific scholarship with peer-reviewed evidence in support of the work; but also, his passion for enhancing the rehabilitation process, helping clinicians provide the best care possible in collaboration with their patients/clients.

Dr. Highsmith, with his extensive academic background and clinical expertise, has compiled a team of contributors who bring diverse perspectives to this text. The combination of theoretical knowledge and practical guidance makes this book a valuable resource for physical therapists at all stages of their careers, from students to seasoned professionals. With its in-depth coverage and clear, evidence-informed approach, *Prosthetics and Orthotics for Physical Therapists* is sure to become a trusted reference with future editions to follow as the world reaps the benefits of Artificial Intelligence and developments in bioengineering. As the scope of prosthetics and orthotics continues to progress, this text will be an indispensable resource for those dedicated to improving the lives of patients and advancing the profession.

The book is divided into two comprehensive sections: Prosthetics and Orthotics. In Section I, the focus is on prosthetics, where the reader is guided through the history, the intricacies of amputation surgery, functional levels of amputees, and the physical therapy required for rehabilitation. From understanding prosthetic componentry to learning about the gait patterns of lower extremity amputees, each chapter is rich with practical insights and evidence-based approaches. Additionally, the psychosocial aspects of amputation—often overlooked in clinical practice—are addressed, ensuring that the emotional and mental health of the patient is given equal attention to their physical rehabilitation.

Section II shifts its focus to orthotics, providing a thorough overview of the pathologies for which orthoses are commonly recommended. The chapters delve into various orthotic devices, from lower extremity orthoses to spinal and chest orthoses, and even extend to cranial and upper extremity orthoses. Each chapter is precisely written, ensuring that practitioners are equipped with the knowledge necessary to effectively manage orthotic treatments and tailor them to the individual needs of their patients.

Prosthetics and Orthotics for Physical Therapists serves as both an educational tool and a practical guide. It invites physical and occupational therapists, prosthetists and orthotists to expand their knowledge, refine their clinical skills, and enhance their ability to work collaboratively with bioengineers and other healthcare professionals in delivering holistic patient care. Educators, especially in physical therapy, will find the text an essential guide for prosthetics and orthotics content; gifted with the educational resources of PowerPoint presentations and teaching tips from seasoned specialists.

Dr. Highsmith, a beloved husband, dedicated father, and frequent runner, has also gone the distance with his co-authors to provide a contemporary, catalyzing resource. Dr. Highsmith's vigilant attention to detail, combined with his passion for both patient care and education, ensures that this book is more than just a textbook—it is a *call to action*. As physical therapists, we have the power to make a profound impact on the lives of those we serve, and this book equips us with the knowledge to do so.

Whether you are a student, an experienced clinician, or a researcher, this book is a valuable resource that will deepen your understanding of the complexities involved in the care of individuals requiring prosthetic and orthotic interventions. Dr. Highsmith's work stands as a testament to the power of collaboration, compassion, and innovation in improving patient outcomes, particularly for those who have borne the weight of service to our nation.

It is with great enthusiasm and gratitude that we recommend *Prosthetics and Orthotics for Physical Therapists*. This book is sure to become a cornerstone resource for the health professions and a lasting tribute to the individuals who have inspired Dr. Highsmith's remarkable career. We wholeheartedly recommend *Prosthetics and Orthotics for Physical Therapists* as an invaluable resource for all professionals involved in the care and rehabilitation of individuals with prosthetic and orthotic needs.

Gina Maria Musolino, PT, DPT, EdD, MSEd
Clinical Professor, Director of Curriculum
University of Florida
Department of Physical Therapy
College of Public Health & Health Professions
Gainesville, FL

William S. Quillen, PT, DPT, PhD, SCS, FACSM
Professor Emeritus
University of South Florida USF Health
School of Physical Therapy & Rehabilitation Sciences
Morsani College of Medicine
Tampa, FL /Key West - retired

Acknowledgements

To the many co-authors and contributors of this comprehensive work. This journey was long, but your commitment, effort, and intellectual contributions have produced a work that will help rehabilitative clinicians to better serve the patients and communities they practice within. Hopefully, their patients are the true benefactors of your efforts. There are no words to adequately show my appreciation. You will always have my deepest gratitude and respect.

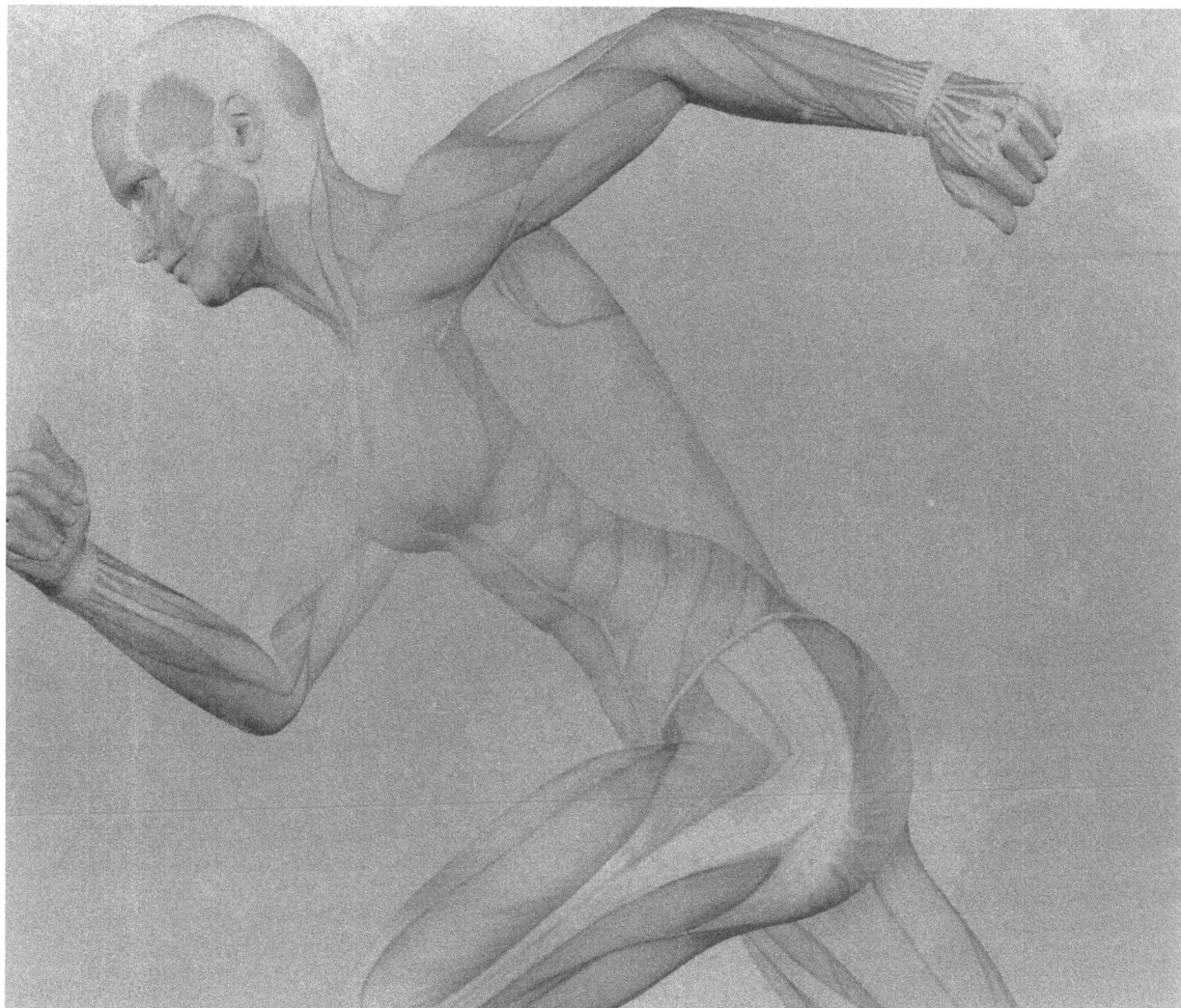

PROSTHETICS

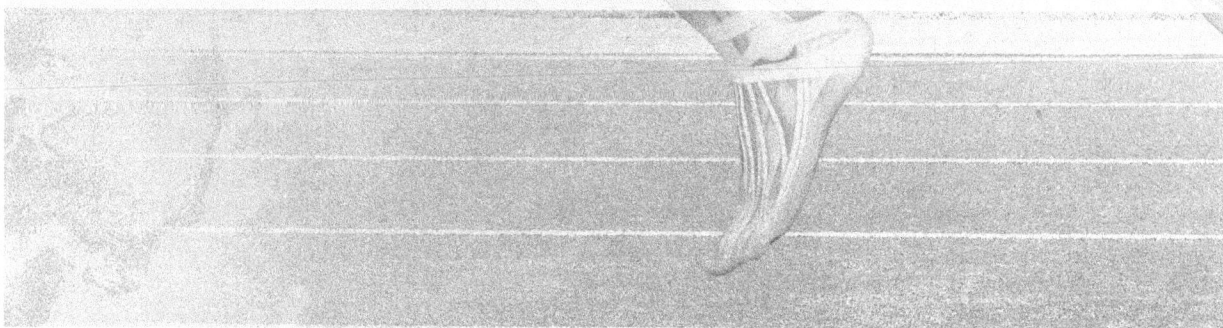

CHAPTER 1

History of Prosthetics and Orthotics

Amanda Lewandowski and Donald Shurr

OBJECTIVES

Upon completion of this chapter, the reader should be able to:
1. Describe the early history of prosthetics and orthotics.
2. Describe various surgical techniques used in early times, and surgical advances over time.
3. Discuss the contributions made to the field during and following major wars.
4. Understand the different professional organizations and professional publications for prosthetists and orthotists.
5. Describe recent advances in prosthetics and orthotics.

EARLY HISTORY

Amputations have been in practice for thousands of years. The earliest known amputations are evidenced by "negative imprints" on the walls of caves in France and Spain. These show paint applied around a hand that was "mutilated," due to the loss of part or all of a finger. These drawings date back to 5000 BC [1]. Amputations were thought to be due to rituals or religious practices of primitive cultures [1].

Amputations were carried out for a variety of reasons. Certain historic tribes would perform ritual amputations in order to ward off evil spirits, and the amputated digits would sometimes be used to create "potions" to prevent evil. Another reason for amputation was as a punishment

for a crime, such as robbery, adultery, or arson. Certain cultures believed that amputation was worse than death, as it affected the "spirit" life after death and, as such, it was used as a punishment. Amputation for judicial reasons was the most common cause of amputation in the Arabic Middle East [1]. Yet another reason for these early amputations was to count prisoners. In this case, the amputation was frequently of a digit or the whole hand, as an amputation of the leg would leave the individual unable to work [2].

Sculptures and pottery from as early as 1500 BC show evidence of individuals with congenital limb loss. Unfortunately, because in some of these cultures congenital amputations were considered a sort of punishment of the child's parents, many of these infants did not survive. One culture in which these infants were allowed to survive was

DOI: 10.4324/9781003526025-2

that of the Aztecs, the inhabitants of Mexico from 900 to 1519 CE. They felt that their god Xolotl produced these "deformities," and consequently paid special attention to these babies [1].

Greek physician and philosopher Hippocrates mentions early amputations being performed as life-saving procedures. Another early mention of amputation for medical reasons concerns the Roman philosopher Celsus, who was thought to have been born around 25 BCE. He felt that amputation was necessary when it was the only option to save a patient's life, and recommended it in cases of severe gangrene and for large fractures where the bones were largely separated from each other [1].

Prostheses date back thousands of years. The earliest written account of a prosthesis is found in the *Histories of Herodotus*, written in 484 BC [1, 2]. It describes a Persian soldier named Hegesistratus, who was captured by enemy forces and shackled by his foot. He escaped by cutting off part of his foot and later replaced it with a wooden prosthesis, similar to the one shown in Figure 1.1. Historical art, such as figurines and vases, sometimes show prosthetics made of wood and other materials [2]. Currently, the oldest recovered prosthesis is a leg made of copper and wood, which has been dated to be from the Samnite Wars in 300 BC (see Figure 1.2).

The early history of orthotics can be found in records of splints being used. Archaeologists have found skeletal remains which show evidence of healed broken bones, but no specific written mention of splints is mentioned in this time. The earliest known period in which splints were used was during the Egyptian dynasty from 2750 to 2625 BC [3]. G. Elliot Smith, a professor of anatomy at the Egyptian Government School of Medicine, wrote in 1908 of examining two sets of splints which were from early Egyptian times. He wrote that "these are certainly the oldest splints

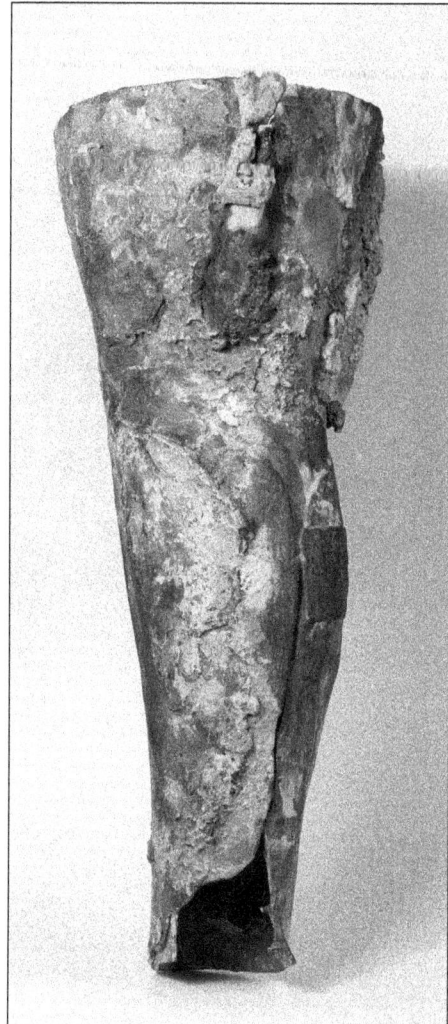

Figure 1.2. The Capua Leg (artificial Roman leg in bronze).

Source: From the Wellcome Collection, https://wellcomecollection.org/works/uegv4fba.

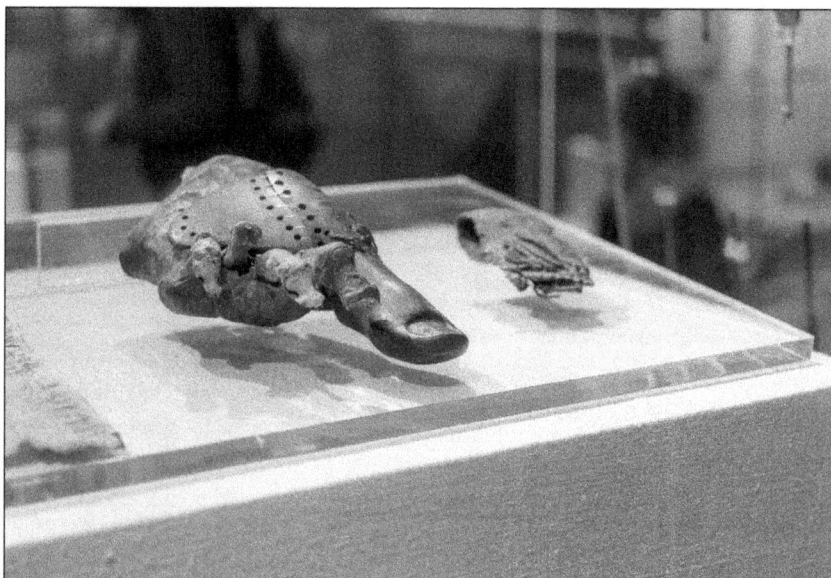

Figure 1.1. "The Cairo Toe."

Source: Shutterstock, 2114761397, Antonio Batinic.

which have come to light in any part of the world." These early Egyptian splints used two or more splints to surround completely the injured limb [3]. The work of Hippocrates also contributed to the early stages of orthotics. Two of the books in the Corpus Hippocraticum, *On Fractures* and *On Articulations*, include discussions on the treatment of fractures, dislocations, congenital deformities, and other orthopedic ailments [4].

Numerous individuals helped to further the field of orthopedics and orthotics in the Middle Ages. Galen (AD 130–210) was the first to use the terms kyphosis, lordosis, and scoliosis. He studied various deformities and is credited with the first attempt at active correction of spinal deformities. He and Hippocrates advocated strapping of the chest, singing, and breathing exercises for the treatment of scoliosis [5]. Another contributor to the field, Antyllus, advocated tenotomy for relief of contractures around joints around 200 AD [6]. Around 400 AD, Caelius Aurelianus recommended passive movement and splints in the treatment of paralysis [7]. In the 1300s, Guy De Chauliac developed the use of traction suspension for the treatment of femur fractures [8].

EARLY SURGICAL TECHNIQUES

There are various surgical techniques described throughout history that show the progression of techniques used in amputations. Anesthetics were rare in primitive times and different cultures used different techniques to calm patients. Europeans used alcohol or opium, whereas South Americans chewed on cocoa leaves and alkali, which released cocaine [1, 2]. Many centuries ago, both Hippocrates (shown in Figure 1.3) and Celsus described the use of ligatures and Celsus also described the use of a flap technique for amputations [1]. Different techniques employed to control hemorrhage during amputation surgery included ligatures, a clamp over the blood vessels to stop bleeding, or cautery via the application of boiling pitch [1]. However, the use of ligatures fell out of practice during the Dark Ages [4]. During this period, surgeons stopped bleeding by applying boiling oil or by crushing the stump; techniques that did not leave a good stump to attempt to fit a prosthesis [2]. Ligatures were reintroduced in the sixteenth century by Ambroise Paré, a French military surgeon [4]. After Paré's time, other methods to stop bleeding include vitriol in the 1670s, cautery (which continued into the twentieth century), and the use of a red-hot knife to cut through soft tissue (as recommended by a German surgeon, Fabricius Hildanus, in 1600) [2].

Ambroise Paré (Figure 1.4) was a French barber surgeon and was the official royal surgeon to four successive kings [9]. He is known for two major advancements in the treatment of wounds. The first is in the way that he dressed wounds. Prior to Paré, many physicians treated wounds, including gunshot wounds, with cauterization—putting

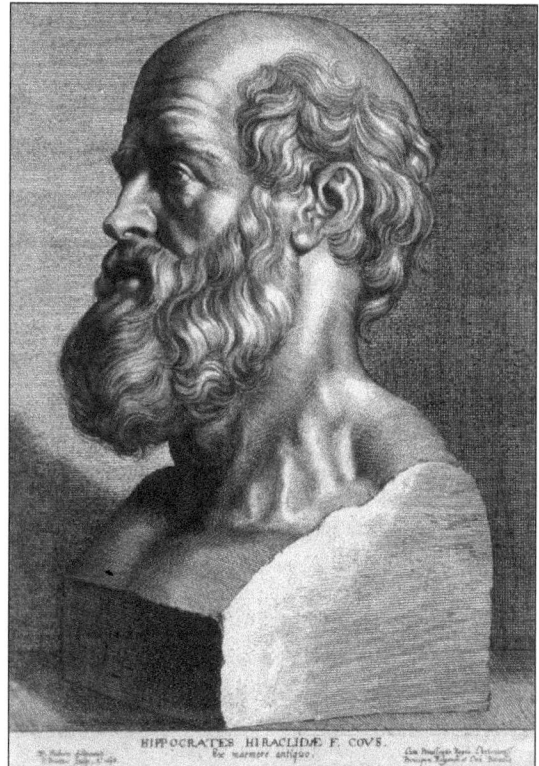

Figure 1.3. Hippocrates.

Source: From National Library of Medicine Digital Collection, https://collections.nlm.nih.gov/catalog/nlm:nlmuid-101418680-img.

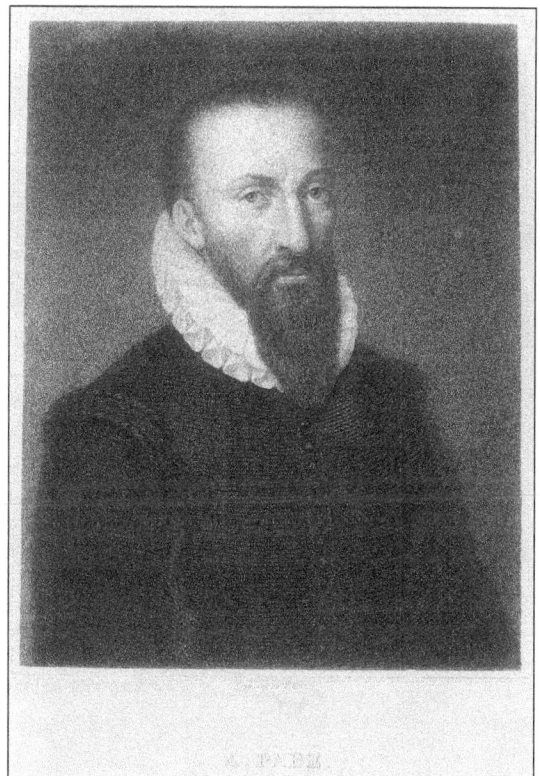

Figure 1.4. Portrait of Ambroise Paré [1510–1590], French surgeon.

Source: From the Wellcome Collection, https://wellcomecollection.org/works/bts6t4wn.

boiling oil on the wound. However, Paré began to dress wounds with a soothing ointment instead of boiling oil, and noticed improvements in his patients. He described this in his work, *Method of Treating Wounds*, in 1545 [9].

Fifteen years later, Paré made his most famous contribution—the use of ligatures for hemostasis in amputations, as shown in Figure 1.5. Ligatures had been described prior to Paré—in fact as early as Hippocrates, mentioned above—yet because of Paré's work, the use of ligatures became widespread. His rediscovery of ligatures has been dated to c.1560; in 1552, for example, he published a book supporting cautery, but in 1564 he wrote another book retracting it [2]. There are various reasons as to why ligatures had not been popular until that time. The two primary reasons were that, first, many surgeries were carried out without anesthesia and, second, that skilled assistants were unavailable to help the surgeon in tying the ligatures [2]. In the former, without the use of anesthesia, surgeons typically tried to perform amputations as quickly as possible and, since cautery took less time than ligatures, cautery was more often used. In the latter, surgeons of the time required assistants to help with holding the patient still while they performed an amputation. This meant that they received less assistance from these helpers for the surgical procedure itself, including the tying of ligatures.

Many "firsts" in amputation technique were developed from the sixteenth century onwards. In 1536 Paré performed the first elbow disarticulation [4], allowing for increased lever arm length. Also, advancements in surgical techniques, such as ligatures, allowed transfemoral amputations to be possible. Notable examples include a successful transfemoral amputation in 1588 by the English surgeon, William Clowes the Elder, who became surgeon to Queen Elizabeth I and served on the fleet that defeated the Spanish Armada; a transfemoral amputation reported in 1614 by Fabricius Hildanus (also known as William Fabry or "the Father of German surgery") [2]; and the introduction of the tourniquet in 1674 by French army surgeon Etienne Morel [4] that was improved upon by another French surgeon, J. L. Petite, in 1718 [2]. In the improved tourniquet, an element of the tourniquet was tied to the abdomen so that it could not slip. Further, it put direct pressure on the major artery of the limb to be amputated [2].

Developments continued apace in the eighteenth century and into the nineteenth. American John Warren, who went on to found the Harvard Medical School, performed an amputation through the shoulder in 1781 and by 1803 Dominique-Jean Larrey, a French surgeon and military doctor, had successfully performed multiple amputations through the shoulder and also through the hip [2]. Another French surgeon, François Chopart, introduced a new partial foot amputation in 1792, where he performed a disarticulation through the talonavicular and calcaneocuboid joints and in 1815 his fellow countryman Jacques Lisfranc de St. Martin described a metatarsal–tarsal disarticulation. In 1843, pioneering Scottish surgeon Sir James Syme described his method for an ankle amputation, which is still called a Syme amputation today [4]. His son-in-law, Lord Lister, went on to introduce the

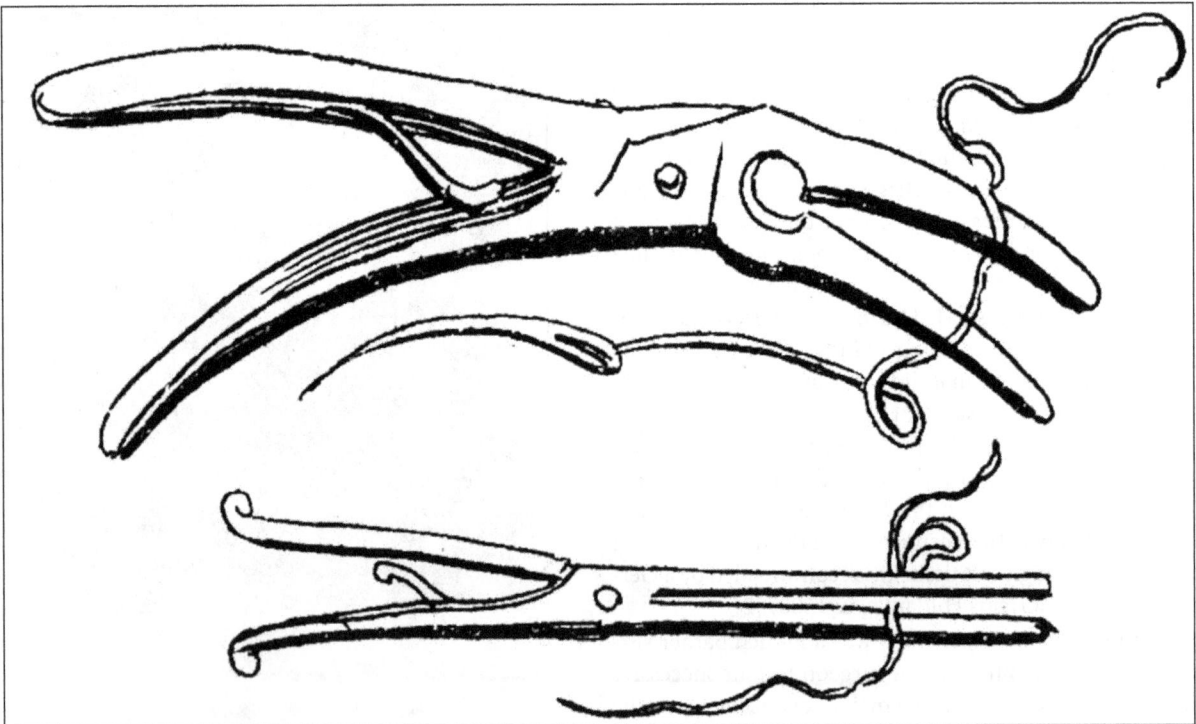

Figure 1.5. Spring forceps and a ligature.

Source: A course of chirurgical operations demonstrated in the Royal Garden at Paris, https://wellcomelibrary.org/item/b28705270#?c=0&m=0&s=0&cv=437&z=-0.
0609%2C0.1398%2C1.7768%2C1.1311.

antiseptic technique in 1867, which improved the overall success rate of amputation surgeries [4]. Also, during the nineteenth century, the Italian Rocco Gritti introduced an operation in 1857 that was designed to give an end-bearing above-knee amputation stump; this was achieved by fixing the patella to the cut surface of the femur, after performing a supracondylar osteotomy of the femur. Gritti's procedure was modified slightly by Irish physician William Stokes in 1870 and subsequently came to be known as the Gritti–Stokes procedure [2].

SURGICAL DECISION MAKING

Historical writings give insight into the decisions made by early surgeons relative to amputations. One such decision is with regard to the level of amputation; Figure 1.6 for instance, depicts an amputation through the tibiofemoral joint which includes numerous implications ranging from the quantity of tissue sparing, end bearing capability, prosthesis style and more. Hippocrates recommended performing the amputation through dead tissue

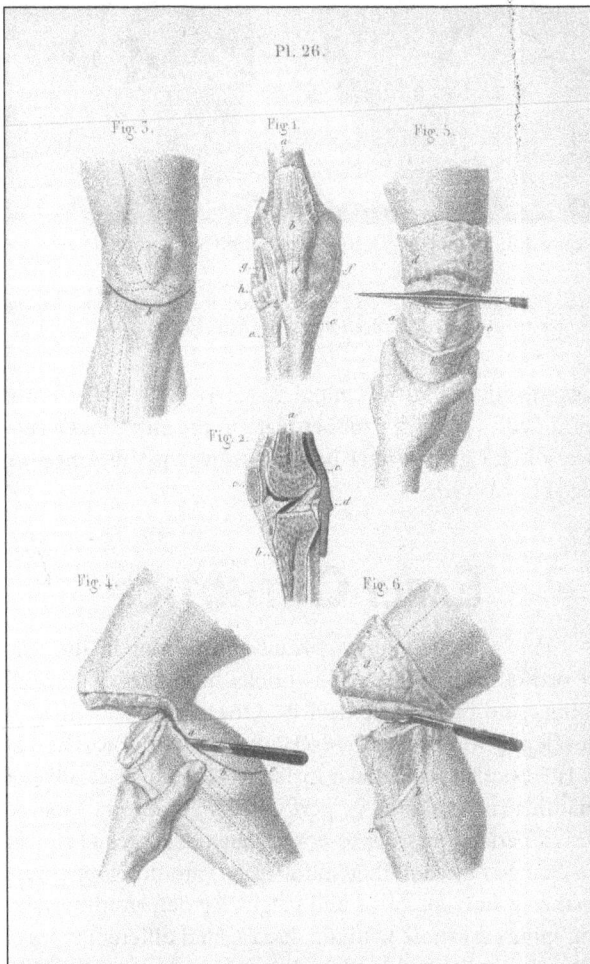

Figure 1.6. Amputation at the tibiofemoral joint.

Source: Plate 26, Amputation at the tibiofemoral joint, The Wellcome Collection, https://wellcomecollection.org/works/cd8487bj.

rather than living tissue to avoid the risk of hemorrhage. Celsus advocated to amputate above the dead tissue, something that was later referenced by Paré, who wrote: it is the practice "to amputate always the part above that [portion] which is mortified and corrupted, as wrote and recommended Celsus, to perform the amputation on that which is healthy, rather than to leave any of the putrefied" [10]. However, even after Paré penned this, not everyone adopted his practices. In 1639 a British surgeon, John Woodall, recommended amputating through the upper end of the dead tissue; he theorized that this would be painless for the patient and that the surgeon could gradually cut away the remaining dead tissue later [2].

Another important surgical decision debated in early literature was whether to perform open or closed amputations. As he amputated through dead tissue, Hippocrates left his amputation wounds open to heal by granulation tissue. Edward Alanson of Liverpool wrote in 1782 of a series of 35 major amputations where all patients survived, an impressive feat for this time period; he left wounds open and approximated the edges with tape [2]. The official *Union Army Manual* of 1861 also recommended leaving wounds open following an amputation, and eventually recommended allowing wounds to heal by granulation tissue. However, others advocated closing wounds after amputation. In the thirteenth century, Hugh of Lucca, his pupil Theodoric, and Henri De Mondeville recommended closing all wounds, even contaminated ones [2]. French surgeons also frequently closed wounds.

The first true flap amputations were credited to James Younge of Plymouth in 1679, although Ambroise Paré had previously recommended retracting skin and muscle proximally before severing the bone in order to leave enough soft tissue to cover the end of the bone [2]. In 1837, British surgeon Robert Liston introduced a flap amputation like the one that continues to be used today [2].

EARLY PROSTHETICS

One of the earliest known prostheses comes from the c.1000 BC in ancient Egypt. In the late 1990s, in Sheikh Abd el-Qurna near Luxor, a mummy was found that had the big toe of the right foot amputated and replaced by a prosthesis made of leather and wood (see Figure 1.1) [11]. The oldest recovered European prosthesis was found in a tomb in Capua, Italy in 1858, and dates from the Samnite Wars in 300 BC (see Figure 1.2) [2]. This prosthesis was made of bronze. Sadly, the original kept in the Royal College of Surgeons was lost during an air-raid in World War II and there is now a brass and plaster replica in the Science Museum, London. Various artists have depicted early prostheses in their works, including on vases and in mosaics. Here, early amputees are depicted using prostheses made of a wooden pylon, a cup-like prosthesis, and a bowl-like prosthesis [1, 2]. Early prostheses were made of wood or wood and metal and could have soft, cloth coverings to protect the stump [1]. In early times, upper limb prostheses were rare, as they were heavy and not functional. If anything, they were used for cosmetic purposes [1]. In the Middle Ages, prostheses were often made of iron for soldiers to wear during battle. These prostheses were mostly likely made to be worn while on horseback as the heavy weight made walking difficult and the shape and structure of the prostheses indicate that they were not made for walking [12].

Over time, the comfort and utility of prostheses improved. Ambroise Paré developed the first known prosthesis with articulated knee and ankle joints [2], as shown in Figure 1.7. Later, James Potts of London developed an above-knee prosthesis in 1800 that had articulated joints, with cords connecting the knee and ankle so that when the knee flexed, the ankle dorsiflexed [2]. This allowed toe lift to coordinate with knee flexion during the swing phase of ambulation. Because the Marquis of Anglesey used this prosthesis after losing his leg in the Battle of Waterloo in 1815, it became known as the Anglesey leg [2] (Figure 1.8). Potts's design was made of wood rather than metal, so it was lighter than Paré's design. The Anglesey leg

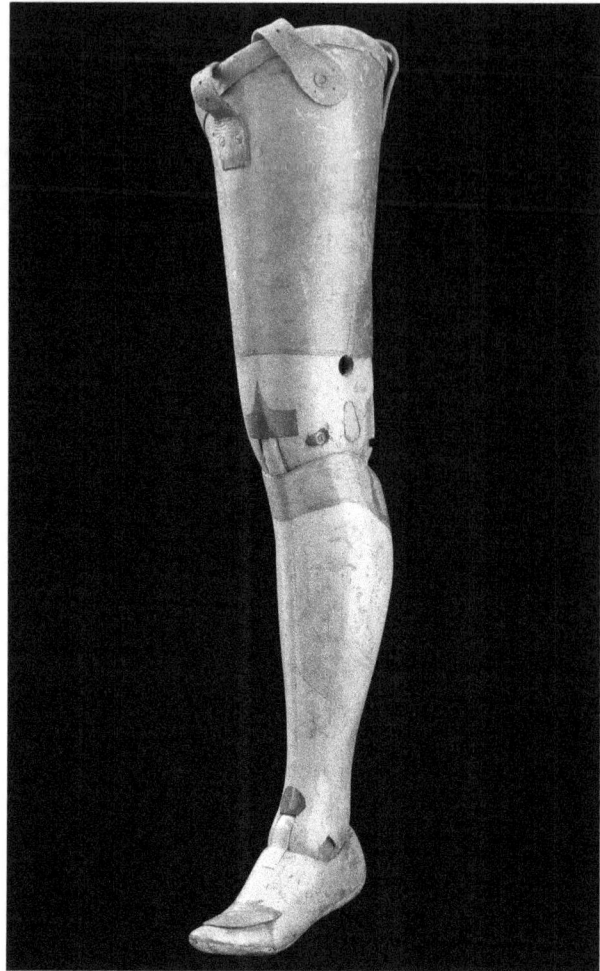

Figure 1.8. The Anglesey leg (an artificial left leg, Europe, 1901–1940).

Source: Science Museum, London, https://collection.sciencemuseumgroup.org.uk/objects/co126870/artificial-left-leg-europe-1901-1940.

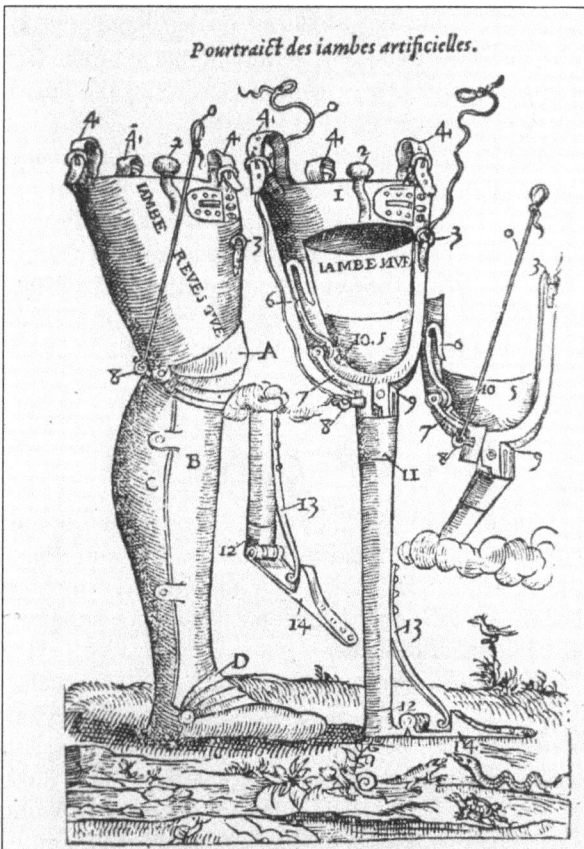

Figure 1.7. Views of a prosthetic leg in 1575.

Source: https://commons.wikimedia.org/wiki/File:Views_of_a_prosthetic_leg_in_1575.jpg.

was introduced in the United States in 1839, where it was modified by adding a rubber plate in the ankle and a rubber sole for grip; it later became known as the American leg [2].

EARLY ORTHOTICS

Paré was also an important contributor in the field of orthotics. In some of his books he described various splints and orthopedic devices. One such device that he developed was a metal corset used "for the correction of twisted bodies," as shown in Figure 1.9 [3]. Paré advised that this corset should be perforated so that it was not too heavy, padded in order to not irritate the skin, and should be changed often. Other splints that Paré developed were leather splints for varus and valgus leg deformities, walking splints for those with hip disease, and different types of shoes for individuals with club foot [3].

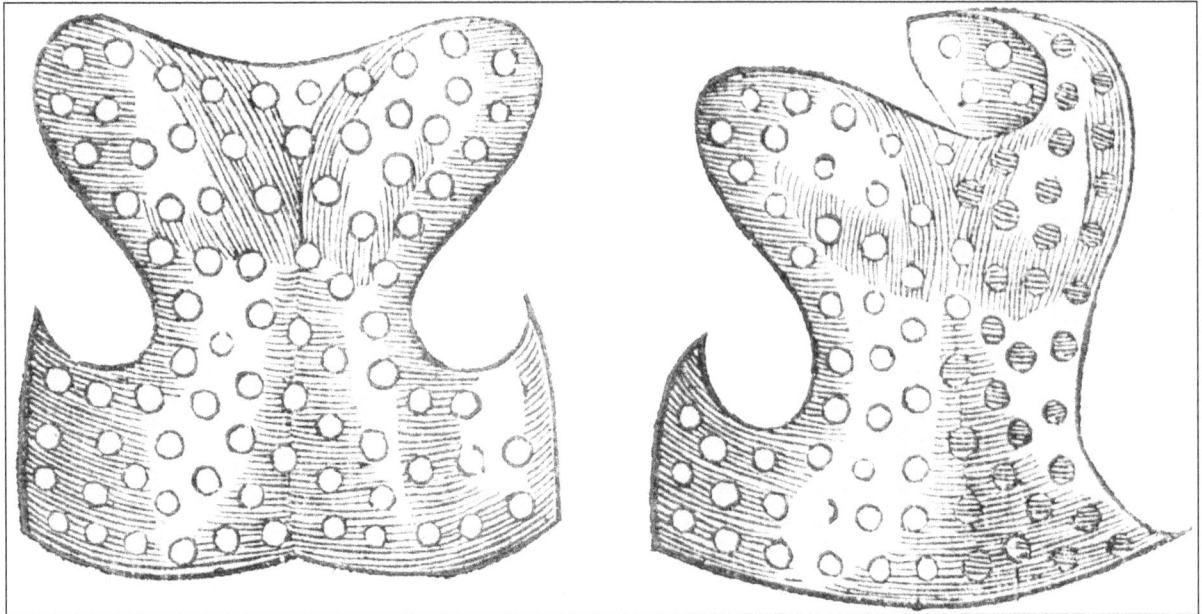

Figure 1.9. The workes of that famous chirurgion Ambrose Paré.

Source: Public domain. See https://wellcomecollection.org/works/pqf232j8/items, page 582.

Another important individual in the field of orthotics during the 1500s was Italian anatomist and surgeon Girolamo Fabrici D'Acquapendente. He stressed gentle manipulation rather than Hippocrates' method of the forceful correction of deformities. Also of interest is Fabricius Hildanus (1560–1624), mentioned earlier, who helped progress the treatment of club foot by developing a corrective brace and stressing the importance of change along with the growth of the child [3]. He also developed the first turntable attachment for the correction of finger deformities. In the seventeenth century, British physician Francis Glisson (1597–1677) used braces, shoes, and splints in his treatment of the deformities of rickets [3] (Figure 1.10). He developed braces for knees and used a suspension apparatus to correct spinal deformities, and added chin and occiput supports.

Further developments were made in the eighteenth century. The German Lorenz Heister (1683–1758) is credited with the introduction of the spinal brace and developed the "Iron Cross" design [3]. In the 1760s, François LeVacher developed a spinal brace with a posterior component that attached to a snugly fitting cap [13]. Examples of early spinal braces are shown in Figures 1.11 and 1.12. Surgical advances were also made during this time, when the aforementioned Lorenz Heister of Frankfort, as well as Jacques Mathieu Delpech and Georg Friedrich Louis Stromeyer all performed surgeries for tenotomies and tendon repairs [14]. In 1803, Antonio Scarpa, an Italian anatomist, developed his famous club foot shoe [3].

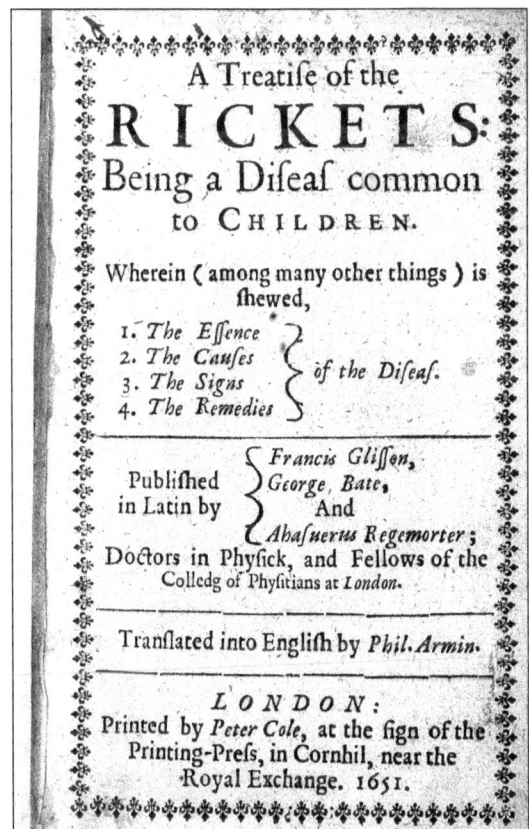

Figure 1.10. F. Glisson, *A treatise of the rickets.*

Source: https://commons.wikimedia.org/wiki/File:Glisson,_A_treatise_of_the_rickets,_1651_Wellcome_L0028412.jpg#/media/File:F._Glisson,_%22A_treatise_of_the_rickets%22_Wellcome_L0013828.jpg.

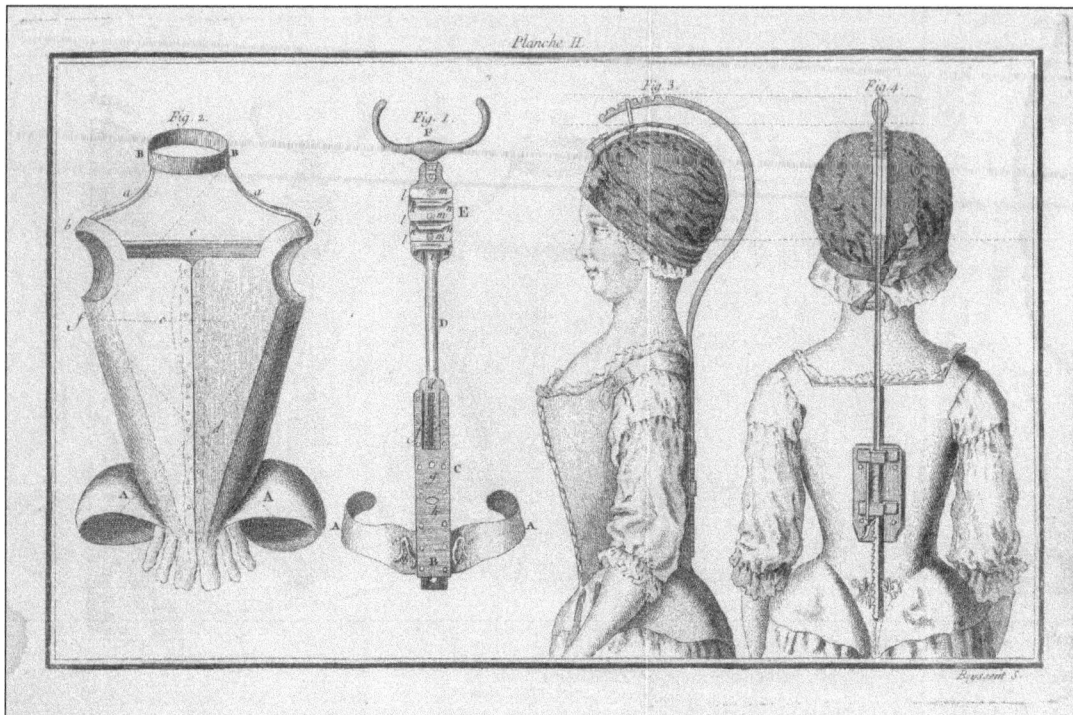

Figure 1.11. Figures showing equipment for the spine and posture of children.

Source: Wellcome Collection, https://wellcomecollection.org/works/hshfpmms.

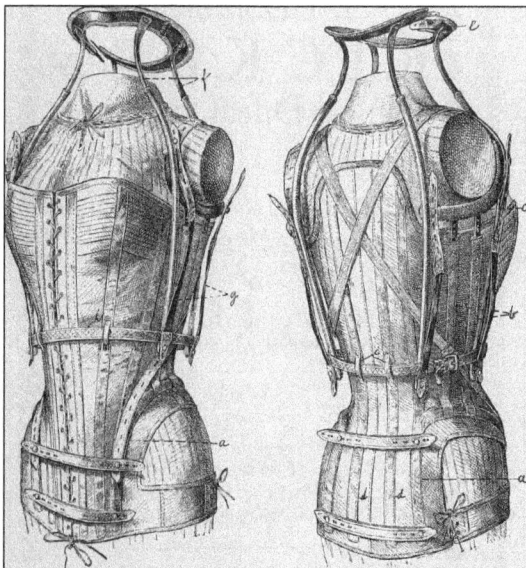

Figure 1.12. Early scoliosis brace.

Source: Dolega, Max (1897). *Zur Pathologie und Therapie der kindlichen Skoliose und über die Unterscheidung einer habituellen und constitutionellen Form derselben—eine kritische und klinische Studie.*

THE AMERICAN CIVIL WAR AND ITS IMPACT

The American Civil War sparked advancements in prosthetics in the United States due to the number of amputees who lost limbs. Approximately 60,000 surgeries performed during the Civil War were amputations—three-quarters of all surgeries performed during the war [15]. A reason for many of these amputations was the introduction of the Minie ball—a bullet made of soft lead that resulted in devastating damage on impact. Bones and limbs were shattered when hit by the Minie ball. Thankfully, anesthesia was developed prior to the start of the Civil War, and during amputation surgery chloroform was often used [16]. However, because so many men were wounded, surgeries had to be performed very quickly by the battlefield surgeons, and dirty instruments were often used. This led to increased levels of infections, some of which were fatal. Surgical infections included pyemia, tetanus, gangrene, erysipelas, and osteomyelitis [16].

The increasing numbers of amputees sparked advancements in the field of prosthetics. Nearly 150 patents were issued between 1861 and 1873 for artificial limb designs [15]. In 1862 the Federal government gave a Union soldier amputee $75 to purchase an artificial leg or $50 to purchase an artificial arm [15]. By 1864, Confederate soldiers also received assistance to purchase artificial limbs. One of the most famous amputees from the Civil War was Confederate army veteran J. E. Hanger. He developed a lower limb prosthesis that included hinged knee and ankle joints, and had rubber bumpers at the ankle that could vary dorsiflexion and plantarflexion [2, 17]. The company that Hanger founded continues to be a leader in the prosthetics industry in the United States today.

Advances in orthotics available during the time of the Civil War include H. G. Davis's 1857 suggestion of using elastic material in a sustained reduction apparatus [3]. Also around then, Gurdon Buck developed a traction system using adhesive or elastic materials; this became widely used in the Civil War.

In other developments, Dutch army surgeon Antonius Mathijsen introduced the plaster of Paris bandage in 1852; however, it was not well received initially due to difficulty in accessing the limb while wearing the cast. In 1882, after the Civil War but related to plaster bandaging, Lewis Sayre became the first to apply a plaster of Paris jacket [18]; Sayre is considered the father of orthopedic surgery in the United States [3]. X-ray results showed that the use of plaster of Paris casts for immobilization were superior to splinting [19], and these casts thus became much more popular.

In the latter half of the nineteenth century, orthopedic surgeons often employed brace makers in their office. This division of medicine was called "mechanical surgery." As the field of orthopedics became more focused on surgery, brace makers moved out of the physician's offices and into their own, where they would work with a number of surgeons instead of just one [3].

The development of orthopedic centers for specialized care for patients dates back to the eighteenth century, when Jean Andre Venel opened the first orthopedic hospital in Orbe, Switzerland. The first orthopedic center in the United States was opened during the Civil War in 1863 under the leadership of James Knight, and was called the Hospital for the Ruptured and Crippled; it was located in New York City [3]. Three years later, Charles F. Taylor led the opening of the New York Orthopaedic Dispensary and Hospital.

ADVANCES IN THE WORLD WAR I AND WORLD WAR II ERAS

The Artificial Limb Manufacturers and Brace Association was founded in 1917 in Washington, D.C. in anticipation of the growing needs of amputees following World War I; this organization would later become the American Orthotics and Prosthetics Association (AOPA) [20]. However, most of the advancements in the field of prosthetics came about following World War II.

Near the end of World War II, amputees began voicing their displeasure with the currently available prosthetics. In response to this, the Surgeon General of the Army, Norman Kirk, contacted the National Academy of Sciences (NAS) [4]. The NAS organized a conference in 1945 of surgeons, prosthetists, and scientists who decided that little current scientific effort had gone into the development of prosthetics and subsequently started a new research project. The group was initially called the Advisory Committee

on Artificial Limbs and assumed its duties on July 1, 1947 [21]. The project was originally funded by the Office of Scientific Research and Development (OSRD), but this was disbanded at the end of World War II. At that time, the Office of the Surgeon General of the Army began to support the project, and later the Veterans Administration took responsibility for it [4]. The group changed its name in 1959 to the Committee on Prosthetics Research and Development (CPRD) and operated within the Division of Engineering and Industrial Research of the National Research Council [21]. The CPRD was a group of 13 individuals, composed primarily of engineers, physicians, and prosthetists [22]. The group met two to three times a year but could meet more often if needed. The committee also formed sub-groups on special topics that could meet outside of the committee; some of these topics that these sub-groups covered included pediatrics, upper extremity prosthesis research, and orthotic design [22].

Both the NAS and the Veterans Administration supervised the program through different universities and laboratories. These programs went through many different names between 1945 to 1959 but eventually became known as the Artificial Limb Program [4]. The Artificial Limb Program was started with the idea that surgeons and physicians could provide engineers with information for prosthetic designs, and then the engineers could actually make these designs using modern materials. However, they soon realized that more research and understanding was needed on how actual human limbs function. Two programs were therefore developed to study limb function: one to study lower limb function at the University of California, Berkeley; and a second to study upper limb function at the University of California at Los Angeles [4]. In 1948, the still then-called Advisory Committee on Artificial Limbs recommended opening an independent evaluation laboratory which was established at New York University. The purpose of this laboratory was to investigate the usefulness of the devices and techniques coming from the aforementioned development laboratories.

Other groups carrying out prosthetic design and developmental projects during this time included Northrop Aviation, Inc.; Cat-ranis, Inc.; the Army Prosthetics Research Laboratory; the U.S. Naval Hospital, Mare Island; U.S. Army Air Force unit at Wright Field; New York University; and the Veterans Administration [4]. The Veterans Administration's laboratory in New York would later become part of the Veterans Administration Prosthetics Center (VAPC) [4].

Many advances were seen in prosthetic design and development during the years following World War II. In 1946, the University of California, Berkeley performed a study of the suction socket for transfemoral amputees [4]. In 1950 they also introduced a new socket design; it became known as the "quadrilateral socket" because of its four well-defined walls. The University of California, Berkeley and San Francisco developed the patellar tendon-bearing

(PTB) prosthesis for transtibial amputees [4]. From experience with the PTB prosthesis, the total-contact quadrilateral transfemoral socket was developed. Foort and Radcliffe were responsible for the development of both the PTB and quadrilateral sockets; they developed the concept of total contact design for both socket types. In the 1980s, groups began to study a new type of socket for transfemoral amputees, and various forms of "ischial containment" sockets were developed [4].

Immediately after World War II, most lower limb prostheses were made of wood and leather [4]. However, these materials were less than ideal, for a variety of reasons. Subsequently, Northrop Aviation, Inc. introduced the use of thermosetting resins to form components of upper limb prostheses. The Veterans Administration Prosthetics Center also began conducting demonstrations to encourage prosthetists to begin using plastic laminates over wood, helping to shift the field towards the use of plastics [4]. The use of plastics to make prosthetics made total-contact sockets practical, and most prostheses currently in use are total-contact sockets made from either a plastic thermoset laminate or thermoformed plastic [4].

Advances in prosthetic knee joints were also made during this time. In 1950, the Navy Variable Cadence Knee Unit was introduced. This was able to increase friction toward the end of swing phase, making it preferable to the constant-friction knee joint [4]. The Northwestern University variable-cadence knee used the same principles. The Stewart–Vickers Hydraulic Above-Knee Leg used hydraulic principles to lock the knee into extension at heel strike and to coordinate motion between the knee and ankle during swing phase [4]. This knee was studied in clinical trials at New York University, and later became available commercially as the Hydra-Cadence. The Hydra-Cadence unit retained the swing phase and hydraulic ankle features but did not include the stance-phase control feature due to high cost [4]. Hans Mauch also developed a knee, the Mauch SnS System, which has both swing-phase and stance-phase control. When speaking before the Prosthetics Research Board, Mauch said,

> Gentlemen, as one of the men who helped to build the first guided missile in the history of the world, I say to you that building that guided missile was simplicity itself compared to building an artificial leg that closely imitates the functions of its human predecessor [23].

Another knee developed by the University of California, Berkeley used pneumatics, and was called the UC-BL Pneumatic Swing Control knee [4].

Prosthetic feet also progressed from being just a single-axis wood foot. The Naval Prosthetics Research Laboratory developed the "Navy ankle," which was an ankle containing a block of rubber with variable stiffness, which could control motions in all three planes [4]. The Greissinger foot also offered three-way motion control, and was developed in Germany. The SACH (solid ankle, cushioned heel) foot was introduced in the 1950s and became very successful,

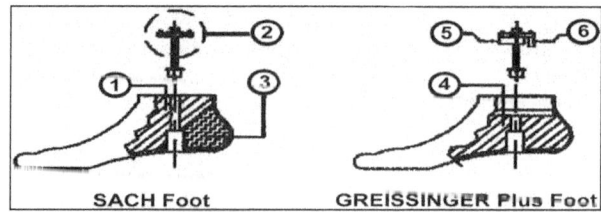
Figure 1.13. The SACH Foot and the Greissinger Plus Foot.
Source: Marinakis 2014 [24].

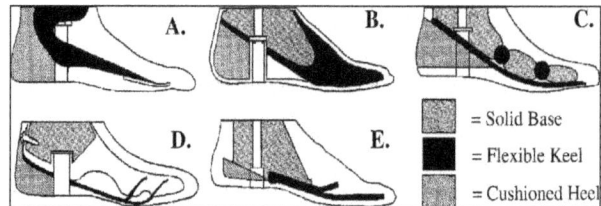
Figure 1.14. Cross-sections of various energy-storing feet.
Source: Hafner et al. 2002 [25].

and is still in use today [4]; both the Greissinger foot and SACH foot are shown in Figure 1.13. In the late 1970s the SAFE (stationary attachment flexible endoskeletal) foot was developed, which was also well accepted. In the early 1980s, the Seattle foot was introduced, which was an energy-storing foot [4]. The Carbon Copy II and the Flex-Foot were later introduced; all three feet are show in Figure 1.14.

Advancements were also made in upper limb prostheses. The Army Prosthetics Research Laboratory (APRL) was tasked with the development of artificial arms, with an emphasis on artificial hands. The APRL hand and APRL hook came out of this effort following World War II [4]. Northrop Aviation developed the alternating-lock elbow unit in 1947. In 1949, Alderson developed the first working model of an electrically powered artificial arm [4]. During the 1980s, the use of externally powered upper limb prostheses increased.

As wars encouraged interest in developing new prostheses, the polio epidemic of the 1950s led to increased focus and developments in the field of orthotics, as shown in Figure 1.15. In the 1970s, it became possible to vacuum-form sheet plastics by adapting industrial techniques, which led to further developments in orthotic designs. As new materials and methods are introduced, the field of orthotics continues to progress and change [26].

Two major developments in the Vietnam War era led to increased attempts by surgeons to preserve the knee joint during amputation surgery. Dr. Robert Barnes, an Iowa vascular surgeon, helped develop the Doppler ultrasound in 1970; an updated version of this machine is shown in Figure 1.16. This paved the way to better detection of blood flow in the lower limb for patients with vascular etiologies. Another important individual during this era was Dr. Ernest Burgess, who published many articles advocating saving the knee joint in lower limb amputations [27]. Combined, these two advancements led to more surgeons opting for transtibial amputations, thus preserving the knee joint.

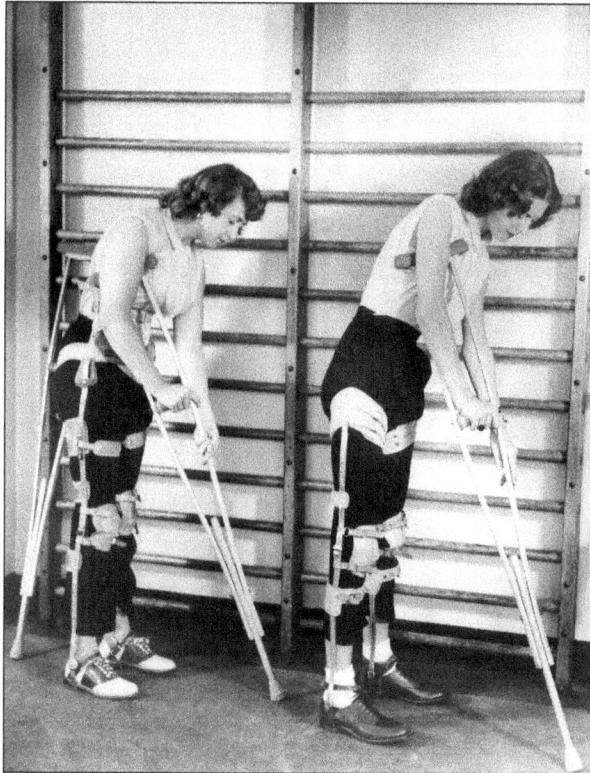

Figure 1.15. Two adult women polio victims with leg braces adjust their crutches.

Source: Available on Shutterstock. https://www.shutterstock.com/editorial/image-editorial/historical-collection-10306767a.

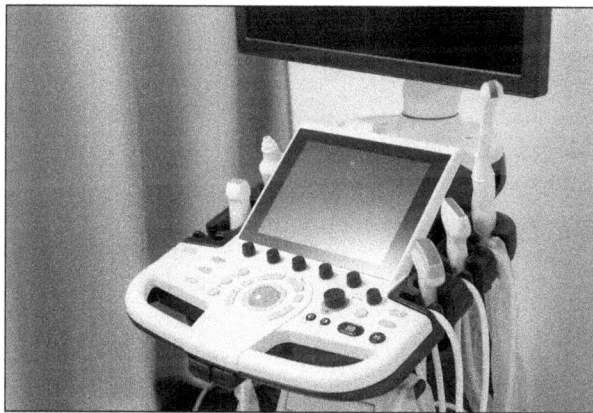

Figure 1.16. Ultrasound equipment.

Source: Shutterstock, 1968567955, Andrey Zhernovoy.

PROFESSIONAL ORGANIZATIONS IN THE UNITED STATES

In 1917, the Artificial Limb Manufacturers and Brace Association was formed to meet the needs of amputees following World War I [20]. In 1946, the name was changed to the Orthopedic Appliance and Limb Manufacturers Association, and then again in 1958 to the American

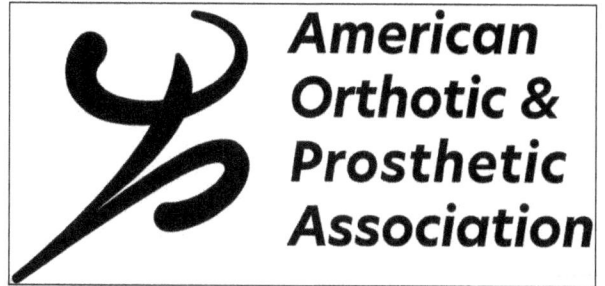

Figure 1.17. AOPA logo.

Orthotic & Prosthetic Association (AOPA) [4] (the AOPA logo is shown in Figure 1.17). According to their website,

> The mission of the American Orthotic & Prosthetic Association is to work for favorable treatment of the O&P business in laws, regulation and services; to help members improve their management and marketing skills; and to raise awareness and understanding of the industry and the association.

The American Board for Certification of the Orthotic and Prosthetic Appliance Industry (now ABC) was created on September 9, 1948 (logo pictured in Figure 1.18). It was founded after the Orthopedic Appliance and Limb Manufacturers Association decided that the orthotics and prosthetics industry needed to develop a plan to certify prosthetic and orthotic fitters and firms [28]. At the first ABC board meeting on December 11, 1948, the terms "Certified Orthotist" and "Certified Prosthetist" were adopted as titles for individuals who met the ABC's requirements for certification; these terms are still used today [28]. Another important date in ABC history is October 3, 1950. On this date, the Board of Directors determined that as of May 1, 1951, no certificate would be awarded without the applicant taking an examination [28].

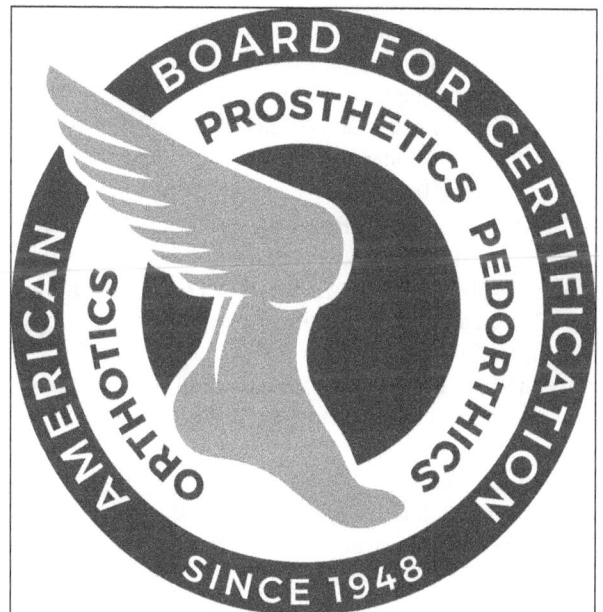

Figure 1.18. ABC logo.

The first ABC examination was given in New York City in May 1951. Sixty-seven applicants sat for the examination, and fifty-one passed the exam and became certified. In 1951, the American Medical Association endorsed ABC's certification program.

In 1954, ABC endorsed receiving a physician's prescription to make a new prosthesis or orthosis [28]. In 1957, the board unanimously voted to have an applicant for examination bring an example of his/her work to the examination [28]. In 1958, many changes were made to the examination procedures. The most notable changes were a requirement that examiners go through an orientation, and taking the Intelligence Quotient and Mechanical Comprehension tests were made prerequisites to taking the ABC examination [28]. Another change made by ABC in 1958 was to establish a rule for facility certification in which a facility that had only one Certified Orthotist or Prosthetist would lose its good standing with the ABC if it did not find a new certified individual within 6 months [28]. In 1959, the board voted to change the organization's name from the American Board for Certification of the Orthotic and Prosthetic Appliance Industry, Incorporated to the American Board for Certification in Orthotics & Prosthetics, Incorporated.

Also in 1959, the board developed standard terminology for the orthotics profession. For many years prior to this, the terms "orthotics" and "orthetics" were used interchangeably in professional literature. However, in 1959 the board determined that standard nomenclature would include "orthosis," "orthotics," and "orthotist" [28]. In October 1960, the board defined the initial designations for practitioners: CP for Certified Prosthetist, CO for Certified Orthotist, and CPO for Certified Prosthetist/Orthotist [28]. In 1970, the board voted that the educational level for an "Assistant" be a 2-year Associates of Arts degree, and that a "Practitioner" had to have a 4-year baccalaureate degree [28]. Prior to the 1970s, the board also decided that the ABC should petition the National Commission on Accreditation for formal recognition as being the group authorized to accredit educational institutions offering programs in prosthetics and/or orthotics. In 1986, the board approved a mandatory continuing education requirement, stating that practitioners would need to complete 75 credit hours in a 5-year period to maintain in good standing [28].

The National Commission on Orthotic and Prosthetic Education (NCOPE) formed as an offshoot from the ABC (the NCOPE logo is shown in Figure 1.19) and in 1972 the ABC formed the Educational Accreditation Commission (EAC) in order to meet the profession's need for an accreditation program for institutions [29]. Major changes in the education requirements for orthotics and prosthetics occurred after this group was formed. In 1973, it was determined that a high school diploma was no longer sufficient to sit for the ABC examination; an associate's degree was required from 1975 to 1979, and a bachelor's degree from an accredited O&P program was required after 1979 [30]. In 1991, the EAC was reorganized and became an independent organization. In 1999, NCOPE

was formed as an incorporated accreditation agency [29]. At the O&P Education Summit Meeting in 2005, it was proposed to move the education requirement for O&P to a master's level [30]. In 2006 and 2007, NCOPE hosted strategic meetings on the movement from a bachelor's to a master's level of education and in 2007 NCOPE approved the requirement that all new programs applying for accreditation as of 2010 must be at a master's level, and all programs had to transition to a master's level by 2012 [30]. NCOPE continues to be responsible for accrediting orthotics and prosthetics educational programs, and maintaining the standards of education in prosthetics and orthotics. NCOPE operates independently from the other three main prosthetics and orthotics organizations in the United States (the ABC, AOPA, and AAOP).

The final major professional organization in the United States is the American Academy of Orthotists and Prosthetists (AAOP). The AAOP is the professional organization representing certified practitioners, state-licensed practitioners, assistants, technicians, fitters, and others affiliated with the O&P profession. The leadership of the AOPA, the sole credentialing agency at that time, agreed on a need for an organized focused on continuing education and research. The AAOP was then founded in 1970 with the support of ABC (the AAOP logo is shown in Figure 1.20). Their mission statement reads: "The American Academy of Orthotists and Prosthetists is dedicated to promoting professionalism and advancing the standards of patient care through education, literature, research, advocacy, and collaboration" [31].

AAOP offers membership to all O&P professionals through eight unique membership opportunities. The Professional Membership category encompasses the voting members of the organization. Professional Membership criteria are as follows:

> The professional membership is open to individuals who are: (i) orthotists and/or prosthetists certified by a nationally recognized credentialing body based in the United States of America; and/or (ii) licensed to practice in orthotics and/or prosthetics in one or more states in the United States of America that require direct and/or indirect formal education from a CAAHEP Accredited Program.

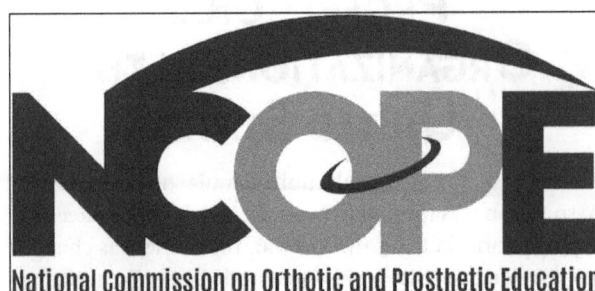

Figure 1.19. NCOPE logo.

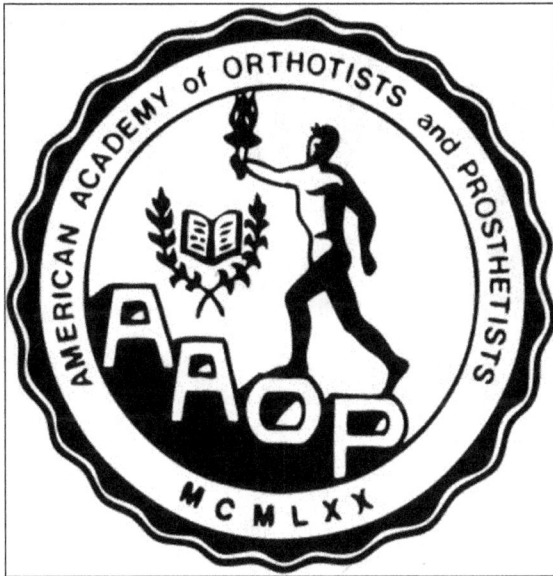

Figure 1.20. AAOP logo.

The AAOP offers a variety of continuing education courses and meetings throughout the year and publishes a variety of O&P research resources including the *Journal of Prosthetics and Orthotics*. This, and other educational and research related tools, are available on its website: www. oandp.org [31].

In 2006, AAOP, AOPA, ABC, and NAAOP (the National Association for the Advancement of Orthotics and Prosthetics) joined together to form the O&P Alliance [31]. The Board of Certification (BOC) later joined the organization. This Alliance enables members from the orthotics and prosthetics field to have one voice as they speak to legislators and the federal government.

PROFESSIONAL PUBLICATIONS

There are multiple peer-reviewed publications relating to prosthetics and orthotics. The first English-language publication for practicing prosthetists and orthotists was the *Orthopedic and Prosthetic Appliance Journal*, first published in 1946 [4]. This journal was published by the Orthopedic Appliance and Limb Manufacturers Association, which later became AOPA. In June 1967, the journal's name was changed to *Orthotics and Prosthetics* [4]. In 1969, the Committee on Prosthetics and Orthotics Education (CPOE) began publication of the *Newsletter—Amputee Clinics* to assist with exchanging information between clinics. This publication continued until CPOE was dissolved in 1976. However, the AAOP initiated publication of the *Newsletter—Prosthetic and Orthotic Clinics* in 1976 [4]. In 1982, the title of this journal was changed to *Clinical Prosthetics and Orthotics* and, in 1988, the AAOP and AOPA combined *Clinical Prosthetics and Orthotics* and *Orthotics and Prosthetics* to create a new journal titled the *Journal of Prosthetics and Orthotics*, which is still in publication today [4].

In 1964, the Veterans Administration began publication of the *Bulletin of Prosthetics Research*; this became the *Journal of Rehabilitation Research and Development* in 1983 [4]. The International Society for Prosthetics and Orthotics (ISPO) began publication of *ISPO Bulletin* in 1972, and published this four times per year until 1976. In 1977, ISPO replaced the *Bulletin* with *Prosthetics and Orthotics International* [4].

RECENT ADVANCES IN PROSTHETICS

Further advances in prosthetics have arisen as a result of Operation Iraqi Freedom and Operation Enduring Freedom. On account of these conflicts, 1,645 major amputations were performed between 2001 and June 1, 2015 due to a battle injury [31]. The increasing number of young, active amputees, coupled with technological advances, has led to innovative new options for prosthetics.

A major advancement in lower limb prosthetics has been the introduction of microprocessor-controlled knee joints. The Otto Bock C-Leg, shown in Figure 1.21,

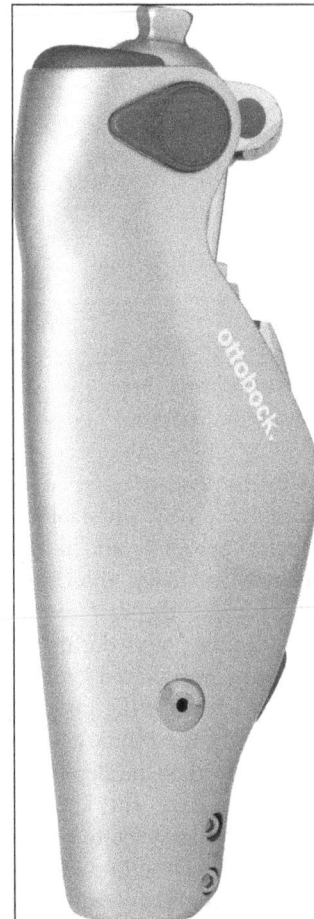

Figure 1.21. The Otto Bock C-Leg.
Source: Permission granted from Otto Bock.

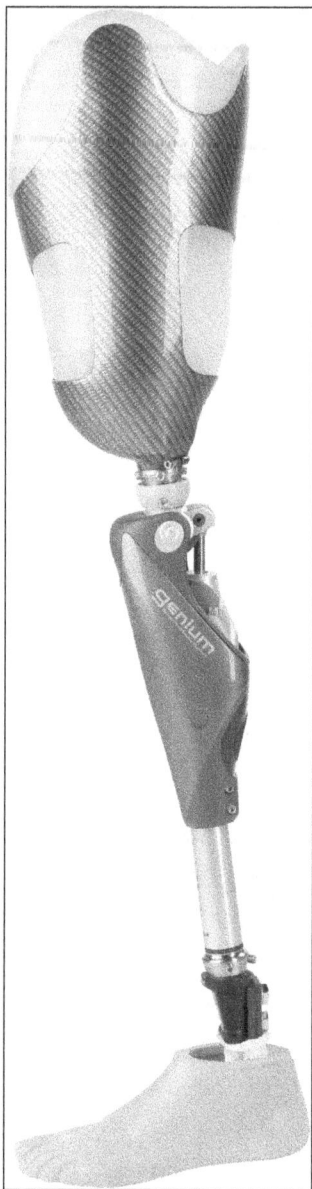

Figure 1.22. The Otto Bock Genium Knee.

Source: Permission granted from Otto Bock.

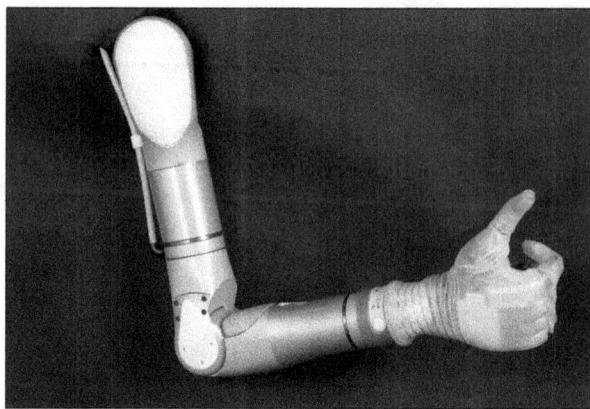

Figure 1.23. The DEKA arm.

Source: https://mobiusbionics.com/luke-arm/.

developed the Genium knee, shown in Figure 1.22, to be sold to the civilian sector.

The most exciting advancement in upper limb prosthetics has been the introduction of the DEKA arm. In 2005, the Defense Advanced Research Project Agency announced the "Revolutionizing Prosthetics" program— a new research project whose goal was to improve the quality of life of upper limb amputees [34]. One of the projects under this new program was the DEKA arm. DEKA was tasked with developing a new prosthetic arm that would drastically improve upon existing prostheses. DEKA worked closely with the Veterans Administration to gain feedback about these prostheses as they moved through different prototypes of these prostheses. The DEKA arm, shown in Figure 1.23, has more degrees of freedom, improved lifting and grasping capabilities, and is available for different amputation levels (transradial, transhumeral, shoulder disarticulation, and forequarter amputations) [34]. The DEKA arm received FDA approval in 2014 and continues to be provided to veterans (https://www.research.va.gov/research_in_action/The-LUKE-DEKA-advanced-prosthetic-arm.cfm).

was introduced in the United States in 1999. It is able to fine-tune the balance between stability and mobility needed by prosthetic knee joints, and has a stumble recovery feature. Still relevant today, the Össur Power knee, released in 2006, became the first commercially available knee able to generate power during ambulation, and to assist the individual in powered knee extension when climbing slopes and when getting up and down from a chair [33]. Subsequently, the Military Amputee Research Program funded Otto Bock to develop the X3 knee, which began clinical testing in 2009. This knee was designed to enable a combat-injured amputee to return to duty, and allows them to walk on uneven ground, walk backwards, carry a heavy load, run without adjusting the settings, and even be submerged in water [33]. Otto Bock has also

SUMMARY

This chapter concerning the history of prosthetics and orthotics is intended to inform the reader of the early developments by many artisans who have attempted to provide orthotic and prosthetic support, assistance, and non-surgical treatment of disease, congenital anomalies, trauma, and the ravages of war. It offers examples of care and of those who provided it, based on the understanding of biomechanics, available materials, and the day-to-day needs of those who survived their afflictions.

Space did not allow us to mention all historical facts and those who contributed to our history. We sincerely hope our readers enjoyed the chapter as much as we did researching it.

References

[1] Friedmann LW. Amputations and prostheses in primitive cultures. *Bull Prosthet Res.* 1972;Spring:105–138.

[2] Sellegren KR. An early history of lower limb amputations and prostheses. *The Iowa Orthop J.* 1982;2:13–27.

[3] *Orthopaedic Appliances Atlas, Vol. I: Braces, Splints, Shoe Alterations.* The American Academy of Orthopaedic Surgeons. Ann Arbor, Michigan, J. W. Edwards, 1952. Book review in: *J Bone Joint Surg Am.* 1952;34(July):758.

[4] Wilson Jr, AB. History of amputation surgery and prosthetics. In: Bowker HK, Michael JW, eds. *Atlas of Limb Prosthetics: Surgical, Prosthetic, and Rehabilitation Principles*, 2002. 2nd edition. Accessed October 19, 2016. http://www.oandplibrary.org/alp/.

[5] Vasiliadis ES, Grivas TB, Kaspiris A. Historical overview of spinal deformities in ancient Greece. *Scoliosis.* 2009;4(6). Accessed September 5, 2024. https://scoliosisjournal.biomedcentral.com/articles/10.1186/1748-7161-4-6.

[6] Grant RL. Antyllus and his medical works. *Bull Hist Med.* 1960; 34(2):154–174.

[7] Fortuna S. Aurelianus, Caelius (Fifth Century AD). In: van den Tweel, JG, ed. *Pioneers in Pathology (Encyclopedia of Pathology)*, 2017. Springer, Cham. https://doi.org/10.1007/978-3-319-41995-4_492.

[8] Hernigou P, Dubory A, Roubineau F. History of traction for treatment of lower limb fractures. *Int Orthop (SICOT).* 2016;40:2635–2641. https://doi.org/10.1007/s00264-016-3272-6.

[9] Hernigou P. Ambroise Paré IV: the early history of artificial limbs (from robotic to prostheses). *Int Orthop.* 2013;37:1195–1197.

[10] Packard F. *Life and Times of Ambroise Paré*, 1926. Paul B. Hoeber, Inc., New York.

[11] Thurston AJ. Paré and prosthetics: the early history of artificial limbs. *ANZ J Surg.* 2007;77:1114–1119.

[12] Hernigou P. Crutch art painting in the Middle Ages as orthopaedic heritage (part II: the peg leg, the bent-knee peg and the beggar). *Int Orthop.* 2014;38(7):1535–1542.

[13] Tarpada SP, Morris MT, Burton DA. Spinal fusion surgery: a historical perspective. *J Orthop.* 2017;14(1):134–136.

[14] Hernigou P, Gravina N, Potage D, Dubory A. History of club-foot treatment (part II: tenotomy in the nineteenth century). *Int Orthop (SICOT).* 2017;41:2205–2212.

[15] U.S. National Library of Medicine. Life and limb: the toll of the American Civil War. U.S. National Library of Medicine. Accessed November 2, 2016. https://www.nlm.nih.gov/exhibition/lifeandlimb/maimedmen.html.

[16] The Ohio State University Department of History. Civil War battlefield medicine. The Ohio State University. Accessed November 2, 2016. https://ehistory.osu.edu/exhibitions/cwsurgeon/cwsurgeon/amputations.

[17] Marshall J. The history of prosthetics. UNYQ. Accessed November 2, 2016. http://unyq.com/the-history-of-prosthetics/.

[18] Sayre LA. *Spinal Disease and Spinal Curvature: Their Treatment by Suspension and the Use of the Plaster of Paris Bandage*, 1877. Smith, Elder, & Co., London.

[19] Ekanayake C, Gamage JCPH, Mendis P, Weerasinghe P. Revolution in orthopedic immobilization materials: a comprehensive review. *Heliyon.* 2023;9(3):e13640.

[20] American Orthotic & Prosthetic Association. History. American Orthotic & Prosthetic Association. Accessed November 3, 2016. http://www.aopanet.org/about-aopa/history/.

[21] Wilson Jr. AB. Committee on Prosthetics Research and Development—a report. *Orthop Prosthet Appliance J.* 1961;March:56–57.

[22] Wilson Jr. AB. Prosthetics and orthotics research in the United States. *Orthop Prosthet Appliance J.* 1963;June:152–160.

[23] Furman B. *Progress in Prosthetics*, 1962. U.S. Department of Health, Education, and Welfare.

[24] Marinakis GN. Interlimb symmetry of traumatic unilateral transtibial amputees wearing two different prosthetic feet in the early rehabilitation stage. *J Rehabil Res Dev.* 2004;41(4):581–590.

[25] Hafner BJ, Sanders JE, Czerniecki JM, Fergason J. Transtibial energy-storage-and-return prosthetic devices: a review of energy concepts and a proposed nomenclature. *J Rehabil Res Dev.* 2002;39(1):1–11.

[26] Shurr D. *Prosthetics and Orthotics*, 2001. 2nd edition. Pearson, London.

[27] Donald Shurr, personal communication.

[28] Singer B. ABC's 40 years of excellence—a retrospective. June–October 1988. *Almanac.*

[29] National Commission on Orthotic and Prosthetic Education. Accessed November 14, 2016. http://www.ncope.org.

[30] NCOPE Timeline. Robin Seabrook, personal communication.

[31] American Academy of Orthotists & Prosthetists. History. American Academy of Orthotists & Prosthetists. Accessed November 3, 2016. http://www.oandp.org/about/history/.

[32] Fischer H. A guide to U.S. military casualty statistics: Operation Freedom's Sentinel, Operation Inherent Resolve, Operation New Dawn, Operation Iraqi Freedom, and Operation Enduring Freedom. Congressional Research Services. 2015. Accessed November 3, 2016. https://www.fas.org/sgp/crs/natsec/RS22452.pdf.

[33] Harvey ZT, Potter BK, Vandersea J, Wolf E. Prosthetic advances. *J Surg Ortho Adv.* 2012;21(1):58–64.

[34] Resnik L, Klinger SL, Etter K. The DEKA arm: its features, functionality, and evolution during the Veterans Affairs Study to optimize the DEKA arm. *Prosthet Orthot Int.* 2014;38(6):492–504.

CHAPTER 2

An Overview of Orthotic and Prosthetic Education and Training for the Physical Therapist

Rebecca M. Miro, Matthew Parente, and Christopher Robinson

OBJECTIVES

Upon completion of this chapter, the reader should be able to:

1. List the different types of providers involved in the delivery of Orthotics & Prosthetics (O&P) services.
2. Review the evolution of O&P education and credentialing.
3. Identify professional organizations associated with the profession of O&P.

The evolution of Orthotics & Prosthetics (O&P) education began post-World War II. Persons who sustained amputations during the war felt that the prosthetic options available lacked function and had excessive weight. While these initial complaints were addressed by engaging Northrup Aviation engineers to design lighter weight prostheses, the initiative's momentum also championed harnessing academia and industry's resources to advance prosthetic education and design [1].

Following World War II, the National Academy of Sciences (NAS) formed the Committee on Prosthetics Research and Development (CPRD) and the Committee on Prosthetics and Orthotics Education. In 1945, NAS organized a meeting in Chicago that brought together surgeons, engineers, and prosthetists with the goal of establishing criteria for upper and lower limb prosthetic design [1]. While this meeting did help achieve some consensus regarding clinical guidelines, a key meeting outcome was the resolution that more scientific studies be performed regarding prosthetic fit, function, and use to address a limited body of evidence.

The first attempt to address the lack of scientific studies regarding prosthetic management was in 1952 when the University of California hosted a 6-week course that essentially consisted of basic studies of human gait and biomechanics. Research-oriented approaches in orthotics did not begin until 1960.

The organized attempt to improve the clinical and scientific aspects of prosthetics also helped spur the creation of managing bodies for the profession. The American Board for Certification in Orthotics, Prosthetics & Pedorthics (ABC) was established in 1948. ABC is responsible for creating, validating, and administering the orthotics, prosthetics, and pedorthics certification examinations. These ABC certification examinations identify the candidates who possess the minimum qualifications to practice as independent practitioners [2]. Today, the ABC also credentials O&P Assistants, O&P Technicians, and several other professions. Over the years, ABC has evolved their standards to attaining certification to match current entry-level educational requirements.

Entry-Level Bachelor's

Until 1965, orthotic and prosthetic education consisted of seminars or certificate programs. In that year, New York University (NYU) became the first institution to offer a formal certificate in orthotics and prosthetics, called a post-baccalaureate long course certificate. As the name implies, students were required to complete a Bachelor's degree prior to enrollment in the certificate. It was NYU that developed the first Bachelor of Science curriculum, including prerequisites in the first 2 years of study and focused prosthetic and orthotic education in the latter 2 years [3].

In 1970 ABC sponsored a conference in which it pressed for reforms of the minimum educational requirements required prior to taking the certification examination. At that time, only a high school diploma was required to apply for certification. The requirements changed again in 1972 when, in addition to a high school diploma, each applicant for certification was required to have successfully completed three short-term courses in either orthotics or prosthetics [4].

In 1975 the requirements were once again raised to include completion of an Associate's degree in addition to the three short-term courses. In 1982, the *Journal of the American Orthotic and Prosthetic Association* released a special education issue. At that time, there were 12 practitioner level education programs in the United States, eight of which were long-term certificate programs and the remaining 4 were baccalaureate programs. By 1983, the minimum educational level acceptable in order to be eligible for ABC certification was completion of a Bachelor's degree or a long-term certificate. By the late 1980s, 12 universities offered orthotics and prosthetics programs. Five of those were baccalaureate programs and the other seven were post-professional certificates in prosthetics, orthotics, or both.

Elevation to the Entry-Level Master's Degree

As early as 1984, the Education Accreditation Commission (EAC), a component of the ABC, recommended the transition to an entry-level Master's degree in Orthotics & Prosthetics [5]. At the 1990 Phoenix Conference, a meeting of orthotics and prosthetics educators re-emphasized the need to transition to the Master's degree, citing the following reasons: (1) increase in the body of knowledge; (2) need for evidence-based practice; (3) need to address marketplace forces; (4) need to meet consumer

expectations; (5) greater demand for accountability; and (6) in order to maintain parity with other allied health professional academic preparation [6]. The National Commission on Orthotic and Prosthetic Education (NCOPE), the organization responsible for accrediting O&P education and residency programs, evaluated and subsequently mandated this change.

As of 2010, any new practitioner programs were required to be entry-level Master's degrees and any existing accredited Bachelor's degree programs transitioned by 2012 [7]. Currently, 15 accredited academic institutions offer Master's degrees in Prosthetics and Orthotics (Table 2.1).

TABLE 2.1 **Accredited Practitioner and Technician programs [8].**	
ACCREDITED PRACTITIONER PROGRAMS	**ACCREDITED TECHNICIAN PROGRAMS**
Alabama State University (Montgomery, AL)	Bluegrass Community and Technical College (Lexington, KY)
Baylor College of Medicine (Houston, TX)	Century College (White Bear Lake, MN)
California State University (Dominguez Hills, CA)	Joliet Junior College (Joliet, IL)
Concordia University (St. Paul, MN)	Spokane Falls Community College (Spokane, WA)
Eastern Tennessee State University (Johnson City, TN)	
Eastern Michigan University (Ypsilanti, MI)	
International Institute of Orthotics & Prosthetics (Tampa, FL)	
Kennesaw State University (Kennesaw, GA)	
Loma Linda University (Loma Linda, CA)	
Northwestern University (Chicago, IL)	
Drexel University (Elkins Park, PA)	
University of Hartford (West Hartford, CT)	
University of Pittsburgh (Pittsburgh, PA)	
University of Texas Southwestern Medical Center (Dallas, TX)	
University of Washington (Seattle, WA)	

EDUCATIONAL STAKEHOLDERS

Much like other practitioner-level rehabilitation professions, the orthotist/prosthetist has a considerable number of stakeholders, each of which is responsible for specific aspects of training, credentialing, and continuing education. The primary role of an educational accreditor is to ensure that institutions which house educational programs develop specific evaluation criteria for said programs and meet acceptable quality levels [9]. Credentialing organizations exist on both a national and state level in order to set standards to ensure quality patient care is provided by the orthotist/prosthetist [11]. Continuing education providers create learning opportunities for the orthotist/prosthetist to stay abreast of the latest standards to ensure patients receive competent care [11]. The primary stakeholders in O&P education are CAAHEP (Commission on Accreditation of Allied Health Education Programs), NCOPE, ABC, state licensing agencies, and two professional organizations that provide continuing education.

NCOPE is a non-profit, 501(c)3 organization whose mission is to improve lives and strengthen the profession through education. NCOPE's earlier responsibilities included [12]*:

- *Promote education in the field of orthotics and prosthetics and raise the standards of education in the field;*
- *Develop standards for, and accredit orthotics and prosthetics programs;*
- *Establish accreditation and evaluation procedures in orthotics and prosthetics education;*
- *Aid the development of new orthotics and prosthetics programs;*
- *Publish an annual report on orthotics and prosthetics education.*

Courtesy of the National Commission on Orthotic and Prosthetic Education.

NCOPE evolved from the EAC which was created in 1972 by the ABC to address the absence of a separate educational accreditation organization. In 1991, the EAC was renamed NCOPE and in 1999 it became a separate incorporated accreditation organization. NCOPE serves as a committee of accreditation under the umbrella of the Commission on Accreditation of Allied Health Education Programs (CAAHEP), which accredits 31 allied healthcare professions including the orthotist/prosthetist, orthotic & prosthetic assistant, and technician programs. Furthermore, NCOPE independently accredits orthotist/prosthetist residency programs, which are a requirement to be eligible for the orthotists/prosthetist certification exams administered by ABC. NCOPE also has the responsibility for credentialing residency training sites, which are a requirement for practitioner level graduates to complete in order to be eligible to pursue their credentialing board examinations. NCOPE works in conjunction with both national and local accrediting bodies to ensure candidates receive appropriate didactic and practical education to pursue certification and/or licensure.

ABC was founded in 1948 in order to credential prosthetists and orthotists on a national level. The ABC fulfills its mission by [2]*:

- *Measuring patient care provider's knowledge and skills through rigorous credentialing programs*
- *Establishing standards of organizational performance through facility accreditation*
- *Mandating professional continuing education to maintain competency*
- *Enforcing a professional ethics program*
- *Communicating the value and importance of ABC credentials.*

Courtesy of the American Board for Certification in Orthotics, Prosthetics and Pedorthics.

Since ABC's inception they have grown to credential other O&P providers and extenders including pedorthists, mastectomy fitters, O&P assistants, and O&P technicians. ABC is also a facility accreditor recognized as a Medicare Deemed Authority recognized for providing Medicare Part B Durable Medical Equipment, Prosthetics, Orthotics and Supplies (DMEPOS) [13]. At present there are more than 12,000 total certified individuals and 5,000 accredited facilities reportedly credentialed by ABC. As of January 2023, there were 5,898 persons holding ABC certification as a prosthetist, orthotist, or prosthetist/orthotists [14]. The ABC practitioner level certification examinations are designed to assess entry-level competency based upon the ABC Practice Analysis scope of practice, which was most recently updated in 2022 [15]. The credentialing examination to become a Certified Prosthetist (CP) or Certified Orthotist (CO) consists of three components: Written Exam, Written Simulation Exam, and the Clinical Patient Management (CPM) Exam. Successfully passing all three components in a single discipline grants the credential of CO or CP. Successfully passing all three components of the exam for both disciplines grants the credential of Certified Prosthetist Orthotist (CPO). In 2012, the ABC earned recognition by the International Society of Prosthetists & Orthotists (ISPO) as meeting their standards for the Category I Credential, which recognizes persons who complete a CAAHEP-accredited orthotist/prosthetist degree, residency training in both orthotic and prosthetic practice, and CPO certification to receive ISPO orthotist/prosthetist recognition [16].

A license to practice prosthetics and orthotics is required in just 16 U.S. states [17]. Licensure benefits patients by giving the profession of O&P official recognition at a state level, identifying a clear scope of practice and by providing recognition as a qualified member of the rehabilitation team [17]. There is an initiative to establish licensure in the remaining states, but the process of creating a licensing bill and subsequently having it enacted into law is a process that requires knowledge, time, and persistence with the judicial process. The vast majority of states with licensure require that individuals pursuing a license hold a credential from ABC in addition to having formal education and practical training.

The American Orthotic & Prosthetic Association (AOPA) was founded in 1917 when it was known as the Artificial Limb Manufacturers and Brace Association (ALMBA). AOPA is considered to be the organization that represents the needs of O&P business [18]. AOPA hosts an annual national meeting in the Fall which provides attendees continuing educational opportunities in clinical, research, and business attributes in addition to an online portal which grants practitioners the opportunity to attain continuing education at the time and place of their choosing. AOPA serves a major role in connecting practitioners and their patients with their local and federal government representatives via their annual policy forum, which enables meetings between elected officials and their constituents engaged in O&P care.

The American Academy of Orthotists and Prosthetists (AAOP) was founded in 1970 under the guidance of AOPA and ABC in order to address the need for continuing education. The AAOP is patient-centered, seeking to improve standards of care via education, literature, and research [19]. The AAOP hosts numerous continuing educational opportunities including the largest library of online O&P resources via the Paul E. Leimkuehler Online Learning Center (OLC), One Day Certificate Programs in addition to local and national level meetings. The academy also recognizes practitioners for significant contribution and attainment in the profession of orthotics via their fellowship program [20]. The Fellow of the American Academy of Orthotists and Prosthetists has two tiers of recognition: the Fellow (FAAOP) and the Fellow with Distinction (FAAOP(D)).

PRACTICAL EDUCATION

Clinical education of orthotists and prosthetists is designed to provide students the opportunity to apply lessons learned in the classroom to real-world patient care settings. Much like other allied rehabilitation professions, O&P students acquire experience as a requirement of their degree program [21]. Unlike physical therapy, where a residency is designed to provide a licensed therapist with additional skills beyond entry-level, the O&P residency is a prerequisite to pursuing national certification and/or licensure. Collectively, the experiences acquired during a practitioner's graduate-level education and residency are essential to preparing an orthotist/prosthetist to provide entry-level O&P clinical services.

During an orthotist's/prosthetist's entry-level schooling, it is imperative that the individual achieve competency and standards defined by CAAHEP in the following three areas [21]*:

Section A—Entry Level Competencies
Section B—Basic Science Curriculum
Section C—Professional Curriculum
    *Courtesy of the Commission on Accreditation of Allied Health Education Programs.

Institutions hosting a CAAHEP accredited O&P education program create formal relationships with clinical sites and define specific learning outcomes for the specific rotations. The students are typically rotated through a variety of settings to enable exposure to a variety of practice settings, diverse patient populations, and different phases of care. Student levels of engagement typically range from being largely observational in nature during initial rotations to assisting and performing during later phases of the clinical experiences.

The contemporary NCOPE O&P residency standards were developed to ensure that resources for clinical education were appropriate, and that residents were required to demonstrate competency in clinical procedures [22]. A list of required competencies is listed below (see Table 2.2) for both O&P residencies.

A residency site can be further defined by the disciplines it offers training in, the residency duration, and whether they offer a clinical or research-oriented residency. At present there are 494 accredited residency sites throughout the United States and abroad offering prosthetic and/or orthotic residencies. While the majority of

TABLE 2.2 **Required competencies for orthotic and prosthetic residencies [22].**	
ORTHOTIC COMPETENCIES	PROSTHETIC COMPETENCIES
Custom Ankle-Foot Orthosis	Post-Operative Care
Custom Foot Orthosis	Symes and/or Partial Feet Prosthesis
Custom Knee-Ankle-Foot Orthosis	Transfemoral Prosthesis
Custom Scoliosis Orthosis	Transtibial Prosthesis
Custom Thoraco-Lumbo-Sacral Orthosis	Upper Limb Prosthesis
Knee Orthosis	
Upper Limb Orthosis	

the sites offer the opportunity to be trained with patients requiring both prosthetic and orthotic care, specialty clinics may dedicate their care to either prosthetics or orthotics depending on the credentials of the practitioners supervising the residency and the patient populations that they service. NCOPE offers two potential residency durations: a single-discipline prosthetic or orthotic residency which lasts 12 months or a dual-discipline prosthetic and orthotic residency which spans 18 months. While a single-discipline residency requires the resident to dedicate their training to either prosthetic or orthotic care, a dual-discipline residency requires that the individual gains comparable exposure to both orthotic and prosthetic patients. The final variable that is determined by the residency site is whether to offer a clinical or research residency. While both clinical and research residencies require the application of evidence-based practice, a research residency requires the resident to generate a research report at a level appropriate for publication in a peer-reviewed journal. Clinical residency positions are more plentiful, whereas research residency opportunities more typically occur in facilities that are part of a larger teaching hospital.

CERTIFICATION

Obtaining certification within any profession provides the consumer with a level of confidence in the individual's knowledge and ability. Becoming certified within O&P provides the patient, physician, and allied health professionals with a level of confidence in the individual's prior training and commitment to maintaining their certification. ABC certification can be obtained in each of the following professional categories: Certified Orthotist/Prosthetist, Certified Pedorthist, Certified Fitter-Orthotics, Certified Fitter-Mastectomy, Certified Fitter-Therapeutic Shoes, Certified Orthotic/Prosthetic Assistant, and Certified Orthotic/Prosthetic Technician [23].

An ABC-certified orthotist and/or prosthetist is an allied health professional specifically educated and trained to make and fit orthoses and prostheses and manage comprehensive orthotic and/or prosthetic patient care. As ABC practitioners, these individuals are certified to independently provide or supervise the provision of patient care [23].

The certification is primarily based upon two documents: ABC's *Certified Orthotist and/or Prosthetist Scope of Practice* and the *ABC Code of Professional Responsibility*. ABC's *Certified Orthotist and/or Prosthetist Scope of Practice* details the specific functions of certified practitioners. This includes patient assessment, formulation of a treatment plan, implementation of a treatment plan, follow-up and practice management [23]. Professional ethics are maintained and ensured as a component of certification by requiring certified individuals abide with the *ABC Code of*

Professional Responsibility. This document promotes and assures the overall welfare of the patient and the integrity of the profession [23].

The *ABC Code of Professional Responsibility* is recognized throughout the profession as the guiding principles which govern the professional, ethical, and moral integrity of individuals and organizations engaged in the delivery of orthotic, prosthetic, and pedorthic care. The *Code of Professional Responsibility* applies to all ABC-credentialed individuals and accredited facilities [23].

Some of the greatest advancements in O&P have occurred around times of conflict and war. One such event occurred after World War II with the formation of the American Board for Certification of the Orthotic and Prosthetic Appliance Industry, Inc. In 1948, a small group of orthotic and prosthetic practitioner and orthopedic surgeons created the country's first O&P standard setting organization [24]. This group realized the need to bring O&P clinicians out of the shadows and into the forefront of patient care within the healthcare community. This could only happen by establishing standards, certification, and a mission. The group's mission—"to encourage and promote the high standards of workmanship and service"— has remained relatively unchanged all these years later. The group also identified the need to be a service organization to assist clinicians (then fitters) to establish themselves within the allied health community [24]. ABC initiated an environment of education and learning through the creation of the Advisory Committee on Educational Standards in 1949. The creation of standards led to the clinician certification process, and provided individuals with ABC certification an opportunity to become a respectable member of the healthcare team.

In 1959 the organization updated its name to the American Board for Certification in Orthotics & Prosthetics, Inc. This change provided the organization with a philosophical shift away from being "leg-makers" and "brace-fitters" to their current role as a clinician. The organization continued to progress as it established the ABC Character and Fitness Committee to review ethical misconduct and oversee the consumer complaint process in 1968 [24]. This committee revised the ABC *Canons of Ethics* [25] which has been updated again to the current version, the *Code of Professional Responsibility and Rules & Procedures* [26]. In addition to considerable ethical standards, ABC and the American Orthotic & Prosthetic Association (AOPA) sponsored the formation of the American Academy of Orthotists and Prosthetists (AAOP) to provide the field with continuing education possibilities [24]. These initial efforts in 1970 provided the field with a path which established mandatory continuing education requirements by 1972.

In 1973, ABC tackled entry-level standards in O&P to require a minimum of an Associate of Arts degree. ABC continued defining roles within O&P by establishing credential programs for Certified Orthotic & Prosthetic Technician and Certified Orthotic & Prosthetic Assistant. Then in 1991 ABC relinquished its responsibility of oversight of primary O&P education to the newly created NCOPE [24]. This coincided with NCOPE's creation of O&P residency programs. One of the most recent changes to ABC occurred in January of 2007 when the Board for Certification in Pedorthics (BCP) was integrated into ABC. This integration brought along a new name, the American Board for Certification in Orthotics, Prosthetics & Pedorthics, Inc. [27]. To date, ABC maintains individual certification for Orthotists, Prosthetists, O&P Assistants, O&P Technicians, Pedorthists, Orthotic Fitters, Mastectomy Fitters, and Therapeutic Shoe Fitters. In addition to individual certification, ABC provides facility accreditation to Patient Care Centers and Central Fabrication facilities [27].

BOC History

In 1984, orthotists and prosthetists were provided with an additional option for certification with the creation of the Board of Certification/Accreditation (BOC). BOC was founded as an independent, not-for-profit agency dedicated to meeting the demands for quality patient care by offering highly valued credentials for professionals and suppliers of comprehensive O&P care and durable medical equipment (DME) services [28]. This credential offered individuals with an alternative pathway to certification [28].

In the early 1990s BOC introduced another credential, facility accreditation, to help facilities independently prove their competency in patient care and sound business practices [28]. Prior to July 2016, BOC offered the following individual professional certifications: orthotists, prosthetists, pedorthists, orthotic fitters, mastectomy fitters and DME specialists [28]. Then in July of 2016 BOC ceased accepting new applications for orthotist, prosthetist, and pedorthist credentials. They will continue to support and maintain certifications for all previously certified individuals. In the future BOC will continue to offer facility accreditation for O&P practitioners, as well as suppliers of DME, pharmacies and chiropractors offering DME and related supplies, respiratory therapy and related supplies, and other facility/practice specialties [28].

Practice Analysis Defining the Board Exams

O&P education is a constantly evolving body of skills and knowledge. Scientific advances and technology have created a "moving target" of knowledge and skills within the field. One way to bring these developments into focus is through utilization of ABC's *Practice Analysis of Certified Practitioners in the Disciplines of Orthotics and*

Prosthetics [15]. This document provides direction for continuing education opportunities for certified clinicians and to educational institutions for supplements to established curriculum criteria, to weight properly the National Board Examinations.

A practice analysis is a psychometrically and legally defensible strategy used to develop or update credentialing examination content and to update the description of the profession [15]. ABC's *Practice Analysis* and its *Orthotic, Prosthetic, & Pedorthic Scope of Practice* [29] document provide direction for candidates completing their ABC Board Exams. The *Practice Analysis* ensures proper balance of content in the examination, while the *Scope of Practice* assists with the determination of inclusion or exclusion of content. These documents work in concert with the *Standards and Guidelines for the Accreditation of Educational Programs in Orthotics and Prosthetics* document created by CAAHEP [21] to formulate the relevance and appropriateness of content on ABC's practitioner certification exams. The utilization of these three documents provide ABC with the ability to monitor the demands of the field, balance them within a clinician's scope of practice, and reference academic standards to create a practitioner certification exam which helps define the credential.

ABC Exam and Sections

There are many places in O&P which seek balance. The most obvious is for our patient. We strive for our treatment to provide the patient with the intricate balance of stability and mobility to give them with the best possible outcomes and ability to meet their goals. One area of balance which can be overlooked relates to the ABC practitioner certification exams. The examinations are designed to allow the candidate to demonstrate a balance of clinical skills and academic knowledge. This is why ABC identifies specific criteria in the *ABC Practitioner Book of Rules and Candidate Guide* [30] to determine a candidate's eligibility to take the exam.

The educational guidelines now require the candidate to complete a CAAHEP-accredited, entry-level Master's degree in orthotics and prosthetics [23]. In addition to educational requirements the candidate must complete a clinical residency which meets NCOPE's requirements as an accredited residency program [23]. When the candidate meets these requirements, they are considered board eligible in a specific discipline.

Maintenance of Credential/ Continuing Education

In 1970 ABC recognized the need to adopt a practice which is required throughout the healthcare community—continuing education. This process was formalized in 1972 with continuing education standards. Remarkably, this process occurred the year before ABC created educational standards to enter the field. Clinicians are required to meet minimum continuing education benchmarks depending on their credential. These minimums provide the clinician with a reminder of a commitment to lifelong learning. This commitment gives patients and the healthcare community a level of comfort that ABC-certified clinicians are engaged in recent trends and technology within the field.

ABC recognized intervals of change occurring within the field, and thus established a 5-year interval of time to complete mandatory continuing education. This interval of time is consistent within the certification industry [31]. ABC recognizes the needs of the patient, payors, and clinicians as a part of the continuing education process, and publishes the *Guide to Maintaining Your Certification* [31] to ensure compliance.

P&O Care Extenders

ABC also offers credentialing examinations for O&P Assistants, O&P Technicians, and Pedorthists. The educational and experience requirements to be eligible for the respective professions' certification examination differ from those for Certified Orthotists and Certified Prosthetists.

Certified O&P Assistants perform orthotic and prosthetic care under the supervision of a certified and/or licensed practitioner. They can perform routine orthotic and prosthetic care such as casting, fitting, fabrication, and related tasks to maximize fit and function for patients under the supervision of an ABC CO, CP, or CPO.

The minimum required educational level to qualify to take the O&P Assistant exam is a high school diploma or General Educational Development (GED) completion. While a college degree is not required, the potential candidate is required to take human anatomy, physics, and medical terminology at an accredited higher education institution [32]. In addition to the educational requirement, a potential candidate must complete 1 year of clinical experience (or 18 months if seeking dual credentialing) under the supervision of an ABC-certified orthotist or prosthetist corresponding to the discipline in which the candidate is taking the examination.

An O&P Technician's main role is to provide technical support in fabricating, repairing, and maintenance of prostheses and orthoses to Certified Orthotists and Prosthetists. Technicians can be credentialed in either or both disciplines, as Certified Orthotic Technician (CTO), Certified Prosthetic Technician (CTP), or Certified Prosthetic-Orthotic Technician (CTPO) [33].

Two educational pathways exist to make a candidate eligible for the O&P Technician certification exam. Via the educational pathway, a candidate successfully completes a CAAHEP/NCOPE accredited technician education program. The alternative pathway is a combination of education (high school diploma, GED, or college degree) and 2 years of technical experience in a particular discipline under the supervision of an ABC-certified practitioner in that same discipline [33].

A Pedorthist is an individual who specializes in footwear and modifications to footwear to address conditions of the foot and lower limb [34]. An ABC-certified pedorthist (C. Ped.) fabricates, fits, builds, and modifies devices for patients with foot and lower limb related conditions.

Eligibility for ABC's Pedorthist certification examination is predicated upon a candidate possessing a minimum of a high school diploma or GED, successfully completing a pedorthic pre-certification course, and completing 1,000 hours of pedorthic experience prior to taking the examination. Unlike O&P Assistants and O&P Technicians, Certified Pedorthists can practice independently, although their scope of practice is limited to anatomy distal to the talocrural joint [34].

Summary

This chapter has provided an overview of educational processes in the O&P professions. The physical therapist should be familiar with O&P education to facilitate interdisciplinary communication and its implications in patient care.

References

[1] Krabich JI, Pinzur MS, Potter BK, Stevens PM, eds. *Atlas of Amputations and Limb Deficiencies: Surgical, Prosthetic, and Rehabilitation Principles*, 2016. 4th edition. American Academy of Orthopedic Surgeons, Rosemont, IL.

[2] ABC. Learn who we are. We're ABC. American Board for Certification in Orthotics, Prosthetics, and Pedorthics. 2024. Accessed September 12, 2024. https://www.abcop.org/who-we-are/about-abc.

[3] Hovorka CF, Shurr DG, Bozik DS. The concept of an entry-level interdisciplinary graduate degree preparing orthotists for the new millennium part 1: history of orthotic and prosthetic education. *J Prosthet Orthot.* 2002;14:51–58.

[4] Fishman S. Preface. *Orthotics and Prosthetics: Special Education Issue.* 1982;36:13–14.

[5] Nielsen CC, Altman RF, Gillespie P, Douglas PD. A model for graduate education in orthotics and prosthetics. *Clin Prosthet Orthot.* 1987;11:63–66.

[6] Malas B. The move toward entry-level Masters. *The O&P Edge.* 2006.

[7] Fairley M. O&P education reaching Master's level and beyond. *The O&P Edge.* 2008.

[8] NCOPE. Accreditation of O&P Education Programs. National Commission on Prosthetic and Orthotic Education. Accessed September 12, 2024. https://ncope.org/index.php/home-page-v2/academic-programs/the-orthotic-prosthetic-profession/.

[9] DAPIP—The Database of Accredited Postsecondary Institutions and Programs. U.S. Department of Education, Office of Postseconday Education. Accessed August 30, 2016. http://ope.ed.gov/accreditation/.

[10] Spath P. The quality cost connection: credential your allied health professionals. 2002. Accessed August 30, 2016. https://www.reliasmedia.com/articles/118002-the-quality-cost-connection-credential-your-allied-health-professionals.

[11] Ferguson A. Evaluating the purpose and benefits of continuing education in nursing and the implications for the provision of continuing education for cancer nurses. *J Adv Nurs.* 1994;19:640–646.

[12] NCOPE. Mission & goals. National Commission on Orthotic and Prosthetic Education. Accessed September 12, 2024. https://ncope.org/index.php/home-page-v2/about/mission-vision-goals/.

[13] American Board of Certification. Facility accreditation: patient care. Accessed August 27, 2016. Current web page leading to Patient Care Standards Guide: https://www.abcop.org/facility-accreditation/why-get-accredited.

[14] *Journal of Prosthetics and Orthotics.* Supplement: *JPO Proceedings: Challenges of and Opportunities for O&P Education and Training: Envisioning Future Needs.* July 2023 July;35(3S):1–55, page 3. https://journals.lww.com/jpojournal/toc/2023/07002.

[15] ABCOP. *Practice Analysis of Certified Practitioners in the Disciplines of Orthotics and Prosthetics.* The American Board for Certification in the Disciplines of Orthotics, Prosthetics & Pedorthics. 2022. Accessed September 12, 2024. https://www.abcop.org/docs/default-source/practice-analyses/abc-practitioner-practice-analysis-2022.pdf.

[16] ABCOP. Individual certification: Orthotist & prosthetist. American Board for Certification in Orthotics, Prosthetics & Pedorthics. Accessed August 27, 2016. Current web page: https://www.abcop.org/individual-certification/get-certified/orthotist-prosthetist/overview.

[17] AAOP. Orthotic & prosthetic licensure: a comprehensive guide. The American Academy of Orthotists & Prosthetists. Accessed August 28, 2016. Current web page: https://www.oandp.org/licensure.

[18] AOPA. About AOPA. American Prosthetic & Orthotic Association. Accessed August 27, 2016. http://www.aopanet.org/about-aopa/.

[19] AAOP. About the Academy. The American Academy of Orthotists & Prosthetists. Accessed August 29, 2016. https://www.oandp.org/about-oandp.

[20] AAOP. Academy Fellows. American Academy of Orthotists & Prosthetists. Accessed August 30, 2016. Current web page: https://www.oandp.org/fellow-program.

[21] CAAHEP. *Standards and Guidelines for the Accreditation of Educational Programs in Orthotics and Prosthetics. Commission on Accreditation of Allied Health Education Programs, 2017.* Accessed August 12, 2024. https://cdn.prod.website-files.com/5f466098572bfe97f28d59df/603da2518a8d7dd3fccdd62b_OPStandardsGuidelines2017.pdf

[22] NCOPE. Standards of Accreditation for The Orthotic/Prosthetic Residency Training Program. National Commission of Orthotic & Prosthetic Education, 2016. Accessed August 30, 2016. http://www.ncope.org/view/?file=2016_residency_standards. Current web page: https://ncope.org/index.php/home-page-v2/residency-program-services/orthotic-prosthetic-residency-standards/.

[23] ABCOP. Orthotist & Prosthetist. American Board for Certification in Orthotics, Prosthetics & Pedorthics. 2016. https://www.abcop.org/individual-certification/Pages/orthotistandprosthetist.aspx. The educational pathways listed were changed January 1, 2020. Current web page: https://www.abcop.org/publication/section/practitioner-candidate-guide/certification-eligibility-requirements.

[24] ABC. *Mark of Merit Newsletter.* September 2013. Special Edition.

[25] Harman JH. Canons of ethical conduct and the law. *Clin Prosthet Orthot.* 1983;7:2.

[26] American Board for Certification in Orthotics, Prosthetics & Pedorthics. The Code of Professional Responsibility: Rules & Procedures. Originally accessed August 2016. Current web page: https://www.abcop.org/docs/default-source/publications/ethics-program/2024_code-of-professional-responsibility.pdf?sfvrsn=e522bac8_1.

[27] American Board for Certification in Orthotics, Prosthetics, & Pedorthics. https://www.abcop.org.

[28] Board of Certification/Accreditation. About BOC. 2016. https://www.bocusa.org/about-boc.

[29] American Board for Certification in Orthotics, Prosthetics, & Pedorthics. *Orthotic, Prosthetic, & Pedorthic Scope of Practice.* 2012. Orginally accessed August 2016. Current web page: https://www.abcop.org/publication/scope-of-practice.

[30] ABC. *Practitioner Book of Rules & Candidate Guide.* 2015.

[31] ABC. *Guide to Maintaining Your Certification.* 2016.

[32] American Board for Certification in Orthotics, Prosthetics, & Pedorthics. O&P Assistant. Originally accessed 2016. Current web page: https://www.abcop.org/individual-certification/get-certified/o-p-assistant/overview.

[33] American Board for Certification in Orthotics, Prosthetics, & Pedorthics. O&P Technician. Originally accessed 2016. Current web page: https://www.abcop.org/individual-certification/get-certified/o-p-technician/overview.

[34] American Board for Certification in Orthotics, Prosthetics, & Pedorthics. Pedorthist. Originally accessed 2016. Current web page: https://www.abcop.org/individual-certification/get-certified/pedorthist/overview.

CHAPTER 3

Epidemiology of Amputation

Tyler D. Klenow, Rebecca M. Miro, Owen T. Hill, and M. Jason Highsmith

OBJECTIVES

Upon completion of this chapter, the reader will be able to:
1. Recall the basic terms and definitions used to explain the demographics of amputation and limb loss.
2. Identify populations most at risk for limb loss.
3. Describe trends in amputation and relative distribution of sub-populations.
4. Differentiate between causes of lower and upper extremity amputation.
5. Explain the impact of diabetes mellitus on the number of individuals with limb loss.
6. Define mechanism(s) of amputation and functional limb loss.

INTRODUCTION

An amputation is a mechanistic removal of the whole or part of a limb from a body by surgery, trauma, or illness. Removal of the fingers and toes or part of a hand or foot are referred to as a minor amputation. Major amputations are those occurring through or proximal to the ankle and wrist. According to the International Standards Organization [1], amputations are referred to by the bone or joint they transect. Congenital amputations are those which occur either in the womb and during or immediately following birth.

Amputations at or distal to the hip are commonly referred to as lower extremity amputations (LEA). Major amputations through the thigh are called transfemoral

amputations (TFA) and through the shank are called transtibial amputations (TTA). Separation at the level of the hip, knee, and ankle are identified as disarticulations of the particular joint. Amputations can also occur through the pelvis and are called transpelvic or through the inferior spine and are called translumbar. When an amputation occurs at the sacroiliac joint on one side it is referred to as hemipelvic (Table 3.1).

Amputations at or distal to the shoulder are commonly referred to as upper extremity amputations (UEA). Major amputations of the arm and forearm are called transhumeral (THA) and transradial amputations (TRA), respectively. Separation at the level of the shoulder, elbow, and wrist are identified as disarticulations of the particular joint. Removal of the arm including part or all of

DOI: 10.4324/9781003526025-4

TABLE 3.1

Names of amputation levels of the lower extremity with transected or separated structures identified

STRUCTURE TRANSECTED	LEVEL NAME
Thigh/femur	Transfemoral
Shank/tibia & fibula	Transtibial
Hip joint	Hip disarticulation
Knee joint	Knee disarticulation
Ankle joint	Ankle disarticulation
Pelvis	Transpelvic
Sacroiliac joint	Hemipelvic
Lumbar spine	Translumbar

the scapula is referred to as interscapulothoracic. Minor amputations are referred to in the same fashion, by the affected joint or segment (Table 3.2).

Historically, amputations were referred to regarding their position relative to (i.e. above or below) a particular joint, named after the introducing surgeon (i.e. eponym), or given other unique names. These terms are antiquated, but are often used as colloquial jargon. For example, the TFA and TTA levels were called above-knee (AK) or below-knee (BK) amputations. The ankle disarticulation was called the Symes amputation. Partial foot amputations were referred to as Chopart, Lisfranc, Pirigoff, or Boyd depending on what part of the foot was removed and the surgeon who is credited with describing the procedure. Similarly, THA and TRA were called above-elbow (AE) and below-elbow (BE). The interscapulothoracic amputation was referred to as the forequarter amputation (Table 3.3).

TABLE 3.2

Names of amputation levels of the upper extremity with transected or separated structures identified

STRUCTURE TRANSECTED	LEVEL NAME
Arm	Transhumeral
Forearm	Transradial
Shoulder	Shoulder disarticulation
Elbow	Elbow disarticulation
Wrist	Wrist disarticulation
Arm and scapula	Interscapulothoracic

TABLE 3.3

Selected examples of amputation levels identified by current ISO accepted terminology and by colloquial and antiquated terminology

LEVEL NAME	COLLOQUIAL/ ANTIQUATED TERM
Transtibial	Below-knee (BK)
Transfemoral	Above-knee (AK)
Ankle disarticulation	Symes
Transradial	Below-elbow (BE)
Transhumeral	Above-elbow (AE)
Interscapulothoracic	Forequarter

Amputations are often combined with limb deficiencies or malformations in public health as their treatment and management methods are similar and their presence can lead to subsequent amputations. Limb deficiencies are referred to as longitudinal deficiencies of the particular long bone, most typically the tibia, femur, radius, and humerus. Although these longitudinal deficiencies can occur in isolation, they often occur in combination with malformation and congenital limb absence of multiple extremities. These conditions are not referred to as amputations, as the limb was never physically removed but failed in utero to form in a typical fashion or to form or at all. Such a condition was historically referred to as a hemimelia or focal deficiency.

A basic review of terms is needed prior to a discussion regarding epidemiology. For the purposes of this chapter and text, <u>incidence</u> is the frequency of occurrence of an event or condition in relation to a given population during a given timeframe. <u>Prevalence</u> is the number of cases of a particular disease or condition in relation to a given population during a given timeframe. Incidence and prevalence are both measures of <u>morbidity</u>: the number of cases of a particular disease present in a given population. <u>Co-morbidity</u> is the presence or relation of two or more diseases or conditions within a given population or in reference to an individual. <u>Mortality</u> is a ratio of the number of deaths within a given population. Mortality is typically presented in relation to a particular cause.

REPORTING METHODS

Amputation trends are known to differ between economically developed and developing parts of the world, but are difficult to compare directly due to variation in reporting methods [2]. These methods include databases, registries, projections, and forecasts. A database is a repository for information collected by a single or a limited number of joint entities and tends to be specialized or regional in nature. The United States (U.S.) Veterans Health Administration manages its own internal Amputee Data Repository CUBE database, for example. Databases are also managed by large clinical providers in the U.S., but these data are designed for internal use and are not commonly published in the literature. A registry is a collection of information regarding all, or a majority of, individuals who undergo a particular procedure in a given area and are typically on a national scale. Currently, no limb loss registry exists in the U.S. However, the Mayo Clinic recently was awarded grant funding by the National Institutes of Health and Department of Defense and is actively developing a limb loss registry [3]. Registries are likely more common in Europe where universal healthcare and smaller relative populations make aggregation potentially more manageable.

When these direct sources are not available, projections must be made based on the morbidity of a limited sample. Forecasts can be made using local incidence rates over a defined horizon. While information regarding the morbidity of individuals with limb loss in developed nations is sparingly available using these methods, statistics are even more rare in developing nations who will typically publish results from one hospital, system, or region. Due to a lack of a registry, public amputation statistics in the U.S. are derived from a few scholarly works which extrapolate from a limited number of states or rely on numerous assumptions. While such forecasts are required when direct sources do not exist, these methods skew results toward a particular region and reduce the power of the statistics for use in funding or public health proposals. However, although such projections may not provide a completely accurate description of the real clinical population, they do at least provide a reasonable estimate of it.

MECHANISM OF AMPUTATION

Amputations are typically caused by some irreparable damage to the bone or vasculature of a limb. The etiologies can be vascular, traumatic, malignant or cancerous, and congenital or developmental in nature. Chronic pain is also a recurrent co-morbidity to elective amputation. The majority of amputations, approximately 82%, are due to vascular etiology [4]. Common forms of vascular dysfunction leading to amputation include peripheral vascular disease, thrombosis, arteriosclerosis, hypertension, and chronic hyperglycemia associated with type 2 diabetes mellitus (DM2) [5]. While many of these ailments may be effectively manageable, some individuals with amputation may be less medically responsible, have less education, or be less compliant with management and treatment.

Chronic wounds are often associated with diabetic cases resulting in major amputation. It is common for patients with DM2 to experience many amputations during their disease process, beginning distally and working proximally in an effort to find viable tissue to heal. Copious amounts of healthcare resources are consumed by chronic wound care and vascular limb salvage in the form of debridement, hyperbaric therapy, minor amputations, etc.

Traumatic etiologies account for 16% of all amputations [4]. They commonly include blunt trauma such as motor vehicle accidents (MVA) or falls from height, occupational injuries, penetrating wounds such as gunshot wounds (GSW) or stab wounds, and blast injuries, but can include a multitude of causes. MVAs are most frequently associated with the civilian population where accidents involving motorcycles or pedestrians more commonly result in LEAs as the legs are unprotected in these situations [6]. MVAs involving only vehicles commonly result in UEAs as the arms are relatively lowered in all types of cars or completely unprotected when hung out of a vehicle window. Blast injuries most commonly occur in the military population and are associated with other bodily injuries. However, they do occur in the civilian population as well, usually from poorly managed firework displays and industrial accidents [7]. GSWs occur commonly in the military and civilian populations and can be purposeful or incidental.

Cancerous and developmental etiologies each make up approximately 1% of all amputations [4]. These etiologies are numerous, but the most common include sarcomas, carcinomas, and amniotic band syndrome. Developmental etiologies can also be caused by in utero maternal consumption of chemicals, such as thalidomide or other drugs.

Etiology of amputation abroad is similar to the U.S. [3]. For example, the primary etiologies of non-traumatic amputation in Denmark in 2011 were arteriosclerosis at 70%, hypertension at 53%, and diabetes at 49% [8]. At the time of these individuals' amputations, 42% were not taking cholesterol-reducing medication, 29% were taking opioids, and 16% were diagnosed with DM2 for the first time. These facts support a common patient profile associated with lack of basic medical knowledge and management as well as noncompliance.

GLOBAL TRENDS

The literature regarding prevalence of amputation is limited and inconsistent. An estimated 185,000 amputation procedures occur in the U.S. annually, resulting in current prevalence of 1.6 to 1.9 M people living with amputation or approximately 1 in 200 people [9–11]. An estimated 80% of these amputations involve the lower extremity and occur secondary to vascular disease. This trend is also noted abroad, where 75–77% of LEAs are secondary to vascular disease [3, 12].

Traumatic amputations do occur regularly, however. From 2000 to 2004, 8,910 patients underwent a traumatic amputation in the U.S. [6]. The majority of these (n = 6,155) were finger amputations and 700 involved toes. The remaining 2,055 patients had major amputations. Of these, 1,904 patients had a single major amputation (782 upper extremity and 1,122 lower extremity). Overall, the most recent reported statistics show that 1.8 M individuals have experienced a lower limb amputation and an estimated 500 k have experienced an upper limb amputation in the U.S. [9, 10].

Nearly half of all LEAs in the U.S., approximately 48.6% or 618,000 people, are of the foot or toes [13]. The prevalence of TTA, the largest population of major amputations in the U.S., is about 29.8% or 378,000 people, as reported in 2016 [9]. The next largest population is TFA,

which accounts for roughly 20% or 254,000 people [14]. The remaining 1% of amputations are at or proximal to the hip or are knee disarticulations. Approximately 97% of all vascular amputations in the U.S. are LEAs. The majority of traumatic LEAs occur at the transtibial level [9].

The incidence rates of LEA between individuals with and without DM2 was published in a systematic review in 2017 [3]. The review included only data on LEA, not UEA, and reported on only a few developed nations which met the study criteria. Incidence rates of LEA were lowest in the Italian population at 4.2 per 100,000 without DM2 and 33.2 per 100,000 with DM2. The highest incidence of LEA was found in the U.S. at 38 per 100,000 people without DM2 and 383.0 per 100,000 with DM2, although these statistics include only those aged 65 years or older. Additional incidence for individuals with and without DM2 were found in various years. Incidence rates per 100,000 without DM2 include 5.9 to 10.6 specifically in Ireland, 8.0 to 16.4 in Germany, 8.0 to 21.0 in the United Kingdom (U.K.), 4.2 to 9.8 in Italy, 9.2 in Spain, 9.4 in Finland, 12.4 in the Netherlands, 13.4 in France, and 28.3 to 38.0 in the U.S. Incidence rates per 100,000 with DM2 include 48.0 to 121.2 in Germany, 48.0 to 160.0 specifically in Ireland, 71.4 in Finland, 114.0 to 370.2 in the U.K., 33.2 to 163.5 in Italy, 147.0 in France, 250.5 to 361.0 in the Netherlands, and 322.8 in Spain. Incidence rates of LEA were also reported in Sweden at 23 per 100,000 people without DM2 and 195 per 100,000 people with DM2, although these numbers include some individuals with partial foot amputations [15] (Table 3.4).

Whereas the primary cause of lower limb amputation is vascular disease, the primary cause of upper limb amputation is trauma. It is reported that 68.6% of individuals with traumatic amputation suffered loss to the upper extremity [10]. In the U.S., prevalence of major upper limb

TABLE 3.4

Incidence of lower extremity amputation with and without diabetes mellitus 2 (DM2) in selected countries

COUNTRY	WITH DM2	WITHOUT DM2
United States	383.0	28.3–38.0
Italy	33.2–163.5	4.2–9.8
Ireland	48.0–160.0	5.9–10.6
Germany	48.0–121.2	8.0–16.4
United Kingdom	114.0–370.2	8.0–21.0
Spain	322.8	9.2
Finland	71.4	9.4
The Netherlands	250.5–361.0	12.4
France	147.0	13.4
Sweden	195*	23*

Note: *Includes partial foot amputations.

amputation is approximately 41,000, only 3% of the total population with amputation. This ratio is found similarly abroad [12].

While the total number of persons living with amputation is expected to double by 2050, the number of amputation procedures both in the U.S. and abroad is in decline. Despite the increased incidence and prevalence of DM2, the decrease may potentially be attributed to better preventive care, though causation cannot be implied [11, 16, 17]. The rate of amputation in elderly diabetic patients dropped 45% in the U.S. from 196 to 119 per 100,000 patients between 1996 and 2011 [17]. It has been suggested that these rates of amputation are underestimated, however [18]. The current global incidence rate of diabetes has increased from 8.8% in 2015 to 10.5% in 2021 [3, 29].

Regardless of the etiology, men are typically at a higher risk of amputation than women globally [3, 12]. Subsequently the incidence of amputation among men is typically higher than women and women tend to have amputations later in life than men [12, 19]. LEAs also occur more commonly globally in those of African or Hispanic ethnicity and less commonly in those of Caucasian or Asian ethnicity. Amputation rates of any etiology have been shown to increase with age [3, 9].

Amputation rates are decreasing most likely due to advances in medical technology including limb salvage and wound care techniques. These advances also lead to increased life expectancy which allows the population living with amputation to progressively increase. Regardless of these advances, the outlook for those with amputation is alarming, especially in those patients with DM2. Perioperative mortality rates have been reported from 9–16% regardless of etiology and 1 year mortality rates from 14–47% [20]. Patients with DM2 interestingly have lower mortality at 1 year, likely a testament to the amount of care they have already received at the time of their amputation. The trend reverses with time, however, as those with DM2 show a 5-year mortality rate of 61% compared with the non-diabetic rate of 54% [21]. The increased rate with DM2 can be attributed to the risk of diabetic foot ulcers, which carry a first-time 5-year mortality rate of 40% [22].

For those who survive, 26% will experience a subsequent amputation within 1 year and roughly 50% will experience a contralateral amputation in 5 years [14, 23]. Walking with a prosthesis requires an increased metabolic expenditure of two- to five-fold, which likely contributes to the 30% of individuals who never walk again following major LEA and the 50% who abandon prosthetic use after 1 year [11, 22]. Ambulation with a prosthesis is protective, however, as the 5-year mortality rate of those who do walk with prostheses is 30% compared with 69% in those who do not [24].

Though the non-military and Veteran population of persons with amputation is larger, amputations acquired due to military service are also seen in the clinical setting. For example, during the most recent allied conflict in the Middle East, the Global War on Terror, it was initially reported that 1,221 U.S. service members experienced 1,631 combat-related amputations from 2001 to 2011 [7, 9]. Of these amputations, 683 were TTA and 564 were TFA. 225 service members with at least one major UEA were also reported [25]. Overall, 366 U.S. service members experienced multiple amputations [7, 9]. An update in 2015 reported 1,645 total service members with traumatic amputation, although the number of amputations were not reported and partial hand or foot amputations were not included [26].

An additional 329 service members from the U.K. suffered traumatic amputations during these conflicts, although casualty data may be suppressed by the Ministry of Defence for strategic reasons [27, 28]. Of these service members, 113 are known to have sustained multiple amputations [27]. The U.K. has reported an additional 159 amputations in areas not associated with the Middle East. Three service members from Australia had major traumatic amputations during these conflicts as well [27, 28]. From these statistics, a minimum of 1,977 allied service members sustained at least 2,076 major amputations associated with the Global War on Terror from 2001 to 2018.

SUMMARY

This chapter reviewed names and naming conventions for amputation levels of the upper and lower extremities and other regions more central in the body. The chapter further surveyed amputation etiologies, prognosis in some cases as well as the incidence and prevalence of amputation in the U.S. and in other countries.

REFERENCES

[1] Standardization IOf. ISO 8549-4:2014(en) Prosthetics and orthotics—vocabulary—Part 4: terms relating to limb amputation. 2014. Accessed January 15, 2019. https://www.iso.org/obp/ui/#iso:std:iso:8549:-4:ed-1:v1:en.

[2] Narres M, Kvitkina T, Claessen H, et al. Incidence of lower extremity amputations in the diabetic compared with the non-diabetic population: a systematic review. *PLOS One*. 2017;12(8): e0182081.

[3] Limb Loss and Preservation Registry (LLPR). nd. https://www. llpr.org.

[4] Ziegler-Graham K, MacKenzie EJ, Ephraim PL, et al. Estimating the prevalence of limb loss in the United States: 2005 to 2050. *Arch Phys Med Rehabil*. 2008;89(3):422–429.

[5] Perkins ZB, Yet B, Glasgow S, et al. Meta-analysis of prognostic factors for amputation following surgical repair of lower extremity vascular trauma. *Br J Surg*. 2015;102(5):436–450.

[6] Barmparas G, Inaba K, Teixeira PG, et al. Epidemiology of post-traumatic limb amputation: a National Trauma Databank analysis. *Am Surg*. 2010;76(11):1214–1222.

[7] Krueger CA, Wenke JC, Ficke JR. Ten years at war: comprehensive analysis of amputation trends. *J Trauma Acute Care Surg*. 2012;73(6 Suppl 5):S438–S444.

[8]   Jensen PS, Petersen J, Kirketerp-Moller K, et al. Progression of disease preceding lower extremity amputation in Denmark: a longitudinal registry study of diagnoses, use of medication and healthcare services 14 years prior to amputation. *BMJ Open.* 2017;7(11):e016030.

[9]   Highsmith MJ, Kahle JT, Miro RM, et al. Prosthetic interventions for people with transtibial amputation: systematic review and meta-analysis of high-quality prospective literature and systematic reviews. *J Rehabil Res Dev.* 2016;53(2):157–184.

[10]   Resnik L, Meucci MR, Lieberman-Klinger S, et al. Advanced upper limb prosthetic devices: implications for upper limb prosthetic rehabilitation. *Arch Phys Med Rehabil.* 2012;93(4):710–717.

[11]   Quality AfHRa. Lower limb prostheses: measurement instruments, comparison of component effects by subgroups, and long-term outcomes. 2018. https://effectivehealthcare.ahrq.gov/topics/prosthesis/research.

[12]   National Amputee Statistical Database. 2004/05 TASDftUK. 2005. http://www.cofemer.fr/UserFiles/File/Amput2004_05.pdf.

[13]   Dillon MP. Partial foot amputation: evidence for device use. In: *Lower Extremity Review* [magazine], 2010. https://lermagazine.com/article/partial-foot-amputation-evidence-for-device-use.

[14]   Dillingham TR, Pezzin LE, MacKenzie EJ. Limb amputation and limb deficiency: epidemiology and recent trends in the United States. *South Med J.* 2002;95(8):875–883.

[15]   Johannesson A, Larsson GU, Ramstrand N, et al. Incidence of lower-limb amputation in the diabetic and nondiabetic general population: a 10-year population-based cohort study of initial unilateral and contralateral amputations and reamputations. *Diabetes Care.* 2009;32(2):275–280.

[16]   Winell K, Niemi M, Lepantalo M. The national hospital discharge register data on lower limb amputations. *Eur J Vasc Endovasc Surg.* 2006;32(1):66–70.

[17]   Goodney PP, Tarulli M, Faerber AE, et al. Fifteen-year trends in lower limb amputation, revascularization, and preventive measures among Medicare patients. *JAMA Surg.* 2015;150(1):84–86.

[18]   Rayman G, Krishnan ST, Baker NR, et al. Are we underestimating diabetes-related lower-extremity amputation rates? Results and benefits of the first prospective study. *Diabetes Care.* 2004;27(8):1892–1896.

[19]   Heikkinen M, Saarinen J, Suominen VP, et al. Lower limb amputations: differences between the genders and long-term survival. *Prosthet Orthot Int.* 2007;31(3):277–286.

[20]   Kristensen MT, Holm G, Kirketerp-Moller K, et al. Very low survival rates after non-traumatic lower limb amputation in a consecutive series: what to do? *Interact Cardiovasc Thorac Surg.* 2012;14(5):543–547.

[21]   Tentolouris N, Al-Sabbagh S, Walker MG, et al. Mortality in diabetic and nondiabetic patients after amputations performed from 1990 to 1995: a 5-year follow-up study. *Diabetes Care.* 2004;27(7):1598–1604.

[22]   Thorud JC, Seidel JL. A closer look at mortality and lower extremity amputation. *Podiatry Today.* 2018;31(4):12–16.

[23]   Boutoille D, Leautez S, Maulaz D, et al. [Skin and osteoarticular bacterial infections of the diabetic foot. Treatment.] *Presse Med.* 2000;29(7):396–400.

[24]   Paquette R, Highsmith MJ, Carnaby G, et al. Duration, frequency, and factors related to lower extremity prosthesis use: systematic review and meta-analysis. *Disabil Rehabil.* 2023:1–19. https://doi.org/10.1080/09638288.2023.2276838.

[25]   Tennent DJ, Wenke JC, Rivera JC, Krueger CA. Characterisation and outcomes of upper extremity amputations. *Injury.* 2014;45(6):965–969.

[26]   Fischer H. A guide to U.S. military casualty statistics: Operation Freedom's Sentinel, Operation Inherent Resolve, Operation New Dawn, Operation Iraqi Freedom, and Operation Enduring Freedom. In: Congressional Research Service, RS22452. 2015.

[27]   U.K. Ministry of Defence. Amputation statistics: 1 April 2013–31 March 2018. Accessed January 12, 2019. https://assets.publishing.service.gov.uk/media/5b55ecebe5274a3fe478c33a/20180612_Amputation_Statistic_O_v2.pdf.

[28]   Wallace D. Trends in traumatic limb amputation in Allied Forces in Iraq and Afghanistan. *Journal of Military and Veterans' Health (JMVH).* 2012;20(2):31–35.

[29]   International Diabetes Federation. *IDF Diabetes Atlas.* 10th edition. International Diabetes Federation, Brussels, Belgium. Accessed June 17, 2024. https://diabetesatlas.org/atlas/tenth-edition/.

CHAPTER 4

Amputation Surgery

Paul Lunseth, Janos P. Ertl, Munjed Al Muderis, Roland Paquette,
and Jason T. Kahle

OBJECTIVES

Upon completion of this chapter, the reader should be able to recall:
1. The role and tasks of the surgeon in terms of
   a. Operative goals;
   b. Tissue management by type;
   c. Limb shape.
2. Select considerations related to the physical examination and clinical tests.
3. Advantages, disadvantages, benefits, drawbacks, and differences in prominent amputation flap closure techniques.
4. Major categories of post-operative dressings along with their respective benefits and drawbacks.
5. Key points related to amputation surgery by amputation level and peri-operative timelines relative to amputation surgery.
6. Key points of major amputation surgical techniques including the traditional Burgess, the osteomyoplastic bone bridge (Ertl), and osseointegration.

OVERVIEW

An amputation of a limb, or portion of a limb, is most often performed to treat complications arising from vascular disease, infections, trauma, or tumor. Children may also have complications from congenital, developmental deformities or deficiencies. Unfortunately, an amputation has historically been viewed as a failure of successful management or therapy, and many physicians may have previously been reluctant to become involved in performing or recommending amputations. Historically, amputation was a field-based procedure performed by a physician after severe injury or to free an individual stuck in a crush injury [1]. Later, as skills and knowledge improved, general surgeons began to perform

DOI: 10.4324/9781003526025-5

amputations within operating theaters using sterile technique. As time progressed, orthopedic surgeons were tasked with the surgical procedures, and follow-up care was carried out with the assistance of prosthetists in rehabilitation facilities. Most recently, vascular surgeons have performed the majority of amputation surgeries and follow-up care has largely been completed through a collaboration between physical therapists and prosthetists.

While skilled, interdisciplinary team-based care is common in certain larger centers such as Veteran and military hospitals, rehabilitation, and university facilities, it is not readily accessible in all medical facilities and systems. The reasoning behind the lack of accessibility to coordinated and interdisciplinary care by all patients is multifactorial. It includes a dispersion of amputation experience across surgical fields, reportable hospital data, economic drive, and interpersonal communication difficulties. In broad terms, general surgeons tend to have less amputation experience due to increasing demands to serve other diagnostic groups and conditions. Orthopedic surgeons may prefer to perform complicated general and limb salvage procedures and may regard amputation as a consequence of a failed limb salvage and an outcome to avoid where possible. Orthopedists likewise may defer amputations due to poor circulation, as in diabetes or other vascular problems, to vascular surgeons. The dispersion of patients requiring amputation across multiple specialties may be leading to a lack of amputation specialization. Economics seems to also be driving a lack of access to skilled, multidisciplinary care. Time to patient discharge is tracked and reported as a measure of hospital success. The desire to decrease patients' time to discharge may be driving hospitals to decrease hospital lengths of stay, which could limit the time needed for post-operative prosthesis utilization. The economics of medicine also benefits from shorter hospital stays which equate to less costs. Likewise, a lack of fee schedules for post-operative prosthetic care could also be leading to a lack of these services being available to the patient. Finally, interdisciplinary communication is now, to a large extent, email or text message dependent. Close communication between services is not as easily accomplished due to a frequent lack of face-to-face or voice-based interpersonal conversations, which can hinder the formulation and execution of a post-operative treatment plan.

Interpersonal and interprofessional communication is essential. Successful treatment of the patient must always start with an evaluation and a well-thought-out plan to assess the seriousness of the problem fully. Discussion with the patient to ensure a full appraisal of the nature and the anticipated seriousness of the process is important. The discussion and planning should also involve all the physicians, nurses, rehabilitation services, and, ideally, the family members, when available. All individuals should be aware of the potential problems and alternatives to be able to decide on an overall treatment plan that seems to be the most appropriate option for each patient's specific needs. If limb salvage is the pathway followed, the patient must be apprised of the need for numerous procedures, imaging studies, skin grafting, bone grafting, prolonged rehabilitation, and the effects of the pain medications that will be administered during treatment. While revision and re-operation may be necessary and numerous complications can occur with all procedures, some treatment pathways have an increased likelihood for revisions [1].

When creating an individualized treatment plan, injuries to other parts of the body and organ systems, such as to the head, chest, abdomen, and neurologic system must be considered. Similarly, the time since the injury or illness began or other causes of inactivity are important factors. The longer a patient remains recumbent or on near complete bed rest, the more complicated wound and fracture healing may be. For example, if a patient is bedridden for even a week, they could likely lose approximately 5% of skeletal mass, and in the case of severe trauma, potentially as much as 25% of their muscle mass [2–4].

Realistic expectations within the treatment team, the patient, and the patient's family are important and should be prioritized before any action is taken. For many, amputation is an emotional experience. It can be difficult for the patient to process emotionally and mentally, which can lead to patients relying on those around them for input. Family members and healthcare staff expectations should remain realistic, as these can be very influential on the patient [1]. Expectation management may be most evident in the case of vascular disease because it may be the most difficult to treat. For instance, patients may present with two or three necrotic toes and expect that, once amputated, the amputation site will certainly heal. Patients hope for and expect no further problems. However, the patient may have claudication, pain, develop problems in the contralateral extremity, or may not adequately heal due to the underlying vascular disease. Moreover, additional procedures may be required.

When treating neoplastic disease, the art of limited resections may be accomplished by excision of a significant portion of the bone with limb salvage or substituting the tumor with an internal prosthetic replacement. The orthopedic surgeon may attempt to perform a "longitudinal amputation," where a muscle compartment or more extensive tissue area is excised. However, the majority of the limb or entire limb does not need to be removed. After "longitudinal amputation," adjunctive treatment with chemotherapy and radiation can and often does continue. The use of this type of amputation and treatment plan can often avoid a transtibial amputation (TTA) or transfemoral amputation (TFA) [5].

PLANNING AND PRE-OPERATIVE CARE

From the patient's point of view, amputation is often one of the most difficult decisions to accept. The non-operative treatment, often thought of as the conservative care option, may in fact be the radical treatment method. Infection or other problem(s) can become systemic and spread, and patients who experience prolonged inactivity and bed rest due to the non-amputation treatment plan can develop deep vein thrombosis leading to cardiovascular risks. As already stated, patients with bed rest and inactivity can experience a high risk of overall loss of muscle mass [2]. It is therefore essential that healthcare staff members must not lose rapport with the patient in order to provide the best patient education possible. Other patients or amputees may also be able to interact with and counsel the patient in reaching the best decision for their overall wellness. Occasionally, it may be appropriate to obtain an independent second opinion.

Ideally, the patient, the prosthetist, the therapist, and the operating surgeon should meet with the patient and family as a single group to discuss the plan and prognosis. As stated, the patient must fully understand the needs and goals of the surgery as well as their feelings about the surgery. The patient should also confer with friends and family, where possible, to ensure understanding and agreement on the way forward [1]. Once the patient approves the amputation procedure, the surgeon, prosthetist, and therapist confer about the likely residual limb length, the location and type of incision, and the post-operative course of care to agree on a plan that represents the patient's best chance of success [1].

Further, all relevant medical history and medication-related data, both in the chart and directly from the patient, must be gathered to clarify potential omissions or misunderstandings of patient information during the creation of the treatment plan [1]. For example, in the case of osteomyelitis, patients have likely been on long-term antibiotics. It is important to note if the patient has been previously informed about alternative treatment methods. Examples of alternative methods include partial foot, mid-foot, and ankle amputations instead of a TTA. The patient must be able to consider alternative management based on the evidence presented rationally. Even though choosing between other treatment alternatives may not be in the patient's best medical, functional, and rehabilitative interests, it is ultimately the patient's choice. They also need to be informed that the need for additional treatments is highly probable. When the surgical plan has been agreed upon, and the patient has provided informed consent, it is time to act and implement the plan. All discussions, interactions, evaluations, imaging, findings, clinical decision-making, and patient consent must be documented in the medical record.

Many patients who undergo amputation have multiple medical problems and can be on numerous medications and undergoing various treatments. These must be thoroughly reviewed and stabilized pre-operatively. All appropriate pre-operative assessments must be completed before the surgery. Pre-operative measures likely include the nasal swab test for staphylococcus aureus, a surgical bath, and preparation of the operative extremity. If possible, oral hygiene should also be accomplished with flossing, brushing, rinsing, and pre-operative antibiotic administration. In most instances, the patient receives anticoagulation treatment post-operatively, although some centers give anticoagulation pre-operatively. As such, contraindications to anticoagulation must also be considered.

Once in the operative theater, anesthesia is begun, and a "time out" occurs in which all members of the staff involved agree and confirm that the correct, planned procedure is to occur and the procedure is to be carried out on the correct limb. In most cases, general anesthesia is accomplished, and a tourniquet is utilized. Furthermore, the limb is elevated and wrapped with an Esmarch or equivalent bandage for surgical hemostasis to facilitate a visually clear operative field. However, in the case of infection and tumor, the limb should not be wrapped but simply elevated before inflation [1]. In most cases, pre-operative antibiotics are administered 60 minutes prior to the initiation. In emergency surgery, antibiotics should be given when appropriate.

SURGICAL CONSIDERATIONS
Amputation Etiology

Amputation etiology includes congenital limb deficiencies, malignancies, trauma, and disease processes. Each etiology has special surgical considerations. Congenitally deficient limbs may be shaped differently than typical anatomy, which alters the limb's surface area and force-producing capabilities, among other attributes. When working with a congenitally altered limb, it is common for surgeons to shape the residual limb in a more typical fashion to accept widely available prosthetic components. However, there are also benefits of not altering the shape and not performing surgery, such as leaving as much of the residual limb as possible or not performing any surgery to avoid anesthesia and the other inherent surgical risks. When working with malignancies, the treatment plan may lead to structural insufficiency, but the alternative could lead to remnants of the malignancy to remain, which inherently lead to skeletal frailty. In patients who experience trauma, surgeons attempt to salvage the limb, but it is important to save as much of the limb as possible in cases where that is not possible. Most traumatic injuries leading to limb loss are life-threatening, resulting in decreased planning time. Finally, in disease-related cases, most related to peripheral vascular disease and diabetes, there is more time for planning, pre-rehabilitation, and peer visitation. In these cases, co-morbidities and age can become large challenges.

Selection of the Amputation Level

The level of amputation is generally chosen to preserve as much limb length as possible. This is particularly true in older patients to preserve balance and residual limb strength. Viable tissue and perfusion are generally top considerations for a surgeon's decision regarding amputation level. However, the decision can be confounded when that level is near a joint. Crossing a joint to amputate more proximally and eliminating the joint will likely lead to diminished ambulatory function. In some cases, the elimination of a joint could be the difference between someone returning to their normal activities of daily living or not being able to ambulate in a meaningful and functional manner realistically. Careful examination of the skin, muscle, and residual neurologic function will assist in determining the incision location and the residual limb length. For the trauma case, the Mangled Extremity Severity Score (MESS) algorithm has been widely accepted to help quickly assist a surgeon in determining limb salvage or amputation [6].

Several assessment methods exist for the vascular surgeon or any surgeon to determine the level of viable ischemic tissue during an amputation. However, none is agreed upon or determined to be the gold standard. The following are physical examination and clinical test findings that may be used in making an amputation limb length determination in limb ischemia.

Physical Examination

- The *color* of the potential amputation site should be comparable to more proximal levels.
- *Capillary refill* should be visible and comparable to more proximal levels.
- *Skin temperature* at the potential amputation site should be approximately that of body temperature.
- A *palpable pulse* should be identifiable at the potential amputation site.
- *Needle stick* at the potential site should be detectable by the patient and provide near normal blood flow compared with a more proximal level.

Clinical Tests

- *Toe blood pressure* is relatively easy to use, is commonly found in vascular labs, and is reliable in patients with calcified tibial vessels. Toe blood pressures of 30–40 mmHg correlate with ~70% wound healing potential [7].
- *Ankle blood pressure* is easy to use and is commonly found in vascular labs; however, it is unreliable with non-compressible, calcified vessels. Pressures > 60–80 mmHg are predictive of 50–90% TTA healing [7].

- *Transcutaneous oxygen pressure* is non-invasive and analyzes the partial pressure of oxygen in the tissue. A sensor warms the skin, creating hyperemia and O_2 diffusion. Oxygen pressure is measured in mmHg with a normal value of >50 mmHg, and < 30 mmHg is considered not viable for healing [7].

Other tests include arteriography, skin percussion pressure, doppler, scintigraphy (gamma scan), infrared thermography, and skin fluorescence. However, these tests have yet to be extensively tested or reported as reliable. In summary, appropriate amputation level determination is currently a clinical decision guided by the surgeon's experience and comfort level, understanding the limitations of reliable physical and clinical exam outcome measures.

Extremity Transection Versus Joint Disarticulation

When tissue viability has been determined to be at the joint, the surgeon can disarticulate the joint instead of transecting the long bone. The advantage of disarticulation is not having to cut a bone, while muscle insertions at that more distal level remain naturally intact. The ability to bear weight through the end of the bone after a disarticulation amputation is also regarded as a potential advantage, at some levels, as is increased limb length relative to transected limb alternatives.

Residual Limb Shape

Ideal residual limb shape begins with the surgical technique. The ideal residual limb shape will help the prosthetist design a socket interface that will equally and efficiently allow distributed weight bearing throughout the entirety of the residual limb. Weight-bearing forces are distributed from limb to socket through the socket's side walls and proximal structures and are minimized at the distal transected section of bone. An ideal shape facilitates optimal fit and weight-bearing forces with the prosthetic socket. There are three common residual limb shapes, illustrated in Figure 4.1.

Conical Residual Limb

When performing a TTA, if the fibula is cut too proximally it will create an undesirable, conical shape (Figure 4.1A). A conical TTA is undesirable because the distal tibia's prominence will lead to more difficult prosthesis fitting [1]. Concerning TFAs, a conical shape is acceptable and even common post-operatively. Additionally, tissue atrophy may create a conical shape to occur naturally over time after TFA. A conical shape is also common among TFAs and can be fit successfully as the primary weight bearing will be achieved through the proximal ischial tuberosity [1].

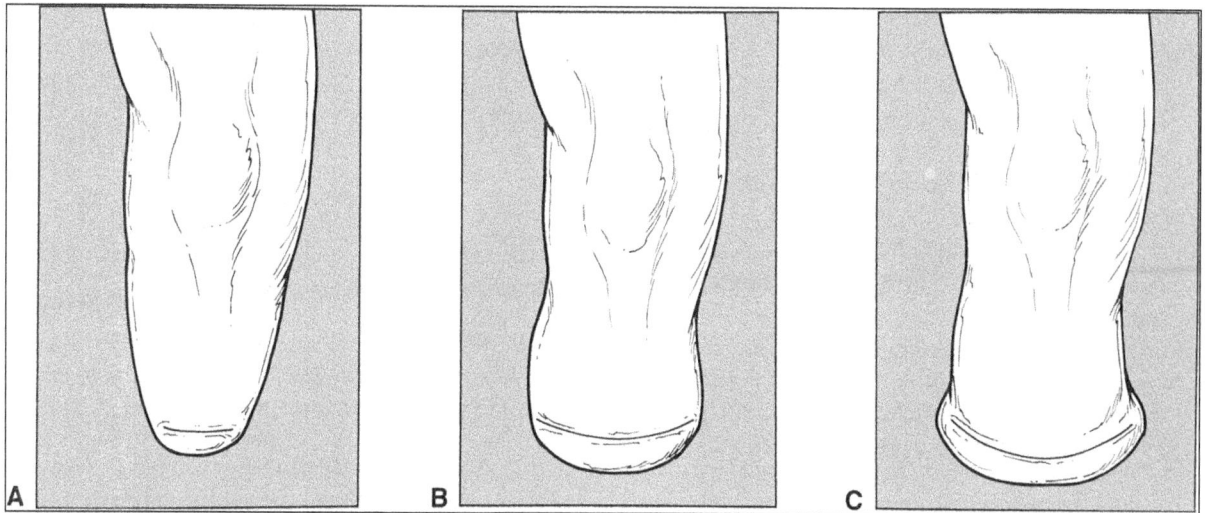

Figure 4.1. Common residual limb shapes demonstrated by A. conical, B. cylindrical, and C. bulbous shaped transtibial amputations.

Cylindrical Residual Limb

A cylindrical residual limb is an ideal shape for both TFA and TTA (Figures 4.1B) and 4.2). A cylindrical shape is achieved at the TTA level when the fibula is transected approximately at or within 1 cm proximal to the transected tibia. If the fibula is transected longer than the tibia, it will cause excessive distal weight bearing on the fibula, which is mobile and can cause additional pressure and pain due to the mobility and crowding of surrounding structures. If the fibula is too short, it will result in a conical shaped limb (Figure 4.1A) with centralization of the tibia. For the TFA, though a bit more difficult, a cylindrical shape may be achieved when there is proper soft tissue coverage over the transected distal end. This coverage is achieved through proper myodesis (securing of muscle to bone) and myoplasty (connecting of different muscles) with centralization of the femur.

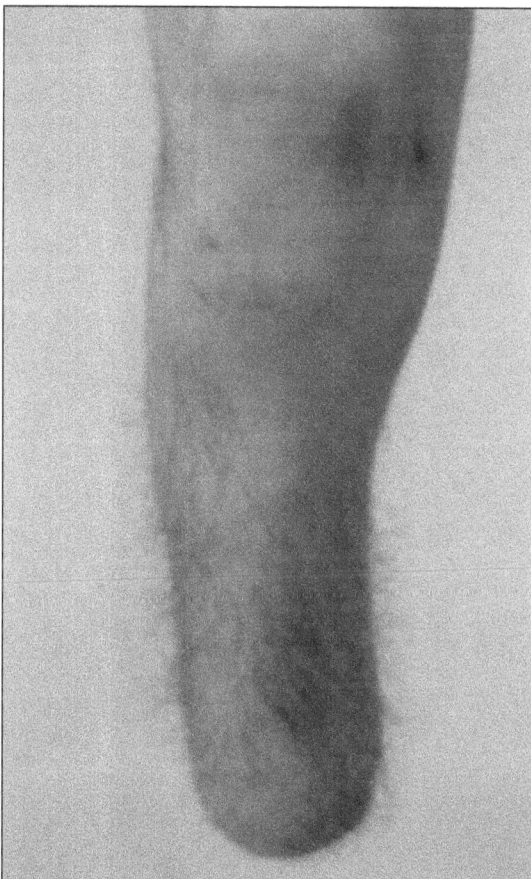

Figure 4.2. Cylindrical shaped transtibial amputation. Photo courtesy of William Ertl, MD.

Bulbous Residual Limb

A bulbous residual limb (Figure 4.1C) can result from poor flap selection and suturing or poor edema management. While most TTAs may have a slightly bulbous shape early on, an excessive bulbous shape will delay and complicate prosthetic fitting. Aggressive volume management strategies such as elastic bandage wrapping, shrinker or liner use, and early and immediate post-operative prostheses may need to be used to reduce and control the bulbous shape. If this shape does not resolve through management, then prosthetic fitting will have to be adjusted to accommodate the fact that the distal circumference is larger than the proximal circumference. This limb shape will inhibit donning and doffing, as the residual limb shape must match the socket interface shape and circumferences exactly, or proper weight bearing will not be achieved.

Soft Tissue Closures

There are four types of soft tissue closures as described below. A combination of these will commonly be used in closing the amputation to provide transected bone coverage, limb control, and an ideal shape.

- *Myofascial* skin closure is used where minimal muscle stabilization or attachment is required. It may be commonly used in joint disarticulation cases.
- *Myoplasty* is the suturing together of opposing muscle groups. Myoplasty provides soft tissue closure of the distal transected bone as well as stabilization and control of the bone.
- *Myodesis* is the suturing of muscles to transected bone through a hole drilled into the bone. Myodesis provides control of the bone with muscle activation. Myodesis is particularly important in transfemoral cases, as most of the adductor muscles will be lost when amputated proximal to the adductor tubercle. The femur must be placed into an adducted position prior to myodesis attachment to allow the remaining adductors the ability to have the required tension to control the femur.
- *Tenodesis* is the suturing of tendon, which can be a reliable anatomic suture anchor to the bone to restore bone control.

Muscles should be trimmed distally to just beyond the end of the bone. Thus, when retention occurs, the muscle can be secured to the bone's periosteum distally and the end of the bone with sutures. Alternatively, formal myodesis can be performed, but either will likely assist with muscle function and ambulation. Muscle trimming should also be performed to prevent bulk. However, a distal conical residual limb should be avoided as it will reduce limb volume and surface area, making socket wear difficult.

TRANSTIBIAL SURGICAL TECHNIQUES

In a TTA, the residual limb can be bulbous if a proper closure is not executed. Scar placement, soft tissue closure, distal coverage, weight bearing, and vascular supply are all considered. There are also less common closures, such as the guillotine, fish mouth, and skewed closure techniques. The three most common amputation types are considered below.

Posterior Flap

The posterior flap is the most common closure and carefully focuses on utilizing a posterior myocutaneous tissue flap comprised of the lateral and medial gastrocnemius and the soleus to cover the distal end of the transected tibia (Figure 4.3). The suture runs from medial to lateral and resides across the anterior aspect of the tibia and fibula. A posterior flap can create a bulbous residual limb if the muscles are not properly debulked. This technique was made popular by Burgess in 1969.

Sagittal Flap

The sagittal flap closure has been reported to have equivalent outcomes to the posterior flap. It is comprised of a lateral flap consisting of anterior and lateral tissue and a medial flap consisting of gastrocnemius muscle and overlying skin to cover the distal end of the transected tibia and fibula. The suture line runs anterior to posterior while careful consideration is given to the anterior flap attachment locating it away from the tibial crest.

The Ertl Bone Bridge

Janos von Ertl developed the Ertl bone bridge in the 1940s as a surgical strategy to maximize the functional outcomes of

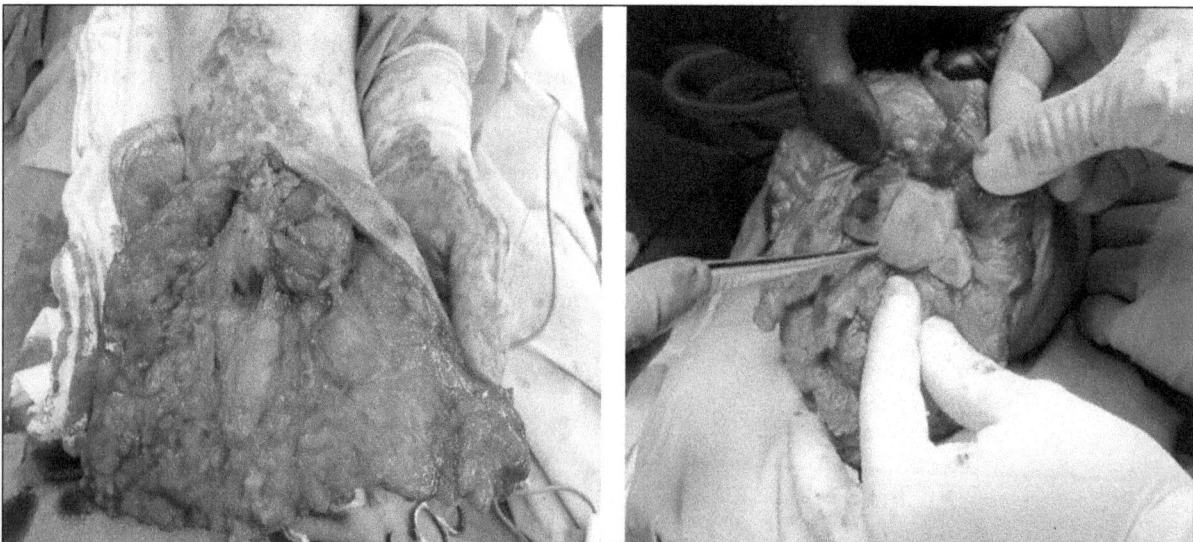

Figure 4.3. A. Posterior flap closure of a transtibial amputation demonstrating the layers of myocutaneous tissue flap closure and myodesis. B. Transected tibia and fibula in a transtibial amputation with bone graft placement. Photo courtesy of CAPT C. Ertl, MD, USN.

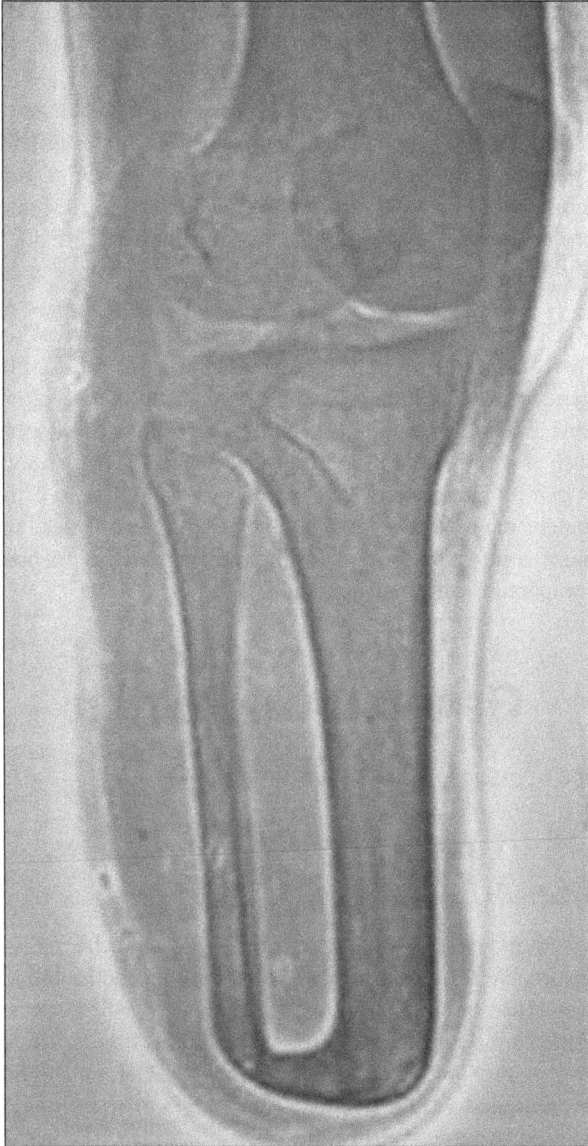

Figure 4.4. Radiographic image of an Ertl bone bridge in a transtibial amputation. Photo courtesy of William Ertl, MD.

amputees. This procedure creates an end-bearing bone bridge between the tibia and fibula (Figures 4.3B and 4.4). The bone bridge allows the use of end bearing, creating a mechanical advantage over traditional transection amputation techniques. It also provides the added advantages of preventing painful movement between the two bones in the prosthetic socket and improved accommodation for volume fluctuation. The distal weight-bearing capability could improve force distribution in the prosthetic socket design [8].

Ertl Transtibial Amputation Detailed Surgical Example

A full description of an amputation procedure is given here to illustrate the comprehensive per-tissue decision-making and management that must be considered during surgery to optimize limb health and function.

The patient is informed of all possible surgical risks and complications. All attempts are made to retain the knee and maximize residual extremity length to spare the burden of increased energy expenditure. The patient is also informed of the possibility of bone graft (Figures 4.3B and 4.4) harvest locally or from the iliac crest. A diagrammatic transverse section of the extremity also assists in anatomic structure identification during surgery. The extremity is prepared in a standard pre-operative fashion. A tourniquet is placed on the upper thigh and used as indicated. However, discretion is used in dysvascular cases. Occasionally a bump is placed under the affected hip to assist in limb rotation. In cases of revision, the previous incision is identified and utilized. In choosing the orientation of the incision, no difference has been found in the result with anteroposterior (AP), medial to lateral, or oblique incisions. The incision is made, and dissection is carried to the muscular layer. Frequently in cases of revision surgeries, the residual extremity has no distal bony muscular coverage as the musculature may have been poorly secured or allowed to retract at the time of initial amputation. In this case, the dissection is carried proximal, and the anterior, lateral, and posterior musculature are identified and isolated. Historically, a long posterior muscle flap has been used and secured anteriorly to the bone. In this situation, care should be taken not to transect the muscle belly and sacrifice muscle length. Revisions could also lead to difficulty in neurovascular structure isolation, as many times these structures are brought forward as well. The posterior flap is isolated and released from its anterior attachment, and fascial scar attachment is maintained on all musculature for later myoplastic reconstruction.

Neurovascular structures are now identified, released from scar tissue, and separately isolated. Depending on the amputation level, the major neurovascular bundles are isolated. These include the tibial nerve, artery and vein, peroneal artery, and vein, superficial peroneal nerve and deep peroneal nerve, artery and vein. Isolation may be difficult as the neurovascular bundle is usually ligated together and embedded in the scar. Palpation for a probable neuroma is performed to assist in neurovascular identification. The saphenous and sural nerves should also be identified. However, at times these may be very difficult to find, and a great deal of time should not be spent searching for them. Once identified, the above-mentioned nerves, arteries, and veins should be isolated and the vascular structures separately ligated. It is important to separate the nerve and artery, so the pulsations of the artery do not constantly irritate or stimulate the nerve. The nerve is separated, distracted, transected as proximal as possible, and allowed to retract into a soft tissue bed. The tourniquet may be released at this time to evaluate and gain control of any sources of bleeding. On reconstruction, the vascular structures are very friable and should be handled gently for fear of tearing or proximal retraction. The artery and associated veins are separately ligated. Once control of the vascular structures has been obtained, the tourniquet may be elevated again.

Attention is now directed to the distal end of the tibia and fibula. The periosteum is incised anterior to posterior longitudinally on both bones. Utilizing a 45°-angled chisel (not osteotome), an osteoperiosteal flap is elevated medially and laterally, maintaining the proximal attachments. Cortical fragments are left attached to the periosteum, which is facilitated by rotating the chisel 180° to assist in cortical elevation. This procedure is also performed on the fibula. Occasionally, it is necessary to split the fibula longitudinally, creating medial and lateral osteoperiosteal cortical flaps. These flaps are sutured together in a tube-like fashion. The lateral tibial flap is sutured to the medial fibular flap, creating a superior barrier. The medial tibial flap is sutured to the lateral fibular flap, creating an inferior barrier. Progressive osteogenesis occurs with eventual bone bridging or synostosis formation and fibular stabilization. Additional bone graft or bone graft extender can be packed into the center of the tube synostosis.

In short or very short residual extremities, free osteoperiosteal grafts are harvested from the proximal tibia, iliac crest, or contralateral limb (tibia) to maintain length. Harvests may also be performed on any length of residual extremities. Free osteoperiosteal grafts harvested from the amputated extremity have been used in primary amputations without difficulty and complete synostosis formation reportedly occurred.

The previously mobilized muscles are brought distally, covering the osteoperiosteal bridge and tibia, forming the myoplasty. The myoplasty may be completed by suturing the posterior to the anterior and lateral muscles under tension, securing the muscle into the osteoperiosteal bridge. The tibialis anterior is rotated over the prominent beveled distal tibia, and the entire bony bridge is covered with the myoplasty. Distal bony coverage and padding are achieved in addition to placing the muscle under tension and reestablishing an insertion. Extremity length may also be gained with distal muscle coverage.

The skin is fashioned to the underlying myoplasty. Care is taken to re-approximate the flaps in a symmetric fashion not to leave dog ears or crevices allowing air leaks. A smooth contour allows for improved total contact socket fit, with a cylindrical residual extremity contour as the goal. Penrose drains are placed through the incision prior to complete incisional closure and before negative pressure wound therapy can be applied.

Post-operatively, the extremity is immobilized in an extension plaster splint, which is removed in one week. A bulky soft tissue dressing is applied with an extended 4- or 6-inch elastic bandage. Sutures are removed in 2 or 3 weeks, depending on wound healing. Temporary total contact end-bearing prosthetic fitting is coordinated with the patient's prosthetist and completed in 4 to 8 weeks.

Physical therapy is initiated for transfers, aerobic and balance training, desensitization, upper body strengthening, and more.

While the Ertl bone bridge procedure does not necessarily increase rehabilitation time, it is important to understand the prosthesis fitting protocol guidelines that must be followed to ensure the optimal outcome. The bone bridge will take several months to mature and heal but does not delay prosthetic socket fitting (preparatory or temporary) compared to other amputation surgical procedures. Mechanical loading applied to the affected site is conducive to bone healing and will increase the chance of a stable bone bridge developing. A stable bone bridge between the tibia and fibula potentially provides important advantages, such as a wide weight-bearing surface and the prevention of painful motion between the bones and soft tissues. Ultimately, many features of a bone bridge potentially lead to more comfortable socket fitting and improved outcomes compared to alternative methods.

GENERAL AMPUTATION PROCEDURES

Neurovascular Structure Management

Blood vessels should be double ligated with either absorbable or non-absorbable sutures. The smaller blood vessels can be singularly tied, and smaller bleeding can be controlled with electrocautery techniques, though these may retract and bleed post-operatively. Nerves should be identified with a hemostat and then cut sharply and allowed to retract within the epineural sleeve. The nerve is allowed to retract into a soft tissue bed to avoid scarring and a static attachment site (i.e., adhesion) which can lead to pain from longitudinal traction on the nerve. This procedure should be performed to avoid painful neuroma development and decrease phantom pain.

Bone Management

Cutting the bone must be accomplished with care to prevent problems. Periosteal stripping is unnecessary and should be avoided, as this may produce heterotopic bone ossification, bone segment necrosis, and osteophyte (bone spur) formation. In transtibial cases, a gentle bevel is recommended to relieve anterior distal pain with prosthetic use and ambulation. In transfemoral cases, a distolateral bevel is recommended to prevent pain with prosthetic weight bearing and ambulation. In the TTA, the fibula should be slightly shorter than the tibia, as previously described.

Skin Management

Skin closure must be done meticulously with adjacent tissue advancement to remove skin asymmetry or small outpouchings of excess skin after closure ("dog ears"). Subcutaneous and subcuticular closure can be done with absorbable sutures. Skin closure includes either interrupted nylon sutures or skin staples. Some surgeons prefer nylon sutures to be combined with skin adhesive and wound closure strips which can be left in place for 3 to 4 weeks for skin closure. Wound closure over two Penrose drains is strongly recommended and can be withdrawn at the first dressing change approximately 72 hours post-operatively. The initial retention of the Penrose drains considerably reduces the likelihood of hematoma formation. Regardless of level, there should be good soft tissue coverage and padding [1]. The skin flap should have good subcutaneous texture and sensation. Redundant soft tissue and irregular skin edges, or dog ears, and variable thickness should be avoided to prevent discomfort and ensure a good fit within the prosthetic socket.

POST-OPERATIVE CARE

Post-operative care is crucial to patient success after an amputation. A post-operative surgical dressing is particularly important in all amputation surgeries. It should be applied methodically. First, a medical mesh gauze dressing should be applied smoothly, followed by four-by-four gauze fluffed open fully and applied without wrinkles to prevent dead space and pressure necrosis. Undercast padding, elastic casting plaster, and finally regular plaster tapes with careful molding of the plaster should be utilized until early plaster setting occurs. A proper post-operative surgical dressing should reduce dead space, create a supportive dressing, and prevent edema or hematoma formation.

Suture Removal

Sutures may be removed in 2 to 4 weeks, and if used, wound closure strips may be changed and replaced as necessary. The residual limb must be patted completely dry before any dressing or edema control device can be applied. Shaving the residual limb is not advised, as this can cause skin irritation, infection, and unnecessary exposure to potential cuts [9].

Post-Surgery Transition

One of the most effective tools in a treatment plan is visitation by other individuals who have successfully undergone amputation and can provide the patient with an incentive to recover. Interaction with other amputees who have shared the same experiences and remain positive and encouraging to the new amputee is important. A physician member of the team must remain active to provide oversight, complete progress notes, and complete prescriptions for the prosthesis as required by insurance. After surgery, the amputee's primary care provider or physiatrist is better positioned to manage long-term care. Interaction between physician, physical therapist, and prosthetist is crucial to get the patient their new prosthesis in a timely fashion. Some electronic health record programs are specially designed to organize and complete all the necessary data and prescription paperwork. When possible, these electronic tools should be utilized to expedite these services and seamlessly provide the prosthesis. As this chapter has discussed, the prosthetist should be involved throughout both the pre-operative and post-operative periods to facilitate peer visitation, plan post-operative devices, and prepare the appropriate prosthesis. The physical therapist should also be involved pre-operatively to oversee and assist with weight bearing, compression, and gait initiation after amputation [10].

After the operation is completed, long-term care must begin to ensure proper healing of the residual limb, which is a key to success after amputation. However, other parts of the body and organ systems must also be addressed during this time. Comprehensive attention to nutrition, fluid intake, anemia, glucose control, and antibiotic use is essential to maximize wound healing and overall rehabilitation [9]. Numerous lifestyle changes may be necessary. These changes include a healthy diet and calorie management, cessation of smoking both by the patient and their family members, maintenance of ideal body weight, and maintenance or implementation of a regular exercise regimen. The prosthetic device must also be carefully fitted to prevent device-related complications.

Joint of Motion and Preventing Contractures

Maintaining a full range of motion in the acute post-operative stage is imperative, as joint tightness and contractures can be challenging to correct. To maintain a full range of motion, early physical therapy intervention is encouraged. Stretching exercises at the remaining joints of both the involved and sound sides are strongly encouraged. The amputee should be provided and instructed on a self-administered stretching routine and schedule. Additionally, the amputee should be encouraged to move and stand with assistance with an assistive device, not lie, or sit, for excessive periods of time. For the TTA, compromised knee joint range of motion is common. To avoid a reduction in range of motion, the amputee should not use a pillow under their knee. Instead, their knee should rest on a firm flat surface and be maintained in full extension. Hip flexion contractors are common in TTAs and TFAs because it is more comfortable for the amputee to lie supine, specifically in an elevated (i.e., recumbent) position. The amputee should spend approximately 15 minutes, at least four times a day, lying prone on a firm surface with a pillow under their chest [9]. Push-ups can be added to increase hip extension during this stretching exercise.

Immediate Post-Operative Prostheses and Dressings

Currently, there is no consensus on post-operative prosthetic dressing care strategies immediately following amputation. Treatment strategies vary from soft wound-dressings to a weight-bearing immediate post-operative prosthesis (IPOP) as shown in Figure 4.5. The strategies can generally be categorized into two groups: soft or rigid [11]. Further, the prosthetic dressing strategies can be stratified into one of four groups: 1) soft dressings (non-weight bearing); 2) semi-rigid soft IPOP (non-weight bearing); 3) rigid IPOP (non-weight bearing) (Figure 4.5A); and, finally, 4) rigid weight bearing IPOPs (Figure 4.5B). These variations can be custom-made by the prosthetist or, more commonly, prefabricated. Prefabricated systems are commercially available and have been contemporarily refined to accommodate expanded weight limits, size, or condition. Newer designs are superior in adjustability, utilize skin-friendly materials, and offer accessibility to the residual limb, as opposed to the first reported older plaster, reticulating foam, and pylon designs [12].

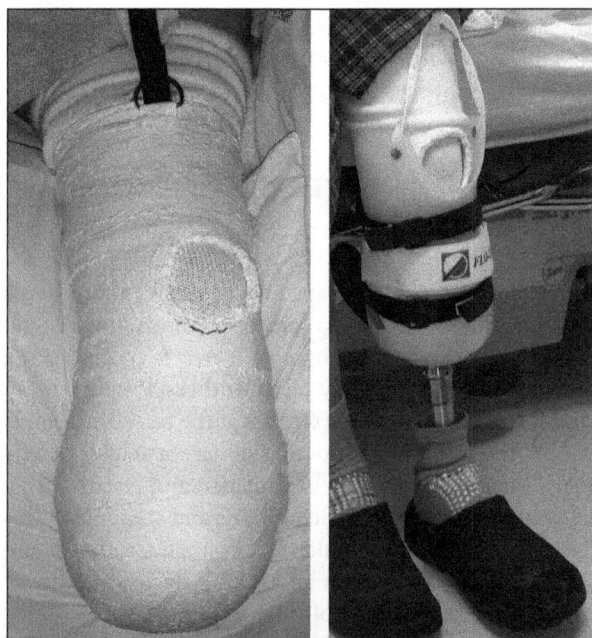

Figure 4.5. A. Non-weight-bearing, rigid and B. rigid weight-bearing immediate post-operative prostheses on transtibial amputations.

Soft Dressings

Elastic bandages and other soft dressing options are widely used because they allow the surgeon and nurse to observe the suture line quickly [1]. Application and removal of soft dressings are also more easily understood, require less time, and are more readily available. An elastic bandage figure-eight wrap has long been considered the standard for edema management. However, the misapplication of elastic bandages, such as wrapping the proximal tighter than the distal portion, will worsen edema. Further, an elastic bandage can be challenging to self-apply. An elastic shrinker sock likely creates more uniform compression, and they are commercially available in many shapes, sizes, and compression levels. Shrinker socks have gained greater popularity because of their ease of donning and flexible options. Soft dressings are breathable and can be worn 23 hours a day, minus dressing changes and cleaning. Elastic sock shrinkers are usually recommended after suture or staple removal. However, with careful donning, a protective suture bandage and a protective thin sock or sheath can be used to prevent edema while the incision continues to heal, and sutures or staples remain. A properly sized and fitted shrinker sock should be tight and encompass all the soft tissue leading up to, or past, the next most proximal joint. For the TTA, the shrinker should extend approximately 10 centimeters proximal to the knee joint. A longer shrinker should be used if edema is collected proximal to the 10-centimeter level. For the TFA, the shrinker sock should contain the adductor tissue. If this medial proximal tissue is not contained, it can form an adductor roll. This formation will create a difficult and painful prosthetic fitting process for the amputee due to the tissue crowding within the adductor area as this tissue needs to be contained inside the socket interface. Disadvantages of soft dressings have been well reported and include prolonged skin healing, development of knee contracture, extended bed rest, limited mobility, stroke, pneumonia, and higher healthcare costs associated with prolonged healing and potential injury (i.e., re-hospitalization) [13–16].

Removable Rigid Dressings

The clinician may prefer prosthetic dressing strategies that offer the healthcare team a conservative approach of a non-weight-bearing option while still providing effective limb protection and edema control. These are more commonly referred to as removable rigid dressings (RRD) [1, 9]. This category of prosthetic dressing has evolved to include many prefabricated options. RRDs have also been proven to reduce overall post-operative pain [1]. They also allow for daily inspection and can be applied in settings other than the operating room, such as the recovery room or a casting room. This flexibility is particularly advantageous in the current healthcare climate, where additional time in the operating room can greatly increase expenses.

Another advantage of RRD use is the prevention of knee flexion contractures. Wound inspection may take slightly longer when compared to soft dressings and, when using an RRD, after removing the dressing and inspecting the residual limb, the RRD should be replaced within minutes to prevent edema development [9]. However, the advantages far outweigh these aspects.

Immediate Post-Operative Prostheses

Finally, IPOPs have been shown to improve residual limb health by controlling edema, promoting ideal shape, desensitizing, and protecting the residual limb. Additionally, some IPOP designs can assist in preventing contracture and accelerating rehabilitation through the benefits of early weight bearing. IPOPs have been reported to provide potentially superior clinical outcomes. The weight-bearing IPOP offers the best optimal potential for edema control, accelerated wound healing, increased blood flow, limb protection, reduction of falls, and the psychological benefit of being able to stand with upper limb support shortly following amputation [16–18]. Weight bearing during this time is limited due to the post-operative status and should always be monitored by the prosthetist or physical therapist. Patients should likely begin with approximately 10% amputated side weight bearing and may gradually increase to 20% by 3 weeks in most cases. The interdisciplinary care team will determine the proper weight-bearing plan and progression.

Early ambulation post-operatively is a contemporary fundamental of "fast-track" surgery protocols and nursing. Early mobilization provides positive outcomes for critical care, cardiovascular, neurological, and orthopedic patient populations [19, 20]. Benefits of post-amputation ambulation include improved functional mobility, decreased pain, enhanced well-being, and shorter hospital stay [21]. While full weight bearing and ambulation are not advised, measured weight bearing of up to 50% of body mass has been determined acceptable in some cases [12]. Falling is an identified major concern among transtibial amputees, potentially resulting in re-injury, re-hospitalization, delayed healing, and revision surgery [22, 23]. During the early recovery and rehabilitation stages, residual limb re-traumatization is common in the acute amputee and can lead to surgical revision, infection, extended hospital stays, re-hospitalization, and delayed rehabilitation. Weight-bearing IPOPs offer the most comprehensive management of the amputee while addressing physiological and psychological concerns of early weight bearing, assisting in transfer and balance, edema reduction, and wound protection [13, 24]. Specifically, regarding falls in amputees, Gooday and Hunter [13] reported a fall incidence of 32%, while Pauley et al. [24] reported a fall incidence of 21%. Most of these incidences can be attributed to poor balance and falling from a wheelchair during an un-assisted transfer. Yu et al. [23] found that falls resulted in a significantly more extended hospital stay than patients who did not experience a fall. Injuries were sustained by 61% of those who fell. Curtze et al. [22] reported that the annual fall incidence in lower limb amputees is approximately 50%, while their elderly, non-disabled, community-dwelling peers have an incidence of 30–40%. A weight-bearing IPOP is a possible fall prevention strategy that could help prevent these injuries. Schon, Short, Soupiou et al. [25] found that patients with prefabricated pneumatic IPOPs had significantly fewer post-operative complications (16%) when compared with patients with soft gauze dressings (65%). The same study found that patients with a pneumatic IPOP required no higher-level revisions, whereas 44% of the patients with soft dressings required higher-level revisions [13, 25]. Unfortunately, the pneumatic IPOP utilized in this clinical study is no longer commercially available. Currently available weight-bearing IPOP designs could expand the utility of the IPOP. A weight-bearing IPOP could potentially benefit the acute amputee by providing maximum residual limb benefit, improved psychological benefit, and reduced overall healthcare costs by reducing falls. The weight-bearing IPOP represents the maximum possible benefits achievable in all current strategies. However, there is presently limited high-quality data substantiating the efficacy of utilizing a weight-bearing IPOP compared with contemporary non-weight-bearing options. Researchers have concluded that falls and associated injuries occur commonly in the post-operative lower limb amputee on the surgical ward. Ultimately, the literature suggests IPOPs and RRDs offer superior outcomes in terms of a potentially reduced infection rate, reduced time to first prosthetic fitting, and therefore, a potential reduction in healthcare costs [26].

AMPUTATION REHABILITATION
Stages of Rehabilitation

Stages, or phases, of rehabilitation are discussed elsewhere in this text but are briefly mentioned here primarily from the perspective of the operative procedure and associated wound healing. Post-amputation rehabilitation is a process generally accepted as having five variably named stages (or phases) of recovery: 1) the *pre-operative* stage; 2) the acute hospital *post-operative* stage; 3) the immediate post-acute hospital (*pre-prosthetic*) stage; 4) the intermediate recovery (*prosthetic training*) stage; and 5) the transition to stable (*lifelong care and maintenance*) stage. Combined, all five stages encompass an estimated 12–18-month period of time but extend out into the patient's lifespan in the fifth stage [24]. Preceding the stable stage, the primary concerns are wound healing, infection, contracture prevention, systemic complications, volume and wound management, further trauma to the residual limb, transfer, and ambulation skills. The immediate post-acute hospital stage begins with hospital discharge and extends 4 to 6 weeks after surgery. This is the time of recovery from surgery, wound healing, and early rehabilitation [13]. The intermediate recovery stage begins when the amputee is ready to progress from their immediate post-acute hospital stage and post-surgical care strategy. This usually extends 4 to 6 months from healing and ends with residual limb volume stabilization, as defined by the consistency of prosthetic fit for several months [13].

Post-Amputation Rehabilitation Timeline

Depending on injury severity and healing processes, an amputee will typically have their first custom prosthetic fitting 8 to 12 weeks post-amputation. Being fit into a custom prosthesis will be dependent on several parameters:

- Has the suture line healed, and can it tolerate some skin compression and tension?
- Does the residual limb shape allow prosthetic fitting?
- Does the patient have the overall physical strength and joint flexibility to begin ambulating?
- Does the patient desire to ambulate with a prosthesis?

During the following process, the rehabilitation team will consider these questions to prepare an amputee for prosthetic fitting.

Initial 2 Weeks Post-Surgery

The amputee may experience swelling and mild to moderate pain, which are both normal parts of the healing process. A vital part of the first few weeks is protecting the surgical site. Most surgeons will use a special dressing to protect the surgical site, and it is recommended to use some type of limb protection device or early postoperative prosthesis. The amputee must do their part to protect themselves and properly train on crutches or a walker. Physical therapists can assist greatly in this phase with assistive device training, balance, bed mobility, transfers, limb positioning, posture, strengthening and more. Amputees are encouraged to position their chairs next to their beds to remind themselves about their recent amputation should they try to stand out of habit. These precautions are necessary to prevent falls. Mental health is a key aspect of the healing process. It is recommended that the amputee takes this time to learn to be active in their own rehabilitation. This autonomous rehabilitation can include continuing physical therapy, for instance. It should be noted that rehabilitation with a physical therapist most likely changes settings from acute hospital-based care to either an outpatient or skilled nursing or other transitional

setting within this period, depending on the patient's function, needs, and other factors. Another way in which patients can be actively engaged in their own rehabilitation is by researching prosthetic options and interviewing many prosthetists to find one with whom they feel confident and comfortable. The Amputee Coalition has many recommended resources, including the Peer Visitation Program, *inMotion* magazine, their expansive website, and the prosthetist finder tool located at prosthetistfinder.org. Networking can also include finding a support group in the area and using social media to meet people and gain knowledge about living with limb loss [8].

2–4 Weeks Post-Surgery

Stitches are removed once the pain has subsided, and swelling is minimal. The suture line should show good signs of healing and minimal drainage. Using a hand towel on the bare skin or over the suture line dressing, begin with gentle compression on the end of the residual limb. An appointment with a prosthetist should be scheduled so they can visually examine the residual limb and discuss individual prosthetic rehabilitation. Physical therapy should also be scheduled and continued because it is an important part of preparing the body to use a prosthesis during the rehabilitation process. The amputee will most likely require multiple weekly visits for 1 to 2 months at a minimum. The intent is to provide the proper degree of preparation, strength training, range of motion, balance, agility, transfer, gait training, other skilled therapeutic exercises, activities, education, and training [8].

4–6 Weeks Post-Surgery

The amputee will likely continue rehabilitation to emphasize and assist with key exercises, stretching, and other therapeutic activities to achieve optimal outcomes. In rehabilitating a patient with an Ertl bone bridge, end-bearing exercises in standing are recommended to stimulate bony in-growth and to assure the best chance of a successful outcome. This exception is unique to the Ertl bone bridge, as it is important to the bone healing and remodeling process. End bearing is contraindicated, for instance, following a Burgess procedure [8].

8–12 Weeks Post-Surgery

The first prosthetic fitting should likely occur around this time and should be done in conjunction with ongoing physical therapy. Rehabilitation likely includes stretching, muscle-strengthening exercises, and prosthetic training. The residual limb will continue to change over the next few months; thus, this first prosthesis is sometimes called a preparatory or temporary prosthesis. In non-Ertl cases, the amputee will likely require another prosthetic socket or a whole new prosthesis in several months, probably due to considerable volume loss [8].

Nutrition During Amputation Rehabilitation

Amputees must be conscious of their dietary choices throughout rehabilitation, as sound nutrition is essential to healing. Sound nutrition includes raw, non-processed fruits and vegetables. Calorie count should be managed, as lower body fat will help improve balance, stamina, and strength. Water is also a key element of healthy living because over 70% of the brain, muscles, and blood and 25% of bone are water. Amputees are advised to drink approximately half their body weight in ounces daily (i.e., if body weight is 180 lbs, drink 90 ounces daily). If there is uncertainty related to nutrition, consultation with a registered dietician may be warranted. A healthy lifestyle will likely improve overall rehabilitation and physical and mental health. Amputees should speak to their physicians about vitamin and mineral supplements in addition to healthy dietary decisions. Supplementation is particularly important after surgery [8].

COMMON AMPUTEE CHALLENGES AND COMPLICATIONS

Members of the healthcare team may note problems and complications. Physician consultation may be necessary as soon as possible in such cases.

Hematoma Formation

Suspected hematomas may necessitate ultrasound or other medical laboratory confirmation. If needed, it should be drained by probing, allowing fluid to egress. If an infection occurs, open drainage merits consideration. If necrosis is present, wedge resection of this region must be accomplished. If good bleeding tissue cannot be identified, the soft tissue and possibly bone must be shortened.

Superficial Abscesses

Abscesses can lead to a draining sinus. If an abscess is present, the depth and bony involvement should be determined using imaging such as X-ray, MRI, or bone scans. Superficial abscesses can also be caused by bone spurs or local osteomyelitis. Commonly, these may require surgical intervention [9].

Bone Overgrowth (Bone Spurs)

Overgrowth can form acutely following surgery. Overgrowth is more commonly seen if the periosteum is stripped. This overgrowth often creates a pressure point under the skin which can be painful, and potentially cause tissue breakdown. Prosthetic socket accommodation and adjustment may reduce or resolve problems related to bone spurs. In more severe cases, surgical intervention may be indicated to resolve these problems [9].

Heterotopic Ossification

Heterotopic ossification (Figure 4.6) is most prevalent at the distal aspect of the cut bone. Heterotopic ossification is commonly seen in high-velocity trauma cases. It can result from inadequate periosteum coverage of the residual bone's cut end. These malformations often appear jagged and antler-like. They can be extremely painful and exacerbated by movement in the socket interface, resulting in pain, inflammation, soft tissue ulceration, and disuse. While adjustments can be made, moderate and severe cases usually require surgical revision.

Bone Pain

Regarding TTA, if the fibula is left longer than the tibia, excessive distal pain and pressure can occur. Additionally, an excessively long fibula can become mobile due to forces generated through the limb from muscular contraction or prosthetic use. This mobility can cause pain.

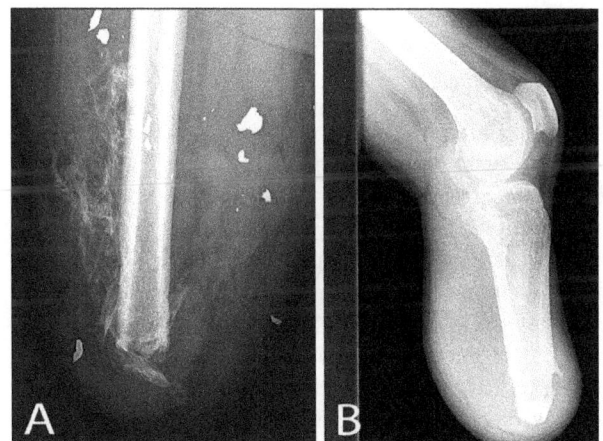

Figure 4.6. Heterotopic ossification after A. transfemoral amputation with concurrent retained foreign bodies and B. a transtibial amputation.

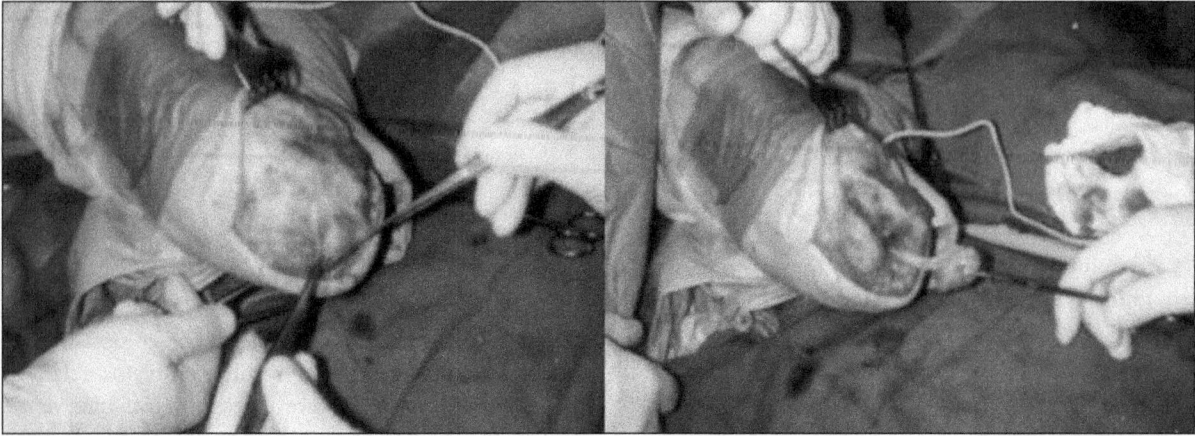

Figure 4.7. Surgical revision and removal of a neuroma to include the distraction of the neuroma and peripheral nerve before excision.

Regarding TFA, an inadequate myodesis procedure, excessive atrophy, or suture failure can cause distal exposure of the femur. This exposure can lead to socket pressure and pain. The first step to rectifying these issues is socket interface adjustment or replacement. Should these changes not resolve the problem, or a failed myodesis creates inadequate femur control, surgical reconstruction may be considered [9].

Incisional Pain

As the residual limb heals, incisional pain should decrease. However, force on an adherent scar can cause pain. Deep massage perpendicular to the scar is recommended to prevent scar adhesion and ensure multidirectional scar mobility. A thick layer of emollient can be used to decrease friction of the massage [9]. This type of massage may begin around 2 weeks after amputation but will depend on the patient's individual tolerance and healing [27]. Gentle massage can also be employed to decrease overall residual limb sensitivity [9].

Neuromas

Neuromas are formed when the cut end of a peripheral nerve continues growing and becomes bundled at the distal aspect. A neuroma is a non-neoplastic proliferation that occurs at the end of an injured nerve and can be seen as early as 1 month post-operatively. There are two types of post-amputation neuromas. Neuromas called terminal neuromas originate at the end of the severed nerve. A terminal neuroma has a normal pattern of healing and is often asymptomatic. A spindle neuroma is localized in the nerve away from the severed nerve ending. It represents the response of a peripheral nerve subjected to micro-trauma due to stretching or compression by the localized scar tissue. Therefore, to the extent healing occurs, it happens at the site of nerve trauma in these cases and not at the severed nerve ending. Pain associated with a neuroma can be misdiagnosed as a phantom sensation. Imaging and lidocaine injection at the painful site can assist in diagnosing a neuroma. A neuroma may require surgical revision if socket interface adjustments or other conservative treatment is ineffective [9, 28]. (See Figure 4.7.)

OSSEOINTEGRATION

Osseointegration (OI) (Figure 4.8) may soon become a prevalent option for prosthetic component attachment. It is an implant that is surgically anchored into the bone of the residual limb, exits through the skin, and attaches directly to the prosthetic components. It is a promising alternative to the current standard of care for the human prosthetic component interface—the prosthetic socket. Unlike the prosthetic socket, OI is intended for use for the rest of the amputee's ambulatory life. OI was first introduced in the late 1990s to clinically address many problems related to wearing a socket, such as skin issues and discomfort. These problems can contribute to lower function, poor quality of life, and possible abandonment, which are all common among amputees who are unable to achieve a good socket fit. OI has become an acceptable alternative to socket prostheses in several centers worldwide, in countries such as Australia, Sweden, and Germany. OI is currently used with non-vascular amputees due to the risk of infection. Etiologies in which OI can be applied include trauma, sarcoma, and congenital etiologies. Limited FDA approval and exemptions have been granted to OI, primarily because the long-term effects on humans are unknown. Clinical trials are underway to determine the efficacy and safety of OI. There are no abundant or definitive studies to date reporting the effects of OI [29].

OI surgery has mainly been performed using two types of implants to date. Cannulated screw-fixation implants, originally developed in Sweden, are used to achieve skeletal integration because of bone in-growth. Treatment is performed in two operations, where an initial procedure

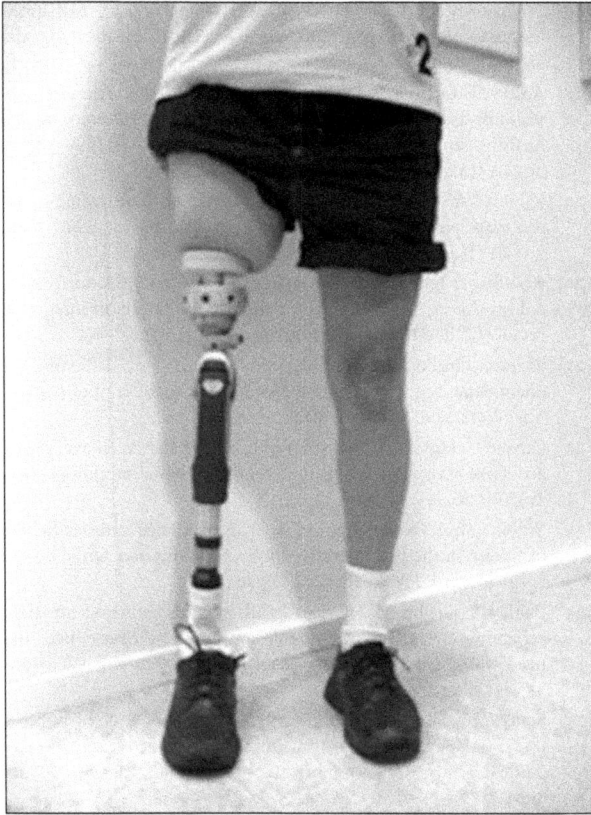

Figure 4.8. Individual with right-sided osseointegration and transfemoral prosthesis.

inserts the intramedullary implant, and a second procedure is performed 6–9 months after the initial surgery to create a percutaneous skin opening allowing abutment attachment and prosthesis fitting [30]. In addition to the screw-fixated implant developed by the Swedish team, alternative press-fitted OI implants with surface structures akin to modern joint arthroplasty implants have been developed by other groups. The macroporous surface coatings of these new implants allow skeletal integration by bone penetration and in-growth, encouraging OI to occur at an accelerated rate and shortening the two-stage operation to a 6–8-week interval between stages [31]. Currently, OI through press-fit technology has been pioneered by the Osseointegration Group of Australia (OGA) based in Sydney, with the world's largest patient cohort of more than 300 cases performed to date. The OGA has developed an accelerated two-stage protocol known as the Osseointegration Group of Australia Accelerated Protocol 1 (OGAAP-1) which enables patients to be mobilized within 3–4 months post-surgery.

Until recently, the majority of OI procedures worldwide have been performed in two stages. From the initial surgery, these procedures require up to 12–18 months for the completion of reconstruction and rehabilitation with screw-fixation implants and at least 3 months even with press-fitted implants under the OGAAP-1 protocol [32]. However, since April 2014, the OGA has refined the OGAAP-1 protocol and developed a single-stage osseointegration procedure referred to as the Osseointegration Group of Australia Accelerated

Protocol-2 (OGAAP-2) [33]. This single-stage approach reduces the overall time required for the definitive osseointegrated reconstruction and rehabilitation of lower limb amputees to approximately 3–6 weeks, which is substantially shorter compared with any currently available two-stage procedure. OGAAP-2 offers a more rapid progression to unrestricted full weight bearing while reducing the need and associated risks of a second surgery and is currently being offered to suitable patients in Sydney, Australia, by the OGA team.

Both OGAAP protocols strongly emphasize implant loading, physical therapy, and prosthetic fitting throughout the entire rehabilitation period. Post-operative rehabilitation occurs in three phases, with Phase 1 starting 3 days after surgery and consisting of the patient applying a static axial load of 20 kg for 20 minutes twice daily. The load is usually increased by 5 kg per day until either 50 kg or half of the patient's body weight is reached. Phase 2 is initiated when the patient has reached the recommended axial loading level and can be fitted with a training prosthesis consisting of a light leg and a stable locked knee. The patient continues to perform core strengthening exercises, balance exercises, as well as gait training aided by parallel bars. Phase 3 is initiated when the patient can safely mobilize with the rehabilitation prosthesis, be fitted with the definitive prosthesis, and proceeds onto daily weight bearing. The weight and speed of loading and prosthetic fitting may be adjusted depending on the patient's bone quality or health conditions. However, overall, this post-operative rehabilitation phase is typically completed within 3–6 weeks following the OI surgery.

In addition, OI reconstruction for amputees was originally developed and indicated to treat transfemoral amputees only. OI reconstruction for transtibial amputees has only begun recently [34]. To achieve rapid bony in-growth in the tibia, the OGA team has specifically developed a customized 3D-printed titanium implant and has successfully performed many below-the-knee reconstruction cases.

In summary, preliminary studies published in the literature suggest that in comparison with standard socket-mounted prostheses, OI provides considerable improvements in both quality of life and functional outcome measures while maintaining very reasonable complication rates [32, 35]. However, many of the studies being performed to date are predominantly observational before and after studies. Large-scale randomized control trials are still necessary to fully establish the efficacy and safety of OI, allowing this novel yet promising technology to help more amputees.

SUMMARY

This chapter overviewed operative goals, tissue management by type, and limb shape. Physical examination and clinical tests were reviewed, along with considerations related to prominent amputation flap closure techniques.

Additionally reviewed were major categories of post-operative dressings along with their respective benefits and drawbacks. Further, key points related to amputation level and peri-operative timelines relative to amputation surgery, rehabilitation, and prosthetic fitting were considered. Finally, fundamental points of major amputation surgical techniques, including the traditional Burgess, the osteomyoplastic bone bridge (Ertl), and osseointegration, were briefly covered.

REFERENCES

[1] Bowker JH, Michael JW, eds. *Atlas of Limb Prosthetics: Surgical, Prosthetic, and Rehabilitation Principles*, 1992. 2nd edition. Mosby Incorporated, St. Louis, MO.

[2] English KL, Paddon-Jones D. Protecting muscle mass and function in older adults during bed rest. *Curr Opin Clin Nutr Metab Care*. 2010;13(1):34–39.

[3] Strax T, et al. *Summary: Effects of Extended Bed Rest—Immobilization and Inactivity*, 2004. Springer Publishing Company, New York.

[4] Stuempfle KJ, Drury DG. The physiological consequences of bed rest. *J Exerc Physiol*. 2007;10(3):32–41.

[5] Lunseth PA, Nelson CL. Longitudinal amputation for the treatment of soft tissue fibrosarcoma. *Clin Orthop Relat Res*. 1975;(109):147–151.

[6] Johansen K, Daines M, Howey T, et al. Objective criteria accurately predict amputation following lower extremity trauma. *J Trauma*. 1990;30(5):568–572; discussion 572–573.

[7] Dwars BJ, van den Broek TA, Rauwerda JA, Bakker FC. Criteria for reliable selection of the lowest level of amputation in peripheral vascular disease. *J Vasc Surg*. 1992;15(3):536–542.

[8] Ertl JP, Kahle JT, Highsmith MJ. The Ertl Bone Bridge. *inMotion*. 2015;25.

[9] Cuccurullo SJ. *Physical Medicine and Rehabilitation Board Review*, 2010. 2nd edition. Springer Publishing Company, New York.

[10] Esquenazi A. Amputation rehabilitation and prosthetic restoration. From surgery to community reintegration. *Disabil Rehabil*. 2004;26(14–15):831–836.

[11] Department of Veteran Affairs and Department of Defense. *VA/DoD Clinical Practice Guideline For Rehabilitation of Lower Limb Amputation*, 2017. pp. 71, 72.

[12] Malone JM, et al. The rehabilitation value and cost effectiveness of immediate postoperative prosthetics for major lower extremity amputation. NovaCare Orthotics and Prosthetics Education Fair, 1998, Orlando, FL.

[13] Gooday HM, Hunter J. Preventing falls and stump injuries in lower limb amputees during inpatient rehabilitation: completion of the audit cycle. *Clin Rehabil*. 2004;18(4):379–390.

[14] Kahle JT. Conventional and hydrostatic transtibial interface comparison. *JPO: Journal of Prosthetics and Orthotics*. 1999;11(4):85–91.

[15] Kahle JT, Highsmith MJ. Transfemoral sockets with vacuum-assisted suspension comparison of hip kinematics, socket position, contact pressure, and preference: ischial containment versus brimless. *J Rehabil Res Dev*. 2013;50(9):1241–1252.

[16] Traballesi M, Delussu AS, Fusco A, et al. Residual limb wounds or ulcers heal in transtibial amputees using an active suction socket system. A randomized controlled study. *Eur J Phys Rehabil Med*. 2012;48(4):613–623.

[17] Highsmith MJ, Kahle JT, Lura DK, Mengelkoch LJ. Transtibial amputee energy expenditure during vertical ice climbing and snowshoeing. *Technol Innov*. 2014;15(4):311–315.

[18] Kahle JT, Orriola JJ, Johnston W, Highsmith MJ. The effects of vacuum-assisted suspension on residual limb physiology, wound healing, and function: a systematic review. *Technol Innov*. 2014;15(4):333–341.

[19] Kibler VA, Hayes RM, Johnson DE, et al. Cultivating quality: early postoperative ambulation: back to basics. *Am J Nurs*. 2012;112(4):63–69.

[20] Pashikanti L, Von Ah D. Impact of early mobilization protocol on the medical-surgical inpatient population: an integrated review of literature. *Clin Nurse Spec*. 2012;26(2):87–94.

[21] Marzen-Groller KD, Tremblay SM, Kaszuba J, et al. Testing the effectiveness of the Amputee Mobility Protocol: a pilot study. *J Vasc Nurs*. 2008;26(3):74–81.

[22] Curtze C, Hof At L, Otten B, Postema K. Balance recovery after an evoked forward fall in unilateral transtibial amputees. *Gait Posture*. 2010;32(3):336–341.

[23] Yu JC, Lam K, Nettel-Aguirre A, et al. Incidence and risk factors of falling in the postoperative lower limb amputee while on the surgical ward. *PM R*. 2010;2(10):926–934.

[24] Pauley T, Devlin M, Heslin K. Falls sustained during inpatient rehabilitation after lower limb amputation: prevalence and predictors. *Am J Phys Med Rehabil*. 2006;85(6):521–532; quiz, 533–535.

[25] Schon LC, Short KW, Soupiou O, et al. Benefits of early prosthetic management of transtibial amputees: a prospective clinical study of a prefabricated prosthesis. *Foot Ankle Int*. 2002;23(6):509–514.

[26] Highsmith MJ, Kahle JT, Miro RM, et al. Prosthetic interventions for people with transtibial amputation: systematic review and meta-analysis of high-quality prospective literature and systematic reviews. *J Rehabil Res Dev*. 2016;53(2):157–184.

[27] Karacoloff LA, Schneider FJ. *Lower Extremity Amputation: A Guide to Functional Outcomes in Physical Therapy Management*, 1986. Aspen Publishers, Boston, MA.

[28] Henrot P, Stines J, Walter F, et al. Imaging of the painful lower limb stump. *Radiographics*. 2000 Oct;20 Spec No:S219–S235.

[29] Kahle JT, Al Muderis M. Osseointegration. *inMotion*. 2016;26:38–41.

[30] Hagberg K, Branemark R. One hundred patients treated with osseointegrated transfemoral amputation prostheses—rehabilitation perspective. *J Rehabil Res Dev*. 2009;46(3):331–344.

[31] Aschoff HH, Kennon RE, Keggi JM, Rubin LE. Transcutaneous, distal femoral, intramedullary attachment for above-the-knee prostheses: an endo-exo device. *J Bone Joint Surg Am*. 2010;92(Suppl 2):180–186.

[32] Al Muderis M, Tetsworth K, Khemka A, et al. The Osseointegration Group of Australia Accelerated Protocol (OGAAP-1) for two-stage osseointegrated reconstruction of amputated limbs. *Bone Joint J*. 2016;98-B(7):952–960.

[33] Al Muderis, M., Yu W, Tetsworth K, et al. Single-stage osseointegrated reconstruction and rehabilitation of lower limb amputees: the Osseointegration Group of Australia Accelerated Protocol-2 (OGAAP-2) for a prospective cohort study. *BMJ Open*. 2017;7(3):e013508.

[34] Atallah R, Li JJ, Lu W, et al. Osseointegrated transtibial implants in patients with peripheral vascular disease: a multicenter case series of 5 patients with 1-year follow-up. *J Bone Joint Surg Am*. 2017;99(18):1516–1523.

[35] Al Muderis M, Khemka A, Lord SJ, et al. Safety of osseointegrated implants for transfemoral amputees: a two-center prospective cohort study. *J Bone Joint Surg Am*. 2016;98(11):900–909.

CHAPTER 5

Lower Extremity Prosthetic Componentry

M. Jason Highsmith and Michael K. Carroll

OBJECTIVES

Upon completing this chapter, the reader will be able to:

1. Understand the relationship between the patient history, functional potential and abilities, goals, and the prosthetic prescription.
2. Recall different classification systems and types of lower extremity prosthetic feet, pylon, knee, and hip systems.
3. Recall different lower extremity prosthetic socket and suspension designs as well as their basic construction.

This chapter addresses the lower extremity prosthetic prescription which includes the selection of the interface, suspension, and necessary components. Key terms are listed at the end of the chapter.

MATCHING LOWER EXTREMITY PROSTHETIC COMPONENTS TO PATIENT FUNCTION

The importance of the patient evaluation cannot be overstated. This should include the patient history and physical examination. Learning about what the patient was involved with and aspired to do prior to the amputation will provide insight into future goals. It must be pointed out that a patient's prior abilities and activities should be considered and discussed. However, it should not be assumed that this will automatically be the patient's current or eventual goals. Some prosthetic components may provide specific functions whereas other componentry may afford a range of functions and activity participation.

Important within the component selection process is evaluating the patient's current functional level and the potential level of function. For patients with lower extremity amputation, the currently accepted system for this is the Medicare Functional Classification Level (MFCL) System [1]. This is a five-level system that briefly lays out as given in Table 5.1.

DOI: 10.4324/9781003526025-6

TABLE 5.1			
Medicare Functional Classification Levels (MFCLs)			
FUNCTIONAL LEVEL	**DESCRIPTION OF WHAT THE BENEFICIARY HAS THE ABILITY OR POTENTIAL FOR**	**PROSTHETIC FEET**	**PROSTHETIC KNEES**
K0	The beneficiary is not a candidate as they do not have the ability or potential to ambulate safely	None	None
K1	Supervised and therapeutic prosthetic use	Basic feet	Basic knees
K2	Limited community ambulation (i.e., low level environmental barriers) and unlimited household ambulation	Multi-axial	
K3	Unlimited community ambulation (most environmental barriers) and variable cadence ambulation	Energy storing and release	Fluid friction
K4	High activity and heavy-duty use; this includes beneficiaries who are bilaterally involved, children, and/or athletes	Any	Any

The challenge with the Medicare functional levels is that they describe the ability or potential to function in accordance with the descriptions and, further, there is no agreed upon measurement for definitive classification into a specific functional level. Again, a thorough patient evaluation including a history, physical examination, and the use of outcome measures is advised. This will provide the best information from which to determine the patient's current functional level, functional potential, and goals. This information will then assist in determining which prosthetic design and components are most appropriate for maximizing function and helping the patient to reach their goals.

Trial Periods and Loaner Programs

Because functional and performance differences between components are unclear, it can be difficult to select the optimal componentry. For example, it may be determined that a foot from a certain class is appropriate for a patient. Within that class however, there may be dozens of components to choose from. Biomechanical attributes or other patient characteristics may be different and lead to a patient's preference [2]. The challenge is that many patients may not have the opportunity to test a component prior to its selection and inclusion in the prosthesis. For this reason, it is encouraged that component manufacturers and prosthetists be queried regarding the ability for a patient to use a component on a trial basis prior to its definitive selection [3].

Finally, before introducing and discussing componentry, it should be pointed out that *not* using a prosthesis may be the best option for some patients even for those who

appear to be eligible based on MFCL criteria. Again, the patient evaluation can assist in making this determination. In such cases, other assistive technologies and devices may be considered such as wheelchairs or other walking aids.

COMPONENTRY

While a prosthesis is made up of multiple components and parts, the term componentry refers to a subset of items that are commonly the non-custom or semi-custom elements of the prosthesis produced by manufacturers as opposed to the patient's prosthetist. These tend to include items such as prosthetic feet, knees, or hips, pylons, rotators, torsion adapters, locking mechanisms, gel liners, and others. When speaking of the prosthetic socket (or interface), these tend to be custom-made for the individual patient by the clinical prosthetist.

A few basic premises to consider when discussing prosthetic componentry include the concept of increased function at increased cost and also the importance of classification. Not always but commonly, when a prosthetic component offers multiple added features over another, there is a good chance that the device may likely have an increased monetary cost, increased mass, and may also require increased maintenance. Again, this should be considered when choosing between different components and discussing options with patients and within the healthcare team.

Regarding the importance of classification, the quantity of available components can be overwhelming. Further, new components become available often and others become obsolete, discontinued, re-named, or re-branded. Therefore, rather than trying to memorize all of the available makes and models of components, it may be more practical to understand the common component classification schemas as a means of matching patient goals and abilities with general component functions. Once a class of component is selected, makes and models of components from within that class can then be considered. Additionally, this step is an excellent point where the physical therapist would benefit from consulting the prosthetist. Prosthetists are routinely versed in the functions of the latest makes and models of components and likely have preliminary experience with many of them. This further highlights the need and value for transdisciplinary healthcare decision making. Prosthetic components are discussed below.

COMPONENTRY: PROSTHETIC FEET

As previously mentioned, the more technically and functionally complex a prosthetic foot is, the more likely it is that the foot will be heavier, more costly, and require additional maintenance relative to alternatives. This may not be true in all cases and may not be an issue in others, but it merits consideration when discussing options with patients, caregivers, and other providers.

Classification Schemas for Prosthetic Feet

A basic component classification system simply describes the primary attribute(s) of prosthetic feet. In some cases this concerns the composition of the foot (i.e. solid ankle cushioned heel [SACH]), in others, the engineering design (i.e. single axis [SA]), and, in still others, the function (i.e. energy storing and return [ESAR]). The component classification schema [4] and a brief description with examples of each foot are described below.

Solid Ankle Cushioned Heel (SACH)

As the name implies, these feet will have a non-articulating ankle constructed upon a cushioned heel. Historically, the solid ankle portion of a SACH foot was made of a wood block for attachment of a through-bolt to fasten to an exoskeletal shin section. Updated coupling mechanisms allow for attachment to endoskeletal systems. The wood block would extend forward to the distal end of the tarso-metatarsal region but not the full length of the foot. The lack of a full-length forefoot (or *keel*) contributes to the premature loss of anterior support during gait (i.e. drop-off). The cushioned heel portion of the foot provides some degree of shock absorption at heel strike which increases comfort and

also hastens attainment of foot flat. Current SACH models may still have foam and wood construction although more contemporary designs may now include composite materials. In either case, these feet are among the least costly classification and are considered basic prosthetic feet suitable for MFCL K1 users. Research shows that patients can use SACH feet successfully for low and comfortable speed walking but are unable to walk fast or run with them [5].

Single Axis Feet (SA)

Still considered a basic foot, SA feet incorporate an articulation for sagittal movement. SA feet are therefore more complex than SACH feet and have an additional wear point to consider. The articulation is a mechanism subject to fatigue and failure that adds mass, cost, and maintenance relative to the SACH foot. The primary benefit of the SA articulation is that, depending upon the dorsi- and plantar-flexion bumper configuration, it can potentially provide a rapid foot flat position during gait which can stabilize the foot and contribute to knee stability. Research shows that SA feet accelerate sagittally in a greater range of motion compared with multi-axial or energy storing feet [6]. Anterior and posterior bumpers act in a similar manner as the plantar-flexor and dorsi-flexor muscles. That is, from heel strike to foot flat, the foot plantar-flexes. Anatomically, the pre-tibial muscles would eccentrically contract to lower the foot. With SA feet, the posterior bumper compresses, preventing foot slap. As the foot progresses from mid-stance into heel off and toe off, the plantar flexors would be stretched, eccentrically contract, and then push off with concentric contraction. Prosthetically in SA feet, from mid-stance to toe off, the anterior bumper compresses to decelerate tibial advancement and dorsi-flexion.

Multi-axial Feet (MA)

MA feet are designed to improve contact between the ground and foot and also to mitigate stress between the patient's skin and the prosthetic interface. Unlike the SA foot which only plantar-flexes and dorsi-flexes about a single axis of rotation, MA feet offer movement in more than one plane. Some designs may offer biplanar motion whereas others offer full triplanar motion. Again, the more complex the function, commonly more wear and maintenance may be expected. For instance, elastomeric bumpers designed to control a plane of motion may begin to squeak and create socially unacceptable noises or may fail altogether requiring repair. MA feet are recommended for MFCL K2 users who are considered to be unlimited household ambulators and who engage the community on a limited basis. This community level of engagement likely creates situations where users will encounter uneven terrain such as grass, slopes, rocks, roots, and others where the accommodation of a MA foot is beneficial. Research shows that MA feet improve involved side propulsion and load symmetry, and are generally preferred relative to comparable feet without MA functionality [6].

Energy Storing and Return Feet (ESAR)

ESAR feet are not considered basic feet. These feet are intended for prosthesis users who ambulate without limitations in the community and who walk with variable cadence, thus making them MFCL K3 level feet. A simplistic way to conceptualize the basic function of these feet is that when an ESAR foot dorsi-flexes after mid-stance, energy is stored. As the patient continues to advance their body over the foot, the energy stored during loading and dorsi-flexion is released as the foot plantar-flexes out of its dorsi-flexed position through toe off. This recoil out of the dorsi-flexed position is thought to provide the patient some degree of push off [5]. Compared with SACH feet, ESAR feet reduce walking energy cost and increase gait efficiency and stride length. ESAR feet increase prosthetic propulsion and stability, and minimize intact joint compensations during gait compared with flexible keel feet. Further, they have been shown to improve stair ascent by reducing ipsilateral hip moment and power requirements compared with SACH feet. Finally, ESAR feet decrease fatigue compared with SA and MA feet [6].

Energy Storing and Return Feet with Multi-Axial Function (ESAR + MA)

Feet that combine energy storage and return with MA function offer prosthesis users improved foot-to-ground contact, accommodation of forces between the device and the limb, plus the benefits of a more dynamic foot that can sustain variable cadence. As previously pointed out however, these feet will likely come at increased financial cost, mass, and maintenance. Additionally, these feet may require increased control on the part of the patient. This could mean that higher levels of balance, strength, proprioception, and kinesthetic awareness are needed to maximally benefit from feet within this class. If the user is an active walker, capable of variable cadence that routinely encounters prevailing and uneven terrain, then an ESAR + MA foot may be indicated and beneficial.

The classification system used here to orient readers is summarized in Table 5.2. It does not include additional important categories of prosthetic feet. Categories of feet not included are described below.

Flexible Keel Feet (FK)

Unlike SACH feet, FK feet have a full-length keel. The keel structure is commonly made from either thermoset

TABLE 5.2			
Categories of prosthetic feet with benefits, drawbacks, and indications			
CATEGORY	BENEFITS	DRAWBACKS	INDICATIONS
Solid Ankle Cushioned Heel (SACH)	Inexpensive. Available in different configurations (i.e. with/ without toes, sandal toe, various heel heights).	Difficult to use at higher ambulatory speeds. Commonly lacks full length keel.	Supervised, therapeutic prosthesis users and household ambulators.
Single Axis (SA)	Decreases time to foot flat.	Difficult to use at higher ambulatory speeds. Commonly lacks full length keel.	Supervised, therapeutic prosthesis users and household ambulators.
Multi-Axial (MA)	Improves foot-to-ground contact. Assists in mitigating skin-to-interface stress.	Does not offer energy storing and return function. Increased mass, cost, and maintenance.	Household and limited community ambulators.
Energy Storing and Return (ESAR)	Improves ability to walk at higher and variable speeds. Can be light weight.	Increased cost.	Unlimited community ambulators who walk with variable cadence.
Energy Storing and Return + Multi-Axial (ESAR +MA)	Improves ability to walk at higher and variable speeds on uneven ground.	Increased mass, cost, and maintenance.	Unlimited community ambulators who walk with variable. cadence and commonly encounter ramps, slopes, or uneven terrain.

laminate materials or plastic materials. This full-length keel prevents a drop off gait deviation which can improve stride symmetry. However, stride length is not improved with FK feet to the extent that an ESAR foot would improve stride length [7]. Because these feet do not store and return energy, they are not intended for unlimited community ambulators, making them appropriate for use at the MFCL K1 and K2 levels of function.

Adjustable Heel Height Feet

Some footwear requires the change of heel height in order to maintain appropriate contact between footwear and the ground. Women's high-heeled shoes for example may include heel heights of 4 to 6 inches. Cowboy, motorcycle, and other occupational footwear (i.e. firefighter boots) may also require elevated heel heights. Conversely, some footwear requires lowered heel heights relative to typical footwear. A common scenario is changing from a man's business shoe with a hard heel which may be ¾″ high to a sandal which requires a neutral height (i.e. 0″). Some adjustable heel height feet are available that allow heights of approximately 2″. Alternatively, other foot options may permit higher heel heights but may not be adjustable. It is important to discuss the patient's footwear and functional goals in this regard. Additionally, upon delivery of the prosthesis, it is important that the therapist and prosthetist evaluate the ability to don and doff the desired shoes, that the shoes and prosthesis function as intended, and that goals have been met (Figure 5.1).

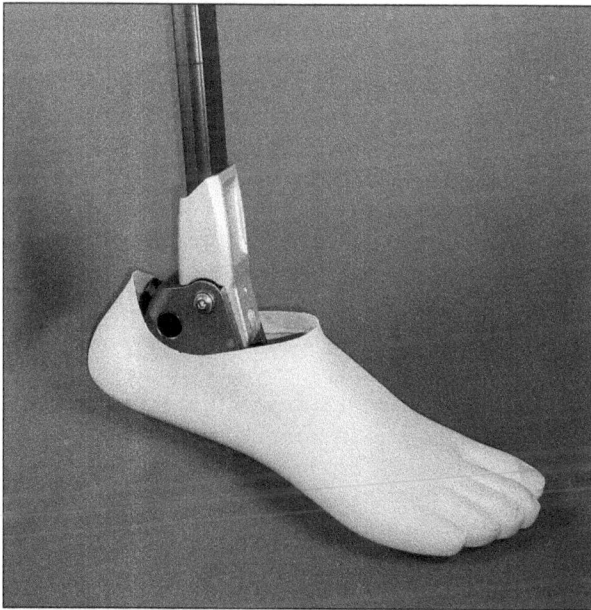

Figure 5.1. Adjustable heel height prosthetic foot.

Light Weight and Heavy Duty Feet

Light weight feet, as the name implies, are intended to be typical sizes but considerably lower mass for users who may have strength limitations. One example may be a person losing mobility, such as the frail elderly. Prostheses constructed with these light weight feet are commonly intended to be low function, possibly supervised use prostheses. If function and strength begin to improve, it may be necessary to change the foot to a component better suited for increased loading. Heavy duty feet components have quite different goals. For example, heavy duty components may be indicated in the presence of high body mass or in other high loading scenarios. Consider, for example, a prosthesis user who lifts weights for exercise. If a patient were performing standing curls, squat exercises, or other activities that transmit loads in excess of those imposed by the body and its own movement, then the prosthetic foot needs to be designed to account for these loads in a way that mitigates peak load failure but that also does not compromise functional performance. Other potential examples of scenarios requiring heavy duty foot construction may include first responder roles (i.e. police officer jumping a fence) or construction roles where loads are carried across rough terrain. There are prosthetic feet exclusively considered heavy duty and others that are not generally considered heavy duty but may be customized upon ordering so that they are constructed to manage higher loads.

Microprocessor Foot/Ankle Systems (MPFAs)

MPFA systems are among the newest technologic advancements in prosthetic feet (Figure 5.2). They include passive systems that dorsi-flex during swing phase or other systems that offer active, powered assist for certain activities such as toe off in gait or stair climbing. These functions are attempts to restore lost muscle and joint functions beyond what is available with non-microprocessor systems. MPFA systems tend to be bulkier than traditional systems, which pose concealment and cosmetic challenges, they require external power (i.e. battery power), are heavier, and are considerably more expensive than non-microprocessor alternatives. Despite their drawbacks, for the right candidate these systems have been found to improve socket comfort, kinetics and kinematics during stair ascent, enhance hill ascent and descent, and reduce back pain [8, 9].

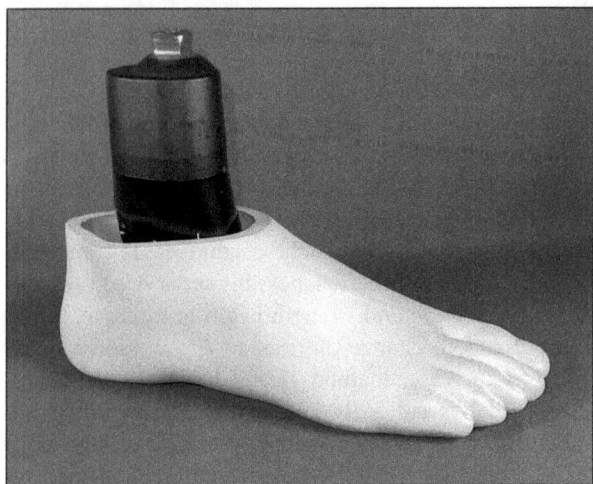

Figure 5.2. Microprocessor foot/ankle system

Athletic and Activity-Specific Feet

Prosthetic feet from this category are generally not intended for basic standing and walking in daily activities. Instead, these feet are designed to maximize function in a particular activity or limited set of activities. Examples include rock-climbing feet and running feet, among others. A rock-climbing foot may likely have a considerably shorter keel that, while smaller than a walking foot, provides increased surface area compared with a basic posting device and decreased mass for climbing. Having a prosthetic foot with a shorter keel for walking would likely result in a premature loss of anterior support (or drop-off gait). A stomper is a basic "terminal device" which means it interfaces the prosthesis to the ground like a foot does but it is not shaped like a foot. It is commonly used as a terminal device for fitting check sockets in clinic to determine socket fit as opposed to walking capability. Stompers have the benefit of high durability which further increases their appeal in this role. One final example of an activity specific foot is a running-specific foot. These tend to be highly durable thermoset materials like those used to construct ESAR feet but the shapes are a bit different. For instance, a C-shape is commonly prescribed for those who desire a foot for distance running whereas a J-shape is more associated with shorter distance sprinting. These running-specific feet lack a heel element making it more difficult to statically stand and balance, which makes clear they are better suited for running as opposed to daily activity. Compared with SACH and ESAR feet, running-specific feet have demonstrated higher running speeds, improved efficiency, and were preferred by transtibial and transfemoral level amputees for regular exercise [10].

Ankle Units

Some prosthetic feet incorporate an ankle and a **shank** portion. Other prosthetic feet do not incorporate either an ankle or shank and are designed to be coupled to other components. In some such cases an ankle unit, designed for the specific prosthetic foot, is used between the foot and the pylon. In some cases, these ankle units are semi-customizable (i.e. durometer or elastomeric bumpers, hydraulic resistance). In other cases, separate ankle units may be available if certain movements or control functions are desired.

Pylons

Commonly, the pylon, or shank, is the structural element connecting, in the case of the transtibial amputee, the prosthetic foot and ankle to the interface. For the transfemoral amputee, the tibial pylon connects the foot and ankle to the knee system. Depending on transfemoral limb length and interface design, an upper pylon section may also be necessary to connect the proximal aspect of the knee to the interface. Routinely, pylons are rigid tubing but they may come in other shapes (i.e. rectangular) or in more compliant materials such as thermoset composites. Beyond basic pylons, there are also options to include vertical or torsional shock absorption units or dual function units. As noted with prosthetic feet, these will likely increase cost, mass, and maintenance. Further, some prosthetic feet integrate these functions into their design. Therefore, if a patient's function is such that vertical and torsional shock absorption is important and beneficial, a foot that already incorporates these units may be worth considering rather than adding separate components to accomplish these functions. Research indicates that compared with rigid pylons, use of telescoping and/or teletorsion pylons does not change the biomechanics of stepping down; step activity or duration; or spatiotemporal, kinetic, and most kinematic measures of level ground walking. Further, shock-adapting pylons result in comparable perceptive measures, and an extended knee position at initial contact [6]. Much of what the literature demonstrates regarding equivalent function of shock adapters compared with rigid pylons accounts for typical function (stair and flat ground gait, circular walking) and does not account for activities with higher vertical and torsional loads. For instance, jumping for recreation or occupation and other activities such as golf and baseball may require vertical and torsional shock absorption beyond basic daily function. If patients participate in these activities with regularity, shock absorbing units may be beneficial.

COMPONENTRY: PROSTHETIC KNEES

The human knee joint is classified as a hinge joint, yet it performs complex triplanar movement beyond simple mechanical hinges which move in a single plane. Exo-prosthetic knee joints for artificial limbs are available in

TABLE 5.3		
Hierarchy of prosthetic knee stability versus control		
HIERARCHY OF PROSTHETIC KNEE STABILITY VS. CONTROL		
Most Inherent Stability/ Least Voluntary Control ⬆ ⬇ Most Voluntary Control/ Least Inherent Stability	1.	Manual Locking Knee
	2.	Polycentric Knee
	3.	Weight Activated Stance Braking Knee (WASB)
	4.	Single Axis Constant Friction Knee
	5.	Outside Hinges

multiple design configurations including single axis, polycentric, and microprocessor-controlled models. As with many other components, prosthetic knees are becoming increasingly complex, making it useful to have means to classify them.

Classification Schemas for Prosthetic Knees

A few classification systems are available to describe prosthetic knees. One classification system describes engineering attributes of knee systems such as the number and type of articulations, the type of friction medium, etc. [11]. A second system describes the media that controls swing phase and stance phase such as hydraulic, pneumatic, etc. [12]. Still another classification system aims to rank knee systems hierarchically in terms of their relative stance phase stability. For instance, a manual locking knee is regarded as highly stable in stance phase relative to a polycentric knee system [13]. Finally, what is missing from all of these systems is a means to classify and differentiate between microprocessor knee systems. One clinical trial evaluated different types of microprocessor systems in perceptive and physical performance measures and offered a subdivision of microprocessor knees that included adaptive and active systems [14]. The MFCL system, previously described, only differentiates between basic and fluid or pneumatic friction knee systems. A brief description of widely used knee classification systems and examples of exoprosthetic knees are described below:

Stability Versus Control

This continuum (Table 5.3) identifies prosthetic knees in order of most inherently stable (i.e. manual locking knee) to least inherently stable (i.e. outside hinges).

This table provides a perspective of more functional value than the MFCL system but it too is not all-inclusive and can be a bit misleading as it is not always hierarchical in terms of matching patient abilities. For example, some polycentric knees (i.e. knees with multiple rotational axes) are designed for individuals with short residual limbs likely needing higher inherent stability and mid-swing ground clearance. Conversely, other polycentric knees are designed for highly active individuals with knee disarticulation level amputations. Such people may prefer a less stable alignment that affords a higher level of voluntary control. If a person's condition improves such that decreased component stability is needed or desired, then changing to a weight activated stance brake knee, as indicated in this hierarchy, would actually be an increase in inherent stability rather than a decrease. The increased function may require switching to a SA knee with fluid friction or outside hinges in order to decrease inherent stability to allow for more fluid gait dynamics. The point is that this method does not fully account for all available products and in select cases, may be hierarchically incorrect.

Attempting to describe microprocessor knees further demonstrates the challenge of classifying different knee systems. According to this classification system, many microprocessor knees may best be described as a SA knee, however the friction is not necessarily constant. Microprocessor knees can be set up or programmed to be much more or less stable than comparably aligned knees from other classes. Microprocessor knees also have the ability to respond to variations in walking speeds and terrains unlike traditional knee systems that operate off of previously set unchanging parameters.

System for Describing Swing and Stance

The role of prosthetic knee units in standing stability, sitting flexion, and two "major and distinct" principal

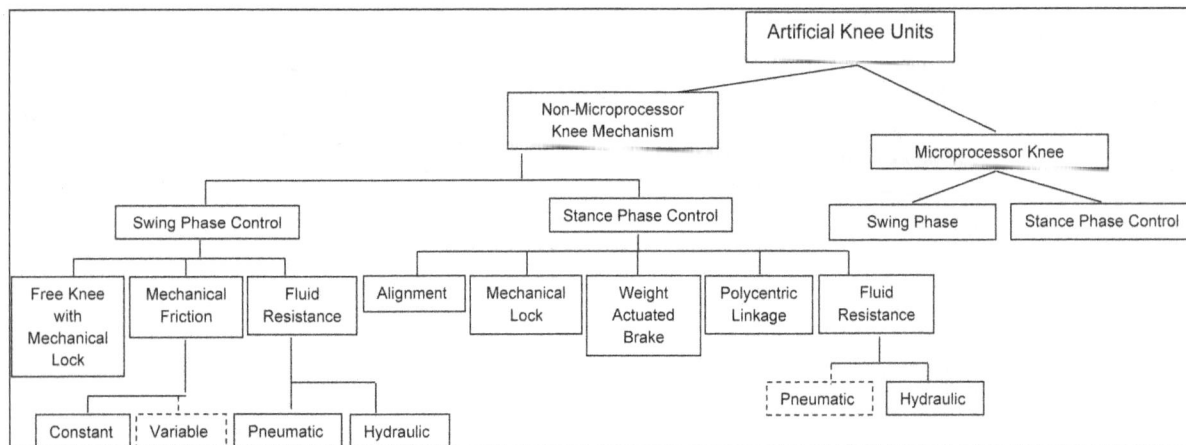

Figure 5.3. Prosthetic knee classification system describing swing and stance control media. At the time this classification system was developed, media in dashed boxes were not represented in commercially available prosthetic knee systems. The system largely holds true currently; however, some components may challenge the original classification system. (Adapted from A.B. Wilson. *A Primer on Limb Prosthetics*. Charles C. Thomas, LTD; Figure 42A.)

functions—1) stance phase joint control and 2) swing phase shank control—have been discussed elsewhere [12]. Wilson presented what he referred to as "a rather simplified" approach to prosthetic knee classification by identifying swing and stance control media [12] (Figure 5.3).

The schematic presentation describes the control options available by swing and/or stance phase but also has limitations. For example, it does not account for extension assist, microprocessor control, the possibility of combined control (i.e. hybrid systems) and so on. Some of this system's shortcomings are likely due to rapid technologic advancement.

Descriptive System for Prosthetic Knees

A descriptive classification system [11, 13] lists the following as knee categories:

1. Axes
2. Friction
3. Braking or Locking Mechanisms
4. Microprocessor Control

An additional category, Extension Aids, has also been described [11, 13]. As the name implies, this schema is more of a descriptive method for discussing and classifying prosthetic knee systems. Most of the five main headings have subheadings. The entire layout, with subheadings is presented in Table 5.4. A brief review of each category is provided in the subsequent text under the same headings and subheadings as in the table.

1. Axes

    A. Single Axis Knees

Prosthetic knee joints are either single or multi-axial. Knees from this class have traditionally had three basic

---

TABLE 5.4

Commonly described aspects of prosthetic knee joints including subheadings

COMPREHENSIVE DESCRIPTIVE CLASSIFICATION SYSTEM OF PROSTHETIC KNEE JOINTS

1. Axes
- A. Single Axis
  - i. Modular/Endoskeletal
    1. Knee Cage
    2. Stand Alone Unit
  - ii. Exoskeletal
  - iii. Outside Hinges
- B. Polycentric

2. Friction
- A. Fluid
  - i. Hydraulic
  - ii. Pneumatic
- B. Sliding
  - i. Constant
  - ii. Variable (not represented prosthetically)

3. Braking or Locking Mechanisms
- A. Manual Locking
- B. Weight Activated Stance Braking (WASB)
- C. Geometric Lock

4. Microprocessor Control

5. Extension Aids
- A. Internal
- B. External

subclasses: modular/endoskeletal, exoskeletal, and outside hinge designs. SA knees were historically among the most simple in design but today can be quite complex. Microprocessor knees, for example, are technically modular, SA knees (Figure 5.4).

Traditional exoskeletal SA knees are among the oldest design of knee units available. They were typically indicated for heavy duty use or when insisted upon by a previous wearer uninterested in using an updated system [13]. They incorporate a simple hinge positioned between the thigh and shin. Exoskeletal thigh and shin sections may be made from wood, foam, or laminate materials (Figure 5.5). Historically, exoskeletal knee units were available with constant friction, fluid friction, manual locks, and extension aids, yet low market demand seems to be decreasing their availability.

Classic outside hinge designs (Figure 5.6) were historically recommended for knee disarticulation length amputees, however they may also be used with transtibial amputees with knee instability [11, 13, 15]. Outside hinges offer no stance control beyond alignment and voluntary residual limb abilities. With classic outside hinges, swing control is also non-existent beyond joint friction, which may be problematic in variable cadence ambulators.

With regard to modular SA knees, there are two designs: the cage design, which houses a separate fluid cylinder; and non-cage, self-contained units. Alone, knee cages may be little more than a hinged frame. Some SA knee cages offer a braking mechanism and others offer a stance flexion feature. Many knee cages provide home to fluid friction cylinder units. Cages combined with hydraulic units provide many options for swing and stance control and some have options for low profile build heights and low resistance motion. This is a popular option for higher functioning users but this is not requisite as they are also available for lower function users.

Self-contained, modular SA knee units may be augmented with various forms of swing and stance control. In a very basic unit, stance control is afforded by alignment and is therefore not technically a knee feature. This is not the rule as other SA units offer a true stance control feature. Examples of stance control afforded by self-contained, SA units include microprocessor control, fluid control, and weight activated braking.

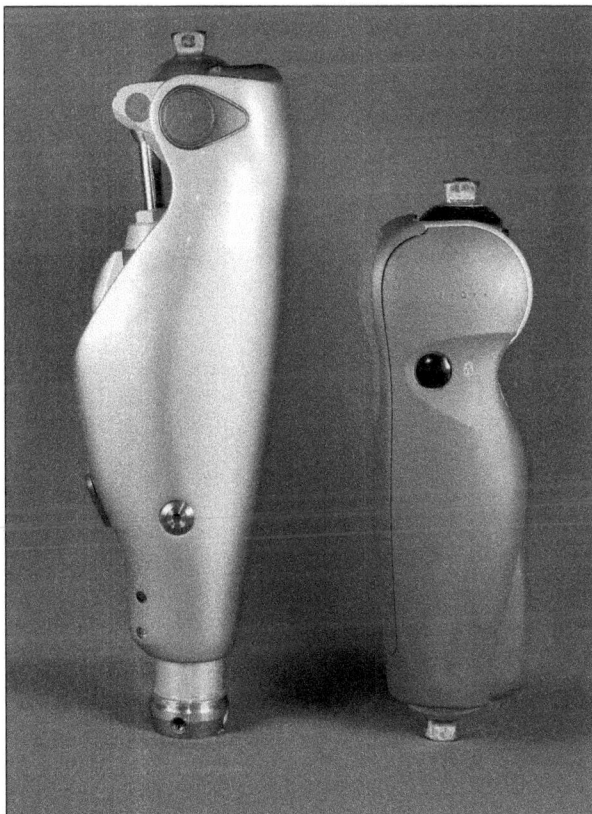

Figure 5.4. Examples of highly technical, modular, microprocessor-controlled knee units that are of a single axis design.

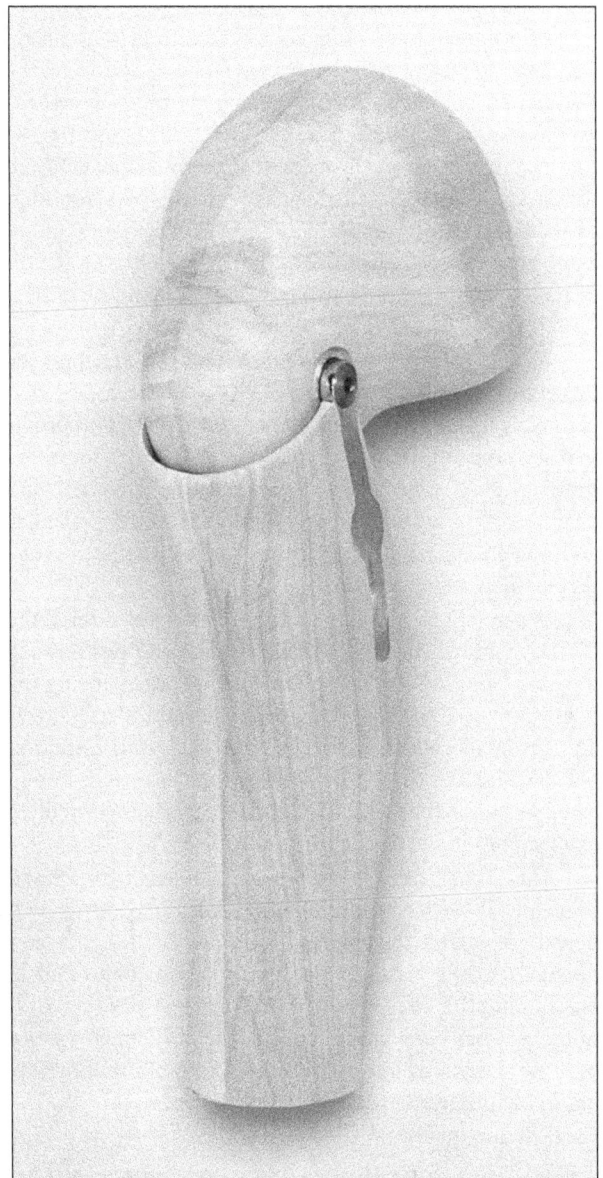

Figure 5.5. Otto Bock exoskeletal single axis constant friction (3P19) knee system. The knee mechanism is integrated into a wooden shin and distal thigh sections. Photo courtesy of Otto Bock Healthcare.

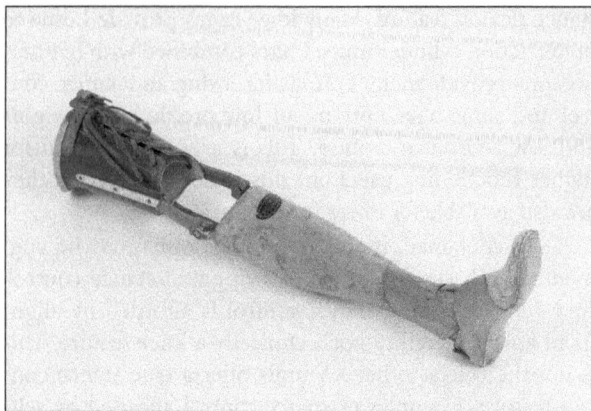

Figure 5.6. Leather socket prosthesis with outside hinges for an individual with transtibial amputation.

B. Polycentric Knees

Multi-axial knee joints are referred to as polycentric (whereas SA units may be referred to as monocentric). Polycentric prosthetic knees mimic anatomic knee arthrokinematics in that both have a center of rotation (COR) that changes position throughout joint movement. When the anatomic knee's COR changes position, it is referred to as an instantaneous center of rotation (ICOR). The COR of a polycentric prosthetic knee is also described as an ICOR. Several benefits are reportedly associated with polycentric knee joints [17, 18, 19].

Polycentric knee joints tend to have multiple bars, or linkages (typically four or five but as many as seven) that connect various pivot points between the distal and proximal segments of the unit. Typically, the ICOR is found by drawing lines, sagittally, that connect the proximal and distal pivot points of the given bars (generally the anterior and posterior bars). The point at which these lines intersect is the ICOR (Figure 5.7).

When typical polycentric prosthetic knees extend, the ICOR position tends to be well proximal and posterior to the distal midline of the mechanical knee axis. Moving the ICOR proximal to the anatomic knee center offers a leverage advantage which eases the task of flexion initiation [12, 16]. Having the ICOR posterior to the weight line in extension affords a stable alignment due to induction of an extension moment about the knee [17].

These knee units are not forced to pivot on a fixed point distal to the residual limb. Therefore, during high degrees of flexion, the proximal aspect of the shin relocates posterior to the distal residual limb. This is beneficial in positioning the knee center and shin while sitting. Additionally, it has been suggested that the polycentric nature of these systems might shorten the length of the shin during swing phase, assisting with toe clearance [18].

2. Friction

Friction, a force that resists motion, is used in prosthetic knee joints to alter the rate of knee cycling. It is incorporated primarily to match side-by-side cycling

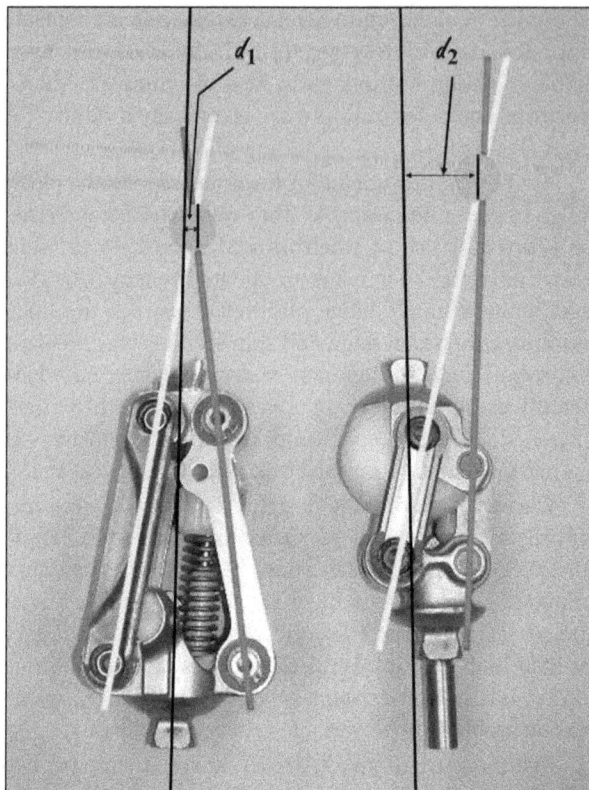

Figure 5.7. Polycentric knees. Otto Bock 3R30 knee unit (left), which is indicated for knee disarticulation amputation level. The ICOR (see the dot—located by intersection of line extending anterior and posterior links) in full extension is close to the distal end of the residual limb (and mechanical knee axis) and only slightly posterior to the body's weight line (d1, the distance between the body's weight line (black line) and the ICOR, is very small). This knee requires a high amount of voluntary control and offers less alignment stability in extension. At right is the Otto Bock 3R36 knee unit. This knee unit's ICOR in full extension is well proximal of the mechanical knee axis (closer to the anatomic hip joint than knee disarticulation models such as the 3R66) and well posterior of the body's weight line (d2, the distance between the body's weight line (black line) and the ICOR, is relatively large). Having the ICOR in such a location offers a higher amount of stability, initially affording less voluntary control.

thereby optimizing the cycling rate on-demand. Two types of friction are present in prosthetic knees: fluid and sliding.

A. Fluid Friction

Fluid friction is provided by pneumatic and hydraulic media. A common goal of both fluid mediums is to provide responsiveness to variable cadence. In order to do this, resistance to movement must generally increase as the velocity of movement increases [11]. With regard to fluid friction, there are differences between pneumatic and hydraulic fluid. The fact that liquids are incompressible and pneumatic fluid (air) is compressible has implications in performance [13, 19].

The compressible nature of air affords an "air-spring effect" at higher cycling velocities [13]. This causes the knee to tend to extend upon being unweighted from a flexed position. Highly active users and those with higher body mass tend to overpower the resistance offered by typical pneumatic systems. This makes hydraulic friction a potentially superior choice in such cases.

Hydraulic friction units do not offer an extension bias due to compression of their fluid. Instead, extension may be augmented with the mechanical assistance of a spring which can induce knee extension upon unweighting [11, 13]. Hydraulic knees tend to weigh and cost slightly more than less technical knee systems but are well known for their cadence responsiveness and ability to assist with stance control [13, 19].

B. Sliding Friction

The second type of friction, sliding friction, is typically used for single speed ambulators [11–13, 15, 19]. By definition, sliding friction may be either constant or variable [12, 13]. These knee units are designed with some form of a pinch assembly that applies friction to an axle (Figure 5.8). Because of this design, once the friction is set, the friction must be manually re-set to affect a change in the knee cycling rate (for example, increasing friction would decrease the cycling rate and vice versa). Therefore, variable sliding friction is not represented in commercially available prosthetic knee units [12]. Sliding friction is constant once the knee is adjusted.

3. Braking or Locking Mechanisms

This knee category provides component options for the lowest and highest functional users. Presently, there are three available systems in this category: the manual locking knee, the weight activated stance control knee, and the geometric lock [13].

A. Manual Locking

The manual locking knee prevents knee flexion by locking the joint in the fully extended position. It includes a manual release to unlock the knee when flexion is desired, such as for sitting. Some manual locking knees incorporate an extension assist to facilitate full extension upon standing.

B. Weight Activated Stance Braking

The next subtype is the braking mechanism. Considered the third most stable on the stability hierarchy (see Table 5.3), this unit is commonly referred to as a weight activated stance braking/control knee. The most popular version of this type of knee is a SA, constant friction joint. When loaded, generally with no greater than 10°–15° of flexion, the knee will lock and flex no further. So long as the knee remains loaded, it will remain locked and resist further flexion. Once the knee is unloaded, it allows flexion for swing phase. This type of knee can also include swing phase control. The knee should be adjusted by the prosthetist regularly as the braking mechanism tends to wear with use and this may lead to falls.

C. Geometric Lock

The final subtype in this category is the geometric lock. Swing control can be via elastic polymer, sliding friction, or fluid media. Several units are available ranging

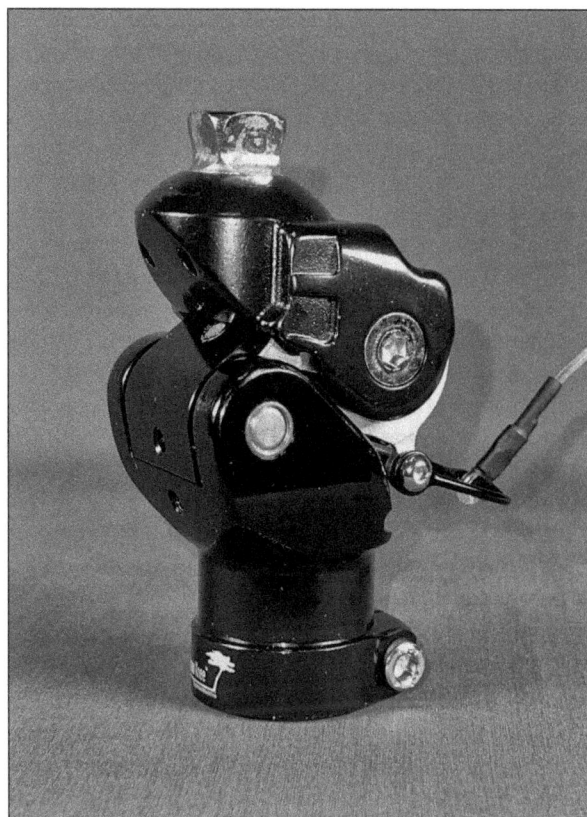

Figure 5.8. A single axis knee unit with sliding, constant friction and single speed cadence per setting. It also features a manual lock. Stance control is via weight activated stance braking. Thus, with threshold load application, the knee will not flex further which could cause buckling. This form of stance control requires prosthetic unloading prior to swing advancement and may lead to gait deviations such as hip hiking and lateral trunk bending.

from pediatric to heavy duty adult options. These options allow coverage of single or variable speed ambulators, as well as children and adults. The geometric lock engages as the knee reaches terminal extension. At that instant, linkage alignment prevents knee buckling. Typically, a knee hyperextension moment is necessary to disengage the lock to permit knee flexion.

4. Microprocessor Control

Presently, several microprocessor controlled knees are available. Options include microprocessor control for swing phase only, or for both swing and stance phases. More options include SA or polycentric designs as well as power actuated systems.

Current microprocessor controlled prosthetic knee units may sample data between 50 and 1,000 times per second for the purpose of making adjustments to flexion/extension resistance or joint angle limits in some cases. In some of these units, multiple alternate modes are available that enable a user to switch from an everyday "walking" mode to activity-specific modes for unique applications such as driving, heavy lifting, or bicycling. The ability to increase or decrease gait velocity from one extreme to another instantaneously without manually adjusting the component or completing a full knee cycle is a very helpful feature for users. Some computerized knees have been shown to enable reciprocal ramp and stair descent more like the anatomic knee [20–23]. Such knees tend to offer a stance feature that is able to sense a break in cadence or rhythm that may be associated with a fall and react by engaging a safe mode that affords users the opportunity to catch themselves [20]. These knee systems require nightly charging, although some systems can run for up to 5 days between charges. The most recent innovation in this area, power actuation, offers the promise of improved biomechanics for activities requiring active knee extension such as that produced via concentric contraction of the quadriceps femoris associated with activities such as stair climbing, ramp climbing, and timed up and go [24, 14]. While these features can be helpful to some groups, these power actuating capabilities may not benefit all groups equally and come with a significant increase in material bulk, mass, and financial cost.

5. Extension Aids

Extension aids or the extension assist feature of a prosthetic knee may be located internally or externally. They may be an integral part of the knee's design or added on "after-the-fact" in some units. Certain aspects of a prosthetic user's gait pattern indicate the need for an extension assist. For instance, extension assist may be considered if the user displays excessive heel rise or delayed knee extension. Knee resistance (friction) against flexion may be too low or friction against knee extension may be too great and thus present similar issues. The extension assist will facilitate knee extension by opposing heel rise and knee flexion in pre-swing and promoting knee extension once the shank begins forward movement in swing phase.

6. The Hybrid Concept

Prosthetic knees may have features from several of the latter categories. This is the basis of the hybrid concept [15, 25]. An example may be as simple as incorporating fluid swing control with weight activated braking for stance control. However, examples may be as complex as combining pneumatic swing control and hydraulic stance control in a polycentric design, controlled by a microprocessor. Hybrid prosthetic knees incorporate unique features from one or more select knee components and combine them with the benefits of features from other knees. The goal of such combinations would be a maximal return to function and, hopefully, participation in activities previously not possible with a less technically complex component.

COMPONENTRY: HIP JOINT SYSTEMS

A relatively small patient population requires external hip prostheses. Those who have undergone a hemipelvectomy or hip disarticulation amputation present with unique challenges, including significantly reduced lower extremity control. The human hip joint provides greater motion than is achievable at any other joint in the body, excluding the shoulder. Though it is impossible to achieve a similar range of motion using external hip prostheses, improvements have been made in recent years to achieve a more natural and physiological gait.

Most prosthetic hip joints operate with a single axis replicating motion only in the sagittal plane. For patients requiring stability, some hip joints incorporate locking mechanisms that limit hip flexion to 5° when walking. Another design uses an adjustable extension assist spring to limit hip flexion. For more active users, hydraulic-controlled hip joints allow greater adjustability for different gait patterns providing greater control during ambulation and a more natural movement [26].

PROSTHETIC SOCKET (INTERFACE) DESIGNS

Exoprosthetic limbs are generally intended to replace as much function of an amputated or congenitally deficient limb as possible. The prosthetic elements such as the knee, shin, ankle, or foot are however substitutes that must ultimately be connected to the body. The predominant means of attachment is currently the prosthetic socket. Other means of attachment, such as **osseointegrated skeletal attachment** [27–33], are becoming increasingly prevalent, however the procedure remains quite rare and has not been universally approved or adopted. Therefore, the prosthetic socket remains the predominant means of exoprosthetic attachment. This section will describe socket designs commonly found in clinical practice in patients with lower limb amputation.

Prior to discussing socket design, it is useful to describe differences between preparatory and definitive prostheses and to introduce options for general construction including material choices. The first prosthesis a patient is fit with is commonly regarded as the *preparatory prosthesis*. This identification has implications in prosthetic, therapeutic, billing, and other domains. For instance, when a patient is using a preparatory prosthesis, it is commonly the case that the patient is not widely familiar with self-care as a person with limb loss and thus may not have a full understanding of what to expect during this time in their rehabilitation. The user may also have considerable post-operative edema that has the potential to reduce rapidly. Therefore, it may be prudent for the prosthetist to select materials and a construction method that enables adjustments to accommodate the significant fluctuations in residuum volume. The exact design is up to the healthcare team in deliberation with the patient but might include softer, more compliant materials such as viscous gels. This may also include a double-walled socket system that includes a flexible interface and a rigid frame.

Therefore, the prosthesis in this case may include first, a viscous gel liner upon the skin. Next, with volume loss, prosthetic socks may be added as needed between the gel liner and the flexible interface. When used, the flexible interface is commonly the innermost wall of the socket and as the name implies may permit small amounts of movement depending upon the construction of the rigid frame (i.e. outer socket wall). Flexible interfaces generally lack the strength for the structural attachment of components, which will thus be attached to the rigid outer frame. This structural outer wall is designed with the strength to protect the residual limb and to resist failure from forces associated with movement. The outer frame is also a place where prosthetists can make adjustments in the event of skin breakdown or other problems.

Prosthetic socket material selection is important with every prosthesis. During the preparatory prosthesis utilization period, material choices are important not only because protective and structural roles are important but, again, because the high degree of volume change coupled with a high likelihood of a lack of self-care mastery as a prosthesis user can demand that the ability to adjust the prosthesis be readily available. For example, thermoplastic materials retain a considerable quantity of adjustability by means of thermoforming whereas thermoset laminates do not retain the same level of adaptability. A preparatory prosthesis may be used by a patient for a period of several months up to a year, depending on the continued fit and structural integrity of the limb.

Once the patient can no longer use the preparatory prosthesis, a *definitive prosthesis* is fit. Definitive prostheses are also individually unique based on patient and healthcare team decision making driven by the patient goals. Definitive prostheses generally differ from preparatory prostheses in that they are anticipated to be used for a longer period of time by the patient, assuming that volume has stabilized somewhat relative to the acute and sub-acute post-operative periods. Therefore, it may be a better option to utilize materials that are as durable and lightweight as possible. The definitive prosthesis still requires adjustability but it may not be as adjustable as the preparatory prosthesis depending upon the construction and choice of materials. Single-walled sockets can of course be used for preparatory or definitive prostheses but they are generally rigid frame designs which would tend to limit adjustability relative to a double-walled alternative. Benefits of the rigid frame, single-walled socket include a reduction in material bulk, mass, and cost.

Transtibial Socket Designs

There are a number of prosthetic socket design options for fitting patients with transtibial amputations. First, the total contact concept should be mentioned. The total contact concept added that sockets need to have contact with the distal end of the residual limb. Some limbs can tolerate greater force through the distal end than others, yet a tolerable level of distal contact is recommended to prevent the limb from **hammocking** or other problems that can emerge from lack of contact, such as **verrucous hyperplasia**. *Specific weight bearing sockets* utilize greater weight bearing through pressure tolerant areas of the residual limb while attempting to minimize loading on pressure intolerant areas. Pressure tolerant areas for preferential loading include areas such as the patella tendon, the medial tibial flare, and the muscle bellies of the gastrocnemius. Pressure intolerant areas that are loaded less in a specific weight bearing or patella tendon bearing (PTB) socket include the tibial tubercle, the fibular head, the distal cut end of the fibula, and others.

An alternative design to the specific weight bearing socket is the *total surface bearing (TSB) socket*. The basic concept of the TSB socket is that if all the anatomy is loaded equally, the load on any one area will be more optimally distributed relative to the higher focal stresses imparted by PTB designs. In addition to the TSB design, there is still another popular design referred to as the *hydrostatic design* (HSD). The HSD uses a loading approach somewhat analogous to the TSB design in that loading is relatively uniformly distributed throughout as opposed to focal loading as in PTB. A key difference in HSD is that, during casting, axial, distally directed tension is applied [34]. This attempts to capitalize on drawing fluid distally into the residual limb. Because fluid is incompressible, the goal is to stabilize tissue within the socket. Because fluid can flow in and out of the residual limb with arteriovenous and lymphatic circulation, it is unclear if a more stable socket results with an HSD socket compared with alternatives; however, these systems have been found to apply pressure more evenly on the residuum [35].

Transfemoral Socket Designs

Transfemoral (TF) residual limbs pose challenges related to end-bearing, mediolateral stability, and transverse rotational control. The post-operative goal for the TF residual limb shape is cylindrical to optimize weight bearing between socket and limb. The transected femur may not accept a high amount of distal loading so other parts of the anatomy or other design features may be called upon for support. One of the earlier designs still used today is the quadrilateral (quad) socket. Named for its four-walled shape, the quad socket is described as maintaining contact between certain parts of the limb anatomy with certain walls of the quad socket. For instance, the anterior wall maintains contact with the quadriceps femoris muscles; the medial wall contacts the subischial triangle including the adductor muscles; the lateral wall contacts the iliotibial band; and the posterior wall contacts the hamstrings [13]. The preponderance of weight bearing is borne through the ischial tuberosity, the gluteal mass, and through total surface bearing across the entire limb. The ischial tuberosity and gluteal mass rest upon a posterior shelf due to posteriorly directed pressure from the anterior wall, preventing the tuberosity and gluteal fold from slipping into the socket.

Unlike the four-walled quad socket, the ischial containment (IC) or ischial ramus containment socket is more triangular shaped and is characterized by muscular channels when viewed transversely. For example, the IC socket has muscular channels for the hamstrings, the rectus femoris, and the adductor muscle group. Another key difference between this system and the quad socket is that the ischial ramus is contained within the socket in IC designs. Load is borne through the ischial tuberosity, the gluteal mass, and through total surface bearing [13].

Finally, another design is the sub-ischial, elevated vacuum assisted suspension design. This design brings the proximal socket wall (or trimline) below the level of the ischial tuberosity. Therefore, no load is borne through the ischial tuberosity. Instead, load is borne through total surface bearing. The elevated vacuum may draw fluid into the distal aspect of the residuum creating a more solid distal fluid–tissue platform and assist in stabilizing fluid all about the residuum. As limb volume is stabilized by the elevated vacuum systems, motion between the user and the prosthesis is reduced, resulting in improved suspension. Data show no differences in gait and balance between IC and sub-ischial sockets; however, patient preference greatly favors the sub-ischial design [36–39].

Suspension Systems

The socket designs previously described predominantly address weight bearing and load distribution for activities such as standing and stance phase during gait. Conversely, it is suspension that retains the prosthesis upon the residual limb when lifted, such as during the swing phase of gait. There are multiple types of suspension systems. A select few will be described here.

For transfemoral (TF) designs, an elastic and Velcro® belt may be used as primary or auxiliary suspension. These belt systems may also serve to minimize transverse rotation. Transtibial (TT) designs may similarly use a knee sleeve as primary or auxiliary suspension. Both TT and TF levels may make use of a gel liner as part of their load distribution and socket design, although liners may also contribute to suspension. Many gel liners have a distal attachment that can be used to secure either a pin or a lanyard for suspension. Pins that attach to liners may be smooth or notched. The pin is pushed into a locking mechanism located in the distal aspect of the socket. Some pins may be drawn down using a key tool and others are simply pushed into their lock. Commonly, a button located on the

distal medial aspect of the socket is pressed to release the pin from its locking mechanism. Some of the notched pins offer an audible click to assist in assuring that the prosthesis is securely attached to the residual limb.

Other types of suspension rely on negative pressure to hold the prosthesis onto the residual limb. In some cases, suction is used. With suction, the limb is usually moved inside the socket distally and air is evacuated providing a secure fit limiting distal migration. A one-way release valve is commonly used so that the user may evacuate additional air during movement or to allow air into the socket for the purpose of prosthesis removal. Vacuum systems rely on pumps. Pumps may be mechanical or electrical. Mechanical pumps require movement whereas electronic pumps do not require movement but may be noisy and require frequent charging.

Another type of suspension is the anatomic fit. These sockets are designed to maintain suspension from the socket design and are based on very unique attributes of an individual's residual limb. They are most commonly used in congenital limb deficiency cases as opposed to acquired amputation cases.

SUMMARY

This chapter addressed lower extremity prosthetic componentry. Specifically, the chapter reviewed component classifications and provided examples of certain makes and models as well as associated indications, contraindications, benefits, and drawbacks. It is important for the physical therapist to be able to recognize major types of componentry and be able to distinguish between them to improve the prognosis, goal setting and rehabilitation intervention selection aspects of therapy.

KEY TERMS

Keel—the keel is analogous to the forefoot. The portion of the prosthetic foot anterior to the ankle joint is referred to as the keel. The portion of the prosthetic foot posterior to the ankle is referred to as the heel.

Shank—anatomically, the shank is analogous to the tibial section of the leg. Prosthetically, this is referred to as the pylon or shank.

Osseointegrated skeletal attachment—using an orthopedic surgical implant as a means to attach an exoprosthesis directly to the skeleton without using a prosthetic socket.

Hammocking—a condition where the residual limb is unable to make distal contact with the socket. It may be that the limb is unable to contact distally because the socket is excessively tight proximally or that the socket is too long for the residual limb.

Verrucous hyperplasia—a skin condition of the amputated residual limb where the residual limb appears warty distally due to proximal constriction and insufficient distal contact.

REFERENCES

[1] Gailey RS, Roach KE, Applegate EB, et al. The amputee mobility predictor: an instrument to assess determinants of the lower-limb amputee's ability to ambulate. *Arch Phys Med Rehabil.* 2002;83(5):613–627.

[2] Raschke SU, Orendurff MS, Mattie JL, et al. Biomechanical characteristics, patient preference and activity level with different prosthetic feet: a randomized double blind trial with laboratory and community testing. *J Biomech.* 2015;48(1):146–152.

[3] Kahle JT, Highsmith MJ, Hubbard SL. Comparison of nonmicroprocessor knee mechanism versus C-Leg on Prosthesis Evaluation Questionnaire, stumbles, falls, walking tests, stair descent, and knee preference. *J Rehabil Res Dev.* 2008;45(1):1–14.

[4] *Prosthetics 621: Transtibial Prosthetics for Prosthetists. Course Manual,* 2004. Prosthetic-Orthotic Center, Feinberg School of Medicine, Northwestern University, Chicago, IL.

[5] Mengelkoch LJ, Kahle JT, Highsmith MJ. Energy costs & performance of transtibial amputees & non-amputees during walking & running. *Int J Sports Med.* 2014;35(14):1223–1228.

[6] Highsmith MJ, Kahle JT, Miro RM, et al. Prosthetic interventions for people with transtibial amputation: systematic review and meta-analysis of high-quality prospective literature and systematic reviews. *J Rehabil Res Dev.* 2016;53(2):157–184.

[7] Underwood HA, Tokuno CD, Eng JJ. A comparison of two prosthetic feet on the multi-joint and multi-plane kinetic gait compensations in individuals with a unilateral trans-tibial amputation. *Clinical Biomechanics (Bristol, Avon).* 2004;19(6):609–616.

[8] Aldridge JM, Sturdy JT, Wilken JM. Stair ascent kinematics and kinetics with a powered lower leg system following transtibial amputation. *Gait Posture.* 2012;36(2):291–295.

[9] Weber EL, Stevens PM, England DL, et al. Microprocessor feet improve prosthetic mobility and physical function relative to non-microprocessor feet. *J Rehabil Assist Technol Eng.* 2022 Jul 11;9:20556683221113320.

[10] Mengelkoch LJ, Kahle JT, Highsmith MJ. Energy costs and performance of transfemoral amputees and non-amputees during walking and running: a pilot study. *Prosthet Orthot Int.* 2016;41(5):484–491.

[11] Seymour R, ed. *Prosthetics and Orthotics. Lower Limb and Spinal,* 2002. Lippincott Williams and Wilkins, Baltimore, MD.

[12] Wilson AB. *A Primer on Limb Prosthetics,* 1998. Charles C. Thomas, Springfield, IL.

[13] *Prosthetics 621: Transfemoral Prosthetics for Prosthetists. Course Manual,* 2004. Prosthetic-Orthotic Center, Feinberg School of Medicine, Northwestern University, Chicago, IL.

[14] Hafner BJ, Askew RL. Physical performance and self-report outcomes associated with use of passive, adaptive, and active prosthetic knees in persons with unilateral, transfemoral amputation: randomized crossover trial. *J Rehabil Res Dev.* 2015;52(6):677–700.

[15] Smith DG, Bowker J, Michael J, eds. *Atlas of Amputations and Limb Deficiencies: Surgical, Prosthetic and Rehabilitation Principles,* 2004. 3rd edition. American Academy of Orthopaedic Surgeons, Rosemont, IL.

[16] Zarrugh MY, Radcliffe CW. Simulation of swing phase dynamics in above-knee prostheses. *J Biomech.* 1976:283–292.

[17] Michael JW. Component selection criteria: lower limb disarticulations. *Clin Prosthet Orthot.* 1988;12:99–108.

[18] Gard SA, Childress DS, Uellendahl JE. The influence of four-bar linkage knees on prosthetic swing-phase floor clearance. *J Prosthet Orthot.* 1996;8:34–40.

[19] Michael JW. Modern prosthetic knee mechanisms. *Clin Orthop Relat Res.* 1999;(361):39–47.

[20] Highsmith MJ, Kahle JT, Bongiorni DR, et al. Safety, energy efficiency, and cost efficacy of the C-Leg for transfemoral amputees: a review of the literature. *Prosthet Orthot Int.* 2010;34(4): 362–377.

[21] Highsmith MJ, Kahle JT, Lewandowski AL, et al. A method for training step-over-step stair descent gait with stance yielding prosthetic knees. *J Prosthet Orthot.* 2012;24(1):10–15.

[22] Highsmith MJ, Kahle JT, Lura DJ, et al. Stair ascent and ramp gait training with the Genium knee. *Technol Innov.* 2014;15: 349–358.

[23] Highsmith MJ, Kahle JT, Wernke MM, et al. Effects of the Genium knee system on functional level, stair ambulation, perceptive and economic outcomes in transfemoral amputees. *Technol Innov.* 2016;18(2–3):139–150.

[24] Highsmith MJ, Kahle JT, Carey SL, et al. Kinetic asymmetry in transfemoral amputees while performing sit to stand and stand to sit movements. *Gait Posture.* 2011;34(1):86–91.

[25] Shurr DG, Michael JW, eds. *Prosthetics and Orthotics,* 2002. 2nd edition. Prentice Hall Health, Upper Saddle River, NJ.

[26] Ludwigs E, Bellmann M, Schmalz T, Blumentritt S. Biomechanical differences between two exoprosthetic hip joint systems during level walking. *Prosthet Orthot Int.* 2010;34(4):449–460.

[27] Al Muderis M, Bosley BA, Florschutz AV, et al. Radiographic assessment of extremity osseointegration for the amputee. *Technol Innov.* 2016;18(2–3):211–216.

[28] Hagberg K, Branemark R, Gunterberg B, Rydevik B. Osseointegrated trans-femoral amputation prostheses: prospective results of general and condition-specific quality of life in 18 patients at 2-year follow-up. *Prosthet Orthot Int.* 2008;32(1):29–41.

[29] Hagberg K, Hansson E, Branemark R. Outcome of percutaneous osseointegrated prostheses for patients with unilateral transfemoral amputation at two-year follow-up. *Arch Phys Med Rehabil.* 2014;95(11):2120–2127.

[30] Carroll M, Rheinstein J. A brief history of bone-anchored prosthetics. *Academy Today.* 2024;20(4):4–7.

[31] Hoellwarth JS, Tetsworth K, Akhtar MA, Al Muderis M. The clinical history and basic science origins of transcutaneous osseointegration for amputees. *Adv Orthop.* 2022;2022:7960559. Published online March 18, 2022. doi: 10.1155/2022/7960559.

[32] Li Y, Brånemark R. Osseointegrated prostheses for rehabilitation following amputation: the pioneering Swedish model. *Unfallchirurg.* 2017;120(4):285–292.

[33] Thesleff A, Brånemark R, Håkansson B, Ortiz-Catalan M. Biomechanical characterisation of bone-anchored implant systems for amputation limb prostheses: a systematic review. *Ann Biomed Eng.* 2018 Mar;46(3):377–391. doi: 10.1007/s10439-017-1976-4. Epub 2018 Jan 11.

[34] Redhead RG. Total surface bearing self suspending above-knee sockets. *Prosthet Orthot Int.* 1979;3(3):126–136.

[35] Moo EK, Abu Osman NA, Pingguan-Murphy B, et al. Interface pressure profile analysis for patellar tendon bearing socket and hydrostatic socket. *Acta Bioeng Biomech*. 2009;11(4):37–43.

[36] Kahle JT, Highsmith MJ. Transfemoral interfaces with vacuum assisted suspension comparison of gait, balance, and subjective analysis: ischial containment versus brimless. *Gait Posture*. 2014;40(2):315–320.

[37] Kahle JT, Highsmith MJ. Transfemoral sockets with vacuum-assisted suspension comparison of hip kinematics, socket position, contact pressure, and preference: ischial containment versus brimless. *J Rehabil Res Dev*. 2013;50(9):1241–1252.

[38] Kahle JT, Orriola JJ, Johnston W, Highsmith MJ. The effects of vacuum-assisted suspension on residual limb physiology, wound healing and function: a systematic review. *Technol Innov*. 2014;15:333–341.

[39] Wernke MM, Albury A, Denune J, et al. American Academy of Orthotists and Prosthetists 43rd Annual Meeting and Scientific Symposium Chicago, IL March 3, 2017. The relationship between limb motion, limb volume, socket comfort, and prosthetic suspension. American Academy of Orthotists and Prosthetists, 2017. http://media.mycrowdwisdom.com.s3.amazonaws.com/aaop/Resources/JOP/2017/2017-F25.pdf.

CHAPTER 6

Physical Examination and Outcome Measurement of the Patient with Lower Extremity Amputation

Christopher A. Rábago, Brian Kaluf, and M. Jason Highsmith

OBJECTIVES

Upon completion of this chapter, the reader will:

1. Recall key elements that should be included in a comprehensive evaluation of a patient with amputation.
2. Understand the role of outcome measures as part of the patient evaluation.
3. Recall properties that make an outcome measure credible and robust.
4. Be familiar with properties that determine the quality of an outcome measure, the general types of outcome measures, and select examples of common outcome measures used with patients with amputation.

INTRODUCTION

The Centers for Medicare & Medicaid Services (CMS) 2017 physician fee schedule introduced three physical therapy evaluation codes replacing the previous one (97001). These codes were meant to reflect the complexity of the evaluation performed: low complexity (97161), moderate complexity (97162), and high complexity (97163). There are four main factors that influence the complexity of the evaluation: 1) patient history to include personal factors and comorbidities; 2) depth and results of examination techniques and use of standardized tests and measures; 3) clinical presentation to include current status and mechanism of condition; and 4) clinical decision making to include goal establishment and prognosis of outcomes [1]. Rubrics have been developed to guide physical therapists in choosing the correct complexity level for their evaluation (Table 6.1). These rubrics not only contain the above-mentioned four factors but also use examples in terms of body structures and functions, activity limitations, participation restrictions, and outcome measures [1].

This new way of characterizing a physical therapist's evaluation actually used a culmination of terminology and elements initially described in the *American Physical Therapist Association's Guide to Physical Therapist Practice 2nd edition* [2, 3] and is still true now in the *Guide's 4th edition, Guide to Physical Therapist Practice 4.0* [4] and the World Health Organization's International Classification of Functioning, Disability and Health (ICF) framework [5]. The Guide defines standard terminology and offers a framework of assessment tools and tests emphasizing the use of outcome measurement in clinical decision making [5]. The ICF framework is the predominant means for

DOI: 10.4324/9781003526025-7

TABLE 6.1					
Physical therapy evaluation codes					
CODE/TYPICAL FACE-TO-FACE TIME	**DURATION**	**HISTORY**	**EXAMINATION**	**CLINICAL PRESENTATION**	**CLINICAL DECISION MAKING**
97161 Low-Complexity Initial Evaluation	20 min	No personal factors and/or comorbidities impact POC	Exam of body systems using standardized tests/ measures for <u>1–2</u> elements of: body structures/functions, activity limitations and/or participation restrictions	Stable and/or uncomplicated characteristics	Low-complexity, using standardized patient assessment instrument and/or measurable assessment of functional outcome
97162 Moderate-Complexity Initial Evaluation	30 min	1–2 personal factors and/or comorbidities impact POC	Exam of body systems using standardized tests/ measures for <u>3 or more</u> elements of: body structures for functions, activity limitations and/ or participation restrictions	Evolving clinical presentation with changing characteristics	Moderate-complexity, using standardized patient assessment instrument and/ or measurable assessment of functional outcome
97163 High-Complexity Initial Evaluation	45 min	3 or more personal factors and/or co-morbidities impact POC	Exam of body systems using standardized tests/ measures addressing <u>4 or more</u> elements of: body structures/ functions, activity limitations and/ or participation restrictions	Unstable and unpredictable characteristics	High-complexity, using standardized patient assessment instrument and/ or measurable assessment of functional outcome
97164 Re-Evaluation	20 min	Review of history and standardized tests/ measures required			Revised POC using standardized patient assessment instrument and/or measurable assessment of functional outcome

Source: Adapted from PT Management Support Systems. Note: POC = plan of care.

understanding function and disability by assessing body functions and structures, activity limitations, participation restrictions, and the influence of environmental and personal factors [5]. Escorpizo et al. [5] stated that,

> as movement specialists, physical therapists can use the Guide and the ICF to address "dysfunction" or disability with prudent consideration, not only of the patient as an individual but also of that individual's role in the larger context of the community and through the continuum of health care—ranging from the acute setting to long-term care—irrespective of the health conditions or associated health-related events.

The ICF framework components can help guide the examination of the individual with amputation [6, 7]. It has been used to aid in the selection of outcome measures in lower extremity amputation rehabilitation [8] and as a benchmark to test classification schemas of new self-reported outcome tools [9]. Given the holistic view of the patient's problems from the perspective of the ICF framework, the evaluation of the patient with amputation ultimately becomes a multidisciplinary endeavor for which the physical therapist plays an important role.

In this chapter, key evaluation elements are presented from the perspective of a physical therapist's assessment of an individual with amputation. The Guide and ICF frameworks are also used to help highlight areas for special consideration as a patient progresses through the five phases of amputation rehabilitation. In addition, outcome measures are introduced with examples given on their use during the care of an individual with amputation. Finally, case examples are presented which include the use of Guide and ICF framework terminology, outcome metrics, and new physical therapy evaluation complexity code guidance.

Key Evaluation Elements

The following elements are often included in a routine patient evaluation, but special recommendations are presented for consideration when evaluating a patient with amputation.

History

A complete history with particular attention to the mechanisms leading to amputation(s) and any co-related factors are at the cornerstone of the patient evaluation. The complete history includes the patient's medical, pharmacologic, surgical, ambulatory, and general functional past. Through this process, the examiner is attempting to understand the patient's participation in occupational, recreational, and educational roles as well as the impact of health and medical factors such as pain tolerance, stressors, drug, alcohol, diet, sleep, and others on recovery, rehabilitation, function, and participation. Familial and social roles and support are also important to explore as these may directly link to a patient's goals for rehabilitation. Mental health and capacity must be considered to determine if a referral is needed, to facilitate optimal communication and to better inform goals [10].

Review of Systems

The review of systems should include all systems including the circulatory, skeletal, muscular, nervous, respiratory, immune, excretory, integumentary, lymphatic, cardiovascular, reproductive, and digestive for their potential impact on rehabilitation and reintegration. For examples, some cardiovascular conditions may limit exercise capacity, and endocrine conditions, such as diabetes, may require monitoring during therapy and exercise.

Observation

Observation is a multi-sensory experience. For instance, having the patient remove their prosthesis may reveal odors that suggest infection or hygiene issues requiring attention. Furthermore, noises produced during prosthetic ambulation may suggest worn or failing components, gait deviations, faulty suspension, or other problems. Visually appreciated phenomena are substantial elements of the physical therapist's observation skills; however, these other senses must be engaged.

In addition, observation includes noting punctuality and attendance of the patient to clinic, which may provide insight to the level of caregiver support, enthusiasm regarding rehabilitation, compliance, or other factors.

Body Regions and Structures

Following the history and review of systems, the patient should be physically examined. There are many differing philosophies regarding the order in which items should be examined. Oftentimes, patient observations will draw attention to concerns that require immediate assessment. For example, odors or abnormal coloring of the stump may need to be addressed first. Thus, visually inspecting the surgical site for healing, infection, swelling, and edema may generate a critical referral before the examination is complete. Additionally, the stump should be assessed for scarring and general limb shape (see Figure 4.1) as these are important and will play a role in rehabilitation outcomes. Similarly, the contralateral limb should be inspected as it will likely experience an increased level of activity and demand while the stump heals. Visually observing the sound limb also allows for a general comparison with the involved limb. Inspecting the skin of all limbs for signs of vascular pathology including ulcers, stasis dermatitis, etc, as well as noting the condition of the nails, can confirm the quality of self-care as well as vascular or other systemic pathology.

Anthropometry

While height and weight are standard measurements along with basic vital signs (i.e. heart rate, blood pressure), regardless of the patient population, patients with amputation likely require recording of additional data from the anthropometric domain. These include stump length and volumetrics. Stump length is important to consider because the shorter the residuum, the greater the bioenergetic demand associated with prosthetic ambulation [11]. Beyond this, recording limb volume enables determination of whether or not the limb is reducing in volume, staying static, or swelling. This can be useful for discussing volume management specifics such as sock ply and the use of shrinkers, or as part of supporting documentation for a prosthetic socket replacement should the need arise.

Palpation

Palpation of involved areas such as the amputation incision and scar areas are important. For example, scars could become "stuck" to deeper layers, or adherent. They may also become hypertrophic, abnormally enlarged or keloid, or even hypersensitive. Additionally, transected muscles could focally contract causing tissue bulking on contraction, requiring relief in the prosthetic socket. Deep tissue discomfort from improper prosthetic setup and alignment can be simulated with palpation. One example of this would be palpation of the lateral distal transected femur in the patient with transfemoral amputation. At times, this area may become exquisitely tender but the tissue may not present visible bruising, discoloration, or ecchymosis; however, palpation can elicit discomfort. This could signify an improperly shaped lateral socket wall or an improper coronal alignment requiring prosthetic intervention.

Sensory Assessment

Regardless of the etiology of the amputation, the patient's stump should be assessed for sensation—specifically, light touch and thermal sensation [10]. The patient's ability to perceive these basic sensory phenomena is requisite to limb protection and preservation. In the case of traumatic amputation, nerve damage could compromise sensory function as could systemic vascular pathology in chronic disease related amputations. Hypersensitivity related to phantom limb sensations or neuromas can also pose significant setbacks during rehabilitation and may require pharmaceutical or surgical intervention to elevate.

Movement

The movement assessment begins with active movement. This provides the examiner with a sense of the patient's abilities in terms of combined strength, endurance, and range of motion for the purpose of producing functional movements with a prosthesis. All extremities and body segments should at least be screened with particular attention focused on joints of involved extremities. Screening non-involved areas for active movement would ideally reveal close to normal values, enabling the provider to focus interventions on more involved areas of the body.

Following identification of areas with active movement limitations, passive movement assessment is conducted. This serves to clarify the potential source of a movement restriction by determining for example if a restriction to movement is capsular, muscular, or caused by some other source such as pain. Common contractures in patients with transtibial amputation are in knee and hip flexion. In patients with transfemoral amputation,

a common contracture pattern is into hip flexion, abduction, and lateral rotation. In those with upper extremity amputations, shoulder capsule and scapular contractures can occur.

Resisted Movements

A very routine part of the physical assessment is resisted movement testing. Commonly, this is performed using isometric testing of a limb segment; however, variations are also common. One consideration if applying manual isometric strength testing is that the cut ends of bone and neighboring tissue may be sensitive to force application. Therefore, maximizing the surface area of the examiner's hand just proximal to the amputation site will likely be more tolerable to the patient. Additionally, since muscles have been cut and the skeletal lever arm is shorter than in the non-amputated limb, it should be noted that the performance will likely differ as well. Thus, functional strength and movement assessment is recommended to complement the manual resisted movement assessment. As with active movement, screening may be useful in non-involved body areas while particular attention is focused on involved body areas.

Functional Movements

Functional movement assessment is a crucial component of the evaluation. These include transfers and transitional movements such as bed mobility, transfers from bed to chair, sit to stand, stand to sit, gait, and others. Sit to stand from a stable chair on a hard floor is quite different than sit to stand from a toilet which tends to be lower than most chairs. Further, standing from a bath tub or a car seat are different still. Thus, functional movement assessment needs to involve specific tasks relevant to the patient in as similar conditions as possible to the patient's environment. Dependence on assistive devices or technology or human support during mobility into the clinic and with transfers provides information about functional independence, strength, and balance. Community mobility will involve the negotiation of multiple environments, surfaces, elevations, etc. As a functional movement, gait is complex in the sense that function at multiple speeds over multiple surfaces should be assessed. Further, turning, accelerating, decelerating, walking while talking or otherwise distracted, walking on ramps and stairs, should all be assessed. Active, passive, and resisted movement assessments are important evaluative precursors to functional movement assessments to provide clues about which component parts of a movement are particularly problematic for the patient. This improves the efficiency, impact, and relevance of intervention for the patient. Finally, noting the patient's posture in standing and sitting along with a history of prolonged sitting and delayed standing post-operatively could provide clues justifying further assessment of possible joint contracture(s) which could lead to difficulty standing and ambulating.

Assistive Devices and Durable Medical Equipment

In addition to observations regarding the patient's anatomy, posture, and function, the patient's assistive technologies, prosthesis, and shoes should also be inspected as applicable. This can begin when the patient presents to therapy by noting if the prosthesis or other technology (i.e. volume management device) is being worn and, if so, whether it is donned and used properly. Furthermore, it should be noted if the shoes and other devices are in good repair and not adversely impacting patient movement, posture, or skin. Equipment and devices in poor condition can be the source of discomfort or pain; and, at worst, cause injury.

Other Assessments

Depending upon the particular case presentation, a review of the patient's intra- or post-operative medical images may be useful. For instance, if a patient's prosthetic socket is causing localized discomfort, a review of diagnostic films could clarify if orthopedic hardware is causing or contributing. Additionally, an assessment of the psychological domain could clarify if a patient is depressed or anxious and requires intervention or referral. Finally, other assessments to consider may include tissue or system specific tests, and/or balance or exercise testing, as indicated.

OUTCOME MEASURES

The use of outcome measures is an important part of the patient assessment as they are often collected during the evaluation. In the rehabilitation of patients with amputation, measurement of patient clinical outcome is needed so plans of care can be adjusted and stakeholders can determine patient progress. The stated goal of the rehabilitation team is typically described in terms of broad constructs, such as returning to pre-morbid levels of function, independence, and participation. Outcome measures are standardized instruments that provide methods of assessing progress toward those rehabilitation goals by quantifying constructs which are difficult to observe directly. Specific examples of such constructs include: pain, balance, ambulatory function, mobility, and quality of life.

A variety of different outcome measure instruments exist for assessing almost any patient population. To apply an outcome measure in clinical care, best practices involve careful selection, consistent administration, interpretation of results, and use of the results to inform clinical decisions [12]. Selecting and administering outcome measures does not have to be a complicated or intimidating process. Many outcome measures consist of simple tasks, minimal equipment, or paper surveys. By becoming familiar with the instructions for use, typically written by the outcome measure developer, and through maintaining consistent techniques or protocols while administering the instrument, a clinician can incorporate an outcome measure into a routine patient appointment. Being prepared to use an outcome measure ahead of time, such as having paper surveys printed or marking out a pre-defined distance on the clinic floor, can help facilitate the administration and documentation process. An important and often overlooked step in consistent use of outcome measures is identifying a location where scores can be documented and readily reviewed for individual or larger group trends.

Outcome measures hold potential for enhancing physical therapy practice and rehabilitation outcomes for patients with lower extremity amputation. For Medicare patients, an "assessment tool" has been required for functional reporting of a G-code modifier to demonstrate continued medical necessity of physical therapy visits [13, 14, 15]. This documentation and the requirement to document functional limitations and progress in therapy can be fulfilled by some of the outcome measures reviewed in this chapter. Also, physical therapy exercises for patients with lower extremity amputation can be prescribed based on weaknesses identified by a functional outcome measure, and rehabilitation programs have been developed following this approach [16]. Finally, outcome measures are necessary for performing comparative effectiveness research to determine the most beneficial physical therapy regimens and to support evidence based clinical practice.

It is important to select the most appropriate outcome measure instrument that has been demonstrated to be reliable, valid, and responsive to the specific patient population and intervention. An outcome measure which is inappropriate for patients with lower extremity amputation or one that does not reflect the intended rehabilitation goal will not provide useful information to a clinician. Selection of an outcome measure requires an understanding of the psychometric properties of an instrument, such as knowing whether there is ample evidence of validity for using a certain instrument to measure mobility in patients with lower extremity amputation.

Psychometric Properties of Outcome Measures

Outcome measures are not created equal, and careful evaluation and selection of the appropriate outcome measure to administer to patients with lower extremity amputation requires an understanding of psychometric properties. Psychometric properties are evaluated through statistical methods in research studies of large patient populations and describe an instrument's reliability, validity, and responsiveness. The reliability of an outcome measure describes whether it is consistent and free from error, or that the score will remain consistent when the instrument is administered repeatedly in the absence of a clinically meaningful change [17, 18]. An outcome measure which has evidence of validity for use in patients with lower extremity amputation can be administered with confidence that the instrument will measure what it intends to measure [17]. Validity is often evaluated statistically by comparing it against another outcome measure considered to be a gold standard [17]. An outcome measure is described as responsive if the score detects a clinically important or meaningful change in the status of the patient [18]. Together, these psychometric properties can help clinicians compare various instruments for patients with lower extremity amputation and ultimately select the most appropriate outcome measure that matches their rehabilitation goal.

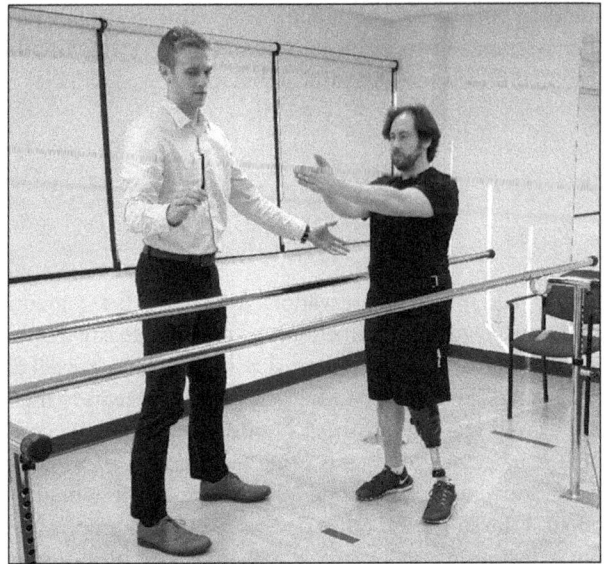

Figure 6.1. Amputee Mobility Predictor item #9: standing reach at 12 inches beyond outstretched arms.

Performance-Based Outcome Measures (PBOMs)

Moving toward more objective instruments, performance-based outcome measures (PBOMs) involve rating or timing a patient's capacity to perform a simulated task in a controlled clinic setting. PBOMs have the advantage of assessing constructs independent of the patient's own perceptions and can provide higher resolution, especially when measured as a ratio such as time or distance. Most PBOMs involve a simple set-up and minimal equipment, such as cones, marks on the clinic floor, a stopwatch, and a measuring tape. Many of the common PBOMs used in other patient populations have also been applied to patients with lower extremity amputation, but other instruments are population-specific to patients with lower extremity amputation.

The Amputee Mobility Predictor (AMP) is a frequently used outcome measure for assessing capacity for functional ambulation in lower limb amputees [19]. The AMP consists of 21 items involving sitting balance, transfers, standing balance (see Figures 6.1, 6.2, and 6.3), gait, stairs, and use of an assistive device, where capacity is rated by a clinician observer and the score on each item is totaled. Evidence of validity and reliability has been established for the AMP [19]. This PBOM is especially useful for managing rehabilitation, because the Amputee Mobility Predictor no Prosthesis (AMPnoPRO) can be administered to patients after their amputation but before they receive a prosthesis, and later once they receive a prosthesis the Amputee Mobility Predictor with Prosthesis

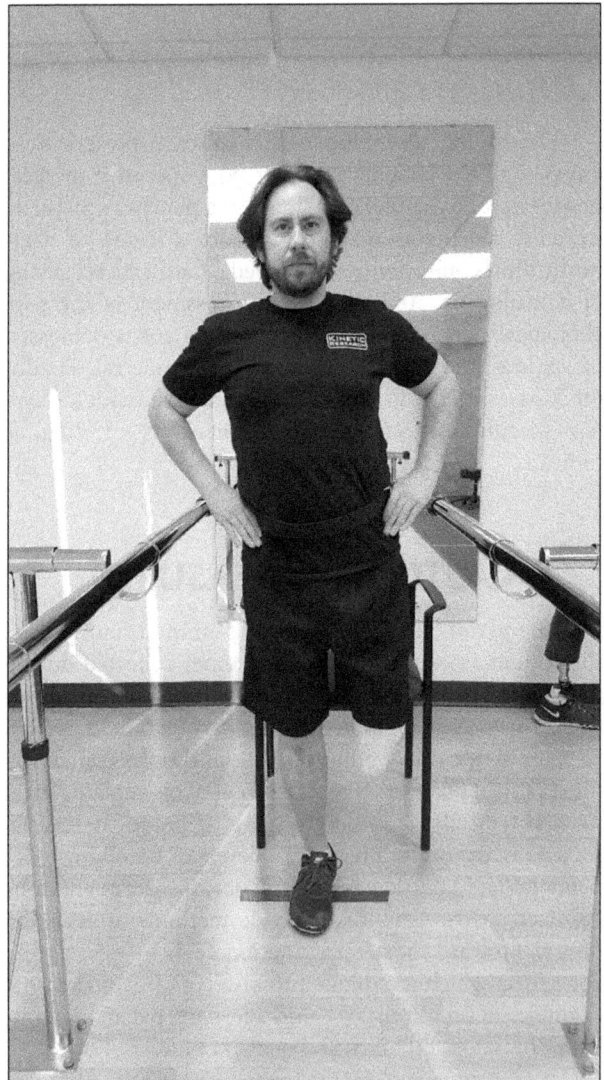

Figure 6.2. Frontal view of Single Limb Stance Test and Amputee Mobility Predictor no Prosthesis item #8: single limb standing balance for 30 seconds.

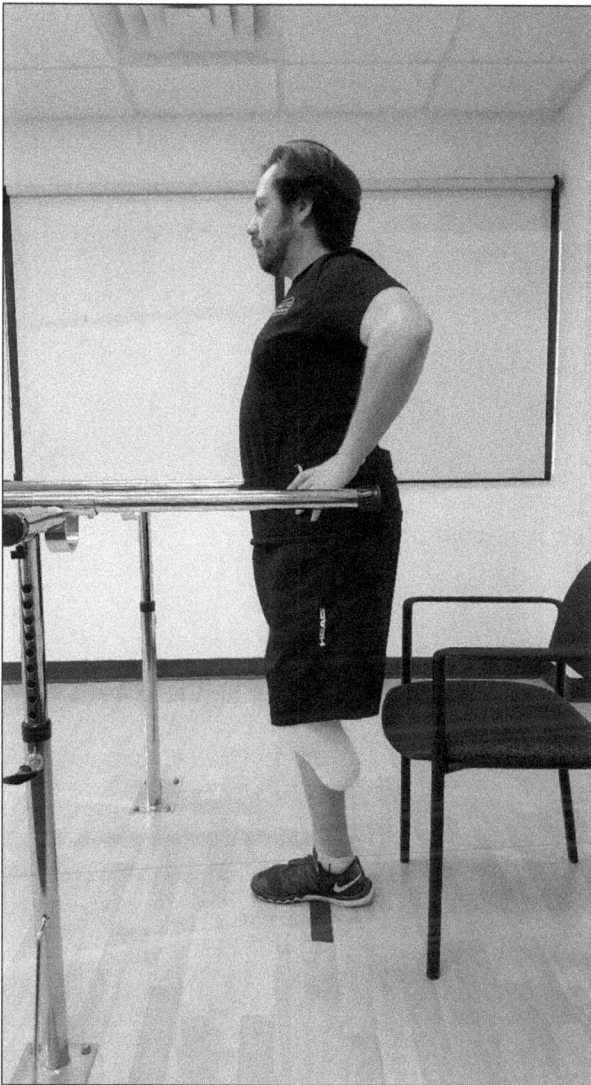

Figure 6.3. Sagittal view of Single Limb Stance Test and Amputee Mobility Predictor no Prosthesis item #8: single limb standing balance for 30 seconds.

(AMPPRO) can be used. The AMP can be administered in approximately 15 minutes and requires the following set-up and equipment: a stopwatch, two chairs with armrests, a 12-in ruler, a pencil, a 4-in-high obstacle (preferably 18–24 in long) (Figure 6.4), and a set of stairs with three steps [19]. As with the Prosthetic Limb User Survey of Mobility (PLUS-M), discussed in more detail below, the utility of the AMP for a clinician treating patients with lower extremity amputation is enhanced by the large study sample population and data tables presented for persons in various groups. For example, Medicare requires all patients with lower extremity amputation to be classified in a K1–K4 functional level (Medicare Functional Classification Level) [20], and mean AMP scores plus or minus one standard deviation (SD) have been presented for groups separated by K-level in several sample populations [19, 21]. This allows the classification of MFCL to be based on objective information of patient capacity for functional

mobility as assessed by the AMP and published data from similar patient populations.

Another PBOM, the Functional Independence Measure (FIM) [22], is more commonly used in the inpatient rehabilitation setting. This instrument is trademarked and requires a license to utilize, but it is already used for assessing other patient populations in many inpatient rehabilitation settings. The FIM scores patient self-reported independence with 18 tasks related to self-care, mobility, sphincter control, locomotion, social cognition, and communication [23]. The FIM has evidence of reliability [22, 24], but evidence of low construct validity and ceiling effects. Due to these limitations, the FIM may not be the most appropriate PBOM for use in patients with lower extremity amputation.

A simple test, the Single Limb Stance Test (SLS) [25], has shown utility in predicting prosthetic rehabilitation [26]. Time is recorded from the instant a patient lifts their foot off the ground with their hands on their hips until their foot is placed back onto the ground. For patients with unilateral lower extremity amputation who have not yet received a prosthesis, the SLS can be administered by starting the time once the patient removes their hands from an ambulatory aid. In elderly patients, a SLS time of 5 s or less was associated with twice the fall risk compared with those who could balance longer than 5 s [25]. Patients with lower extremity amputation due to trauma were able to balance twice as long (22.3 s) than those due to dysvascular causes (10.9 s) [27]. A study of patients with lower extremity amputation found that the SLS measured with the intact limb 2 weeks post amputation was the most important factor that predicted rehabilitation outcome [26]. Furthermore, patients who could balance unassisted for more than 10 s had a much higher likelihood of gaining functional use of a prosthesis [26]. The SLS is often included as an item as a part of other PBOMs, such as the AMP. The test can be performed on both sides at the clinicians' discretion.

The Timed Up and Go (TUG) (Figure 6.5) is another PBOM that has evidence supporting reliability and validity for use in patients with lower extremity amputation [28, 29], and it is easily set up in a clinical setting. In the TUG, time is measured while a patient stands from a chair (seat 46 cm, arms 67 cm), walks 3 m, turns around, walks back, and sits back down in the chair [28]. The TUG assesses functional ambulation better than straight line walk tests because of the inclusion of standing, turning, and sitting. A cut-off score of 19 s was found to identify those who suffered multiple falls from a sample of patients with lower extremity amputation [30]. Also, patients with transtibial amputation were shown to perform the TUG quicker than those with transfemoral amputation, at 23.8 s and 28.3 s, respectively [26]. TUG times for healthy community dwelling adults have also been reported based on decade of life (60–69 yo = 8.1 s, 70–79 yo = 9.32 s, 80–89 = 11.3 s) [31]. This information helps clinicians to interpret

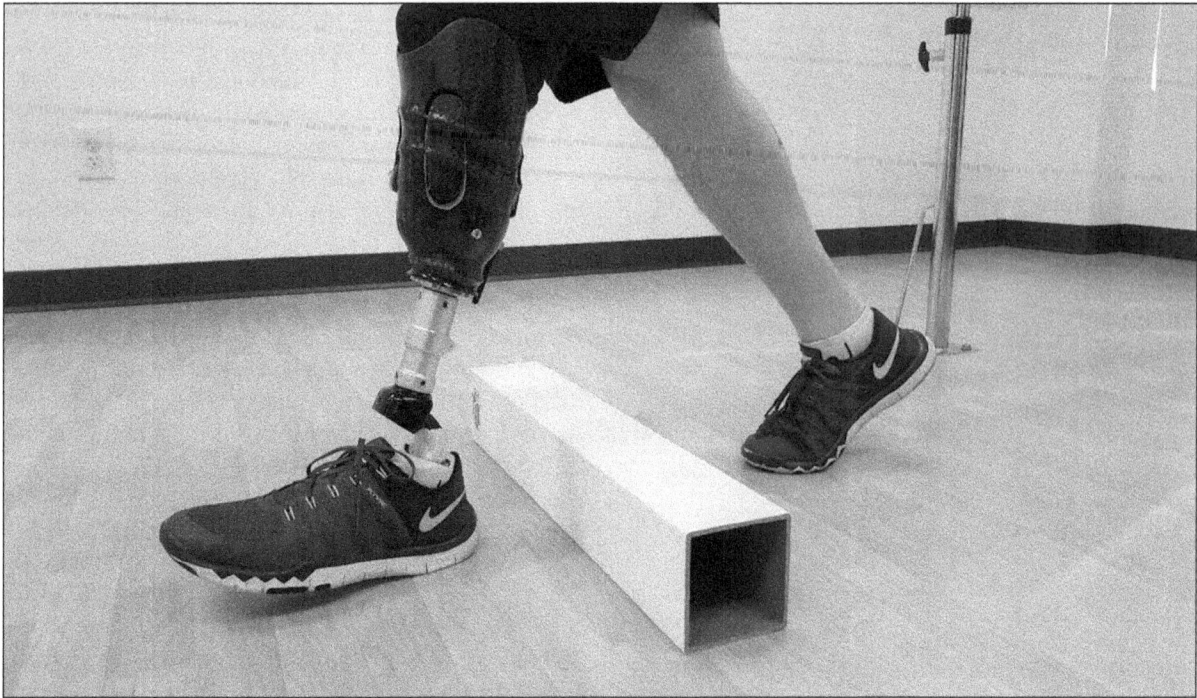

Figure 6.4. Amputee Mobility Predictor item #19: stepping over a 4-inch-tall obstacle.

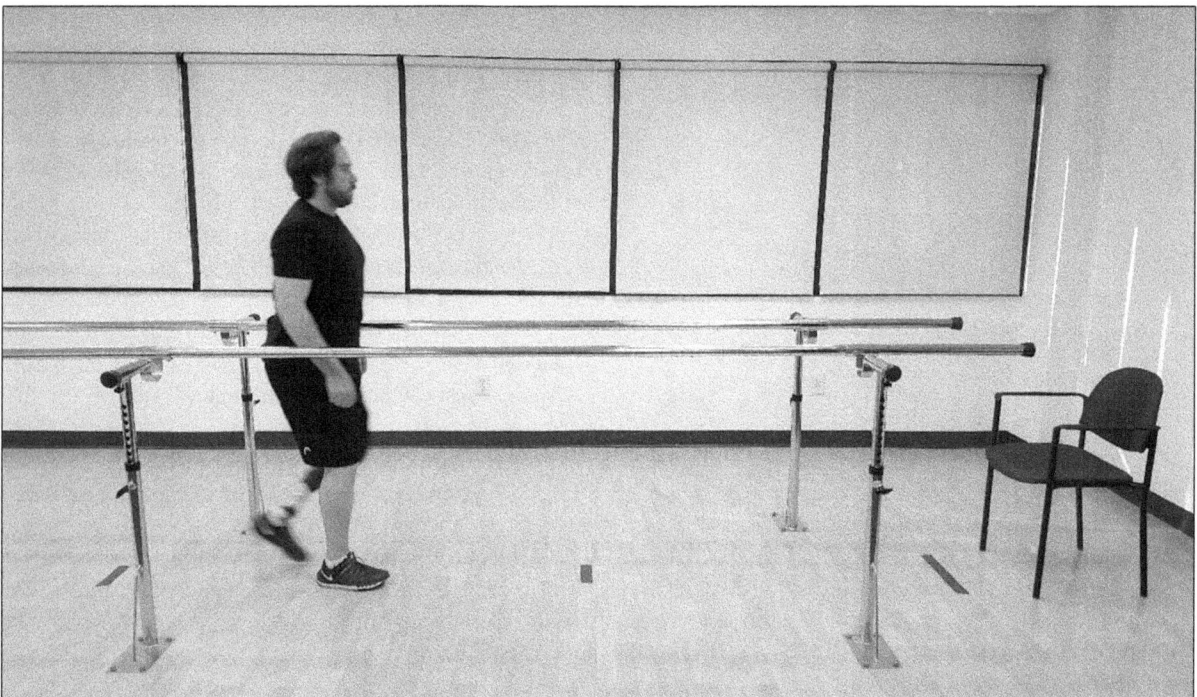

Figure 6.5. Set-up for Timed Up and Go with standard height armchair and a mark on the floor at 3 m from the chair.

individual patient TUG times when assessing patients with lower extremity amputation.

More PBOMs than the ones summarized above have evidence supporting reliability and validity for patients with lower extremity amputation. A variety of Timed Walk Tests can be applied, including the 10-meter Walk Test (10 m WT) [32], 2-minute Timed Walk Test (2 min TWT) [33], and 6-minute Timed Walk Test (6 min TWT) [34–36]. The Berg Balance Test (BERG) [37] and the Four-Square Step Test (FSST) [38] can be useful for quantifying balance. Other publications support the use of the Hill Assessment Index (HAI) and Stair Assessment Index (SAI) for assessing these specific modes of mobility in patients with lower extremity amputation [39, 40]. Further PBOMs can be applied for quantifying gait deviations with visual observational gait deviation scores, such as the Prosthetic Orthotic Gait Score (POGS) [41]. Finally, to address instances where patients can experience a ceiling effect by approaching the highest score possible on the AMP, the Comprehensive High-level Activity Mobility Predictor (CHAMP) was developed [42].

Patient Reported Outcome Measures

For a patient-centric approach, self-rated rehabilitation progress is often quantified with patient reported outcome measures (PROMs). These survey instruments have the advantage of being easy to administer in paper form and allow clinicians to quantify constructs that are difficult to simulate in the clinical setting. For patients with lower extremity amputation, a frequently used PROM is the Activities Specific Balance Confidence (ABC) scale [43]. The ABC scale assesses a patient's confidence that they will not lose their balance when performing 16 specific tasks. Evidence of reliability and validity have been established for the ABC scale in a population with lower extremity amputation [43]. A fall risk cut-off score of 67% has been established for the ABC scale [44], although not specific for patients with lower extremity amputation, and the cut-off score can be useful in identifying patients at risk of suffering a fall. Another study found that a lower balance confidence score on the ABC scale was associated with fewer steps taken in a day among a sample of patients with lower extremity amputation [45].

For quantifying patient mobility in the community, the Prosthetic Limb User Survey of Mobility (PLUS-M) is recommended and supported by evidence of reliability [46] and validity [47]. Due to the extensive sample population used in the development of the instrument, this measure provides utility to the clinician in interpreting results. For example, the PLUS-M T-score is reported for the 50th percentile patient in the following groups separated by amputation cause and level: transfemoral dysvascular 42.6, transtibial dysvascular 47.2, transfemoral trauma 50.1, transtibial trauma 55.4 (a T-score of 50 represents the mean of all patients in the study sample) [48]. Additionally, the PLUS-M user guide provides many visual tools and data tables from the large sample population to reference for interpretation. This level of interpretation allows the PLUS-M to be very useful in assessing mobility in patients with lower extremity amputation.

PROMs can also be useful for measuring a variety of other constructs including: comfort of the prosthetic socket with the Socket Comfort Score (SCS) [49], and functional status, quality of life and satisfaction with orthotic and prosthetic devices with the Orthotic Prosthetic User Survey (OPUS) [50]. Further PROMs may be of interest, but their results cannot be interpreted with the same level of confidence as those reviewed above until

they are evaluated for reliability, validity, and responsiveness in patients with lower extremity amputation. While these measures provide advantages for use in clinical care, there are also limitations related to measuring the patient perspective such as the influence of the patient demeanor, cognitive ability, and survey fatigue. Some best practices to improve data collection with PROMs include instructing the patient to answer the questions as completely and honestly as possible, providing an opportunity to have the questions read aloud to the patient, allowing the patient to ask for clarifications, and most importantly taking the time to review the survey results with the patient to highlight the importance that the clinician places on the results of the PROMs.

Virtual Reality-Based Outcome Measures

Functional outcome measures like the FIM have a patient perform simulated tasks that they would encounter during daily activities. The intent is that independent performance of these tasks would indicate and potentially predict independence upon discharge. The simulation of functional tasks for the purpose of assessment and treatment is not a new concept to rehabilitation. Clinicians must attempt to simulate the environment, equipment, and circumstances for each task (e.g. car transfer). Virtual reality environments are novel tools that can be used to simulate tasks that an individual may encounter. Assessments within virtual reality environments have been created complete with embedded outcome measures to determine an individual's ability to maintain stability during physical and visual perturbations [51]. As with most outcome measures, minimal detectable change values were first established in healthy individuals together with reference values for patient comparisons [52]. Military specific tasks have also been simulated within virtual reality environments to determine a service member's ability to function cognitively and physically following severe extremity trauma such as amputation. With the cost of virtual reality tools decreasing and becoming more portable and accessible, many physical therapists may find them in common use during their routine evaluation.

Outcome Measures and Clinical Decision Making

There are many instances when interpreting results of an outcome measure can be vital for making clinical decisions. The FIM [22], comprised of different function tasks, may be used to identify the most appropriate discharge destination for a person with lower extremity amputation following an inpatient rehabilitation hospital encounter. The AMP [19] can inform the prediction of rehabilitation potential required for assigning the MFCL [20], which dictates the prosthetic technology a patient is eligible to receive. A SCS [49] can be used to judge whether a lower limb amputee requires a prosthetic replacement socket before continuing with physical therapy. Interpretation of outcome measure results can be informed by published research data that may present normative data, cut-off scores or means and ranges of scores from specific patient groups. The results of a virtual reality-based assessment, for example, can help determine if a service member has maximally rehabilitated and may be ready to be discharged back to their unit.

ASSESSMENT CONSIDERATIONS BY REHABILITATION PHASE

There are five general phases (or stages) of rehabilitative care for the individuals with limb amputation: 1) Pre-operative; 2) Post-operative (also referred to as acute hospital post-operative); 3) Pre-prosthetic (also referred to as immediate post-acute hospital); 4) Prosthetic (also referred to as intermediate recovery); and 5) Lifelong care (also referred to as maintenance). The physical therapist may become involved pre-operatively, acutely post-operatively, or at any time thereafter. The focus of the evaluation may vary depending upon which phase of rehabilitation the patient is in, what their impairments are, the extent of their functional limitations, and what their goals are. Regardless of the particular phase of rehabilitation, proper introductions of the provider and their staff to the patient and the patient's support network are vital for establishing a mutually beneficial rapport [53]. Initial conversations set the tone for the course of care that follows and their importance cannot be overstated.

Pre-Operative Phase

Physical therapy intervention is not always possible pre-amputation. For example, accidents leading to amputation do not commonly afford the opportunity for pre-operative rehabilitation in the way that a planned amputation resulting from failed limb salvage or dysvascular-diabetic conditions might. However, when the opportunity for rehabilitation is available prior to amputation, a pre-operative evaluation should be conducted. Information and outcome measures collected during the evaluation can be used to establish a baseline for comparison as the patient progresses through each rehabilitation phase. Additionally, this evaluation will allow the physical therapist to create an initial plan of care. Using the ICF framework as a guide, there are specific elements that should be assessed and documented pre-operatively.

A review of the health condition (e.g. disorder or disease) which may have contributed to the decision to amputate is crucial to understand. For example, patients with diabetes and vascular disease are at the most risk for an initial amputation and progressive amputations (e.g. additional proximal amputations). Often, certain behaviors (i.e. smoking, poor blood glucose control) lead to the worsening of these conditions which in turn lead to a need for amputation. The physical therapist and/or other disciplines on the clinical team must assess the severity of these contributing behaviors. The patient should be asked about their quantity of smoking (packs/day, cigars/day, etc.) and their daily blood glucose levels. Smoking and poor glucose control can slow wound healing following amputation. Thus, patient education on smoking cessation and diabetic nutrition should be initiated prior to amputation. This may necessitate referrals to a behavioral therapist, diabetes educator, and nutritionist. Not determining if these and other contributing behaviors exist could prevent intervention at a time when a patient may be most receptive to lifestyle changes.

A physical examination of body structures and their function must be done and be thorough to include all parts; not just the limb to be amputated. Oftentimes, the contralateral limb may have pathology or dysfunction that could slow a person's return to independence following amputation. Unhealed wounds, painful joints, and paretic limbs could all concurrently present with the individual who requires an amputation. These conditions could limit independent performance of bed mobility, transfers, balance, and gait and should thus be assessed. The length of time since the patient was last able to perform these activities is also important to document as this can help establish practical short- and long-term goals.

The patient's post-amputation goals and expectations must be assessed together with their pre-amputation function. A patient's desire to participate in vocational, recreational, and other social roles will influence their rehabilitation goals and expectations. At times, a return to independent mobility, gait, and work may all be achievable post-amputation. Maximizing function, at whatever level, should always be a goal. However, new challenges like phantom sensation, stump pain, and the use of prostheses must be discussed early in the rehabilitation process. The physical therapist should determine the accessibility of a patient's home and the existence of environmental barriers that may need to be addressed via durable medical equipment. The availability of family members or caregivers to assist at home and in the community must also be documented. These factors will influence the physical therapist's assessment and rehabilitation prognosis.

Based on findings, a treatment plan to address deficits will be warranted, which will likely include a vast amount of patient and family education. Specific education regarding skin health, stump protection, and flexion contractures may be beneficial, but care must be taken not to overwhelm the patient with information. If possible, it may also be helpful to consider introducing the patient to a credentialed peer-visitor, a peer support group, and a certified prosthetist. This may facilitate improved understanding of the assistive technologies, gait, mobility, and rehabilitation to come and better prepare the patient prior to amputation.

Post-Operative Phase (Acute Hospital)

Early concerns commonly assessed in this phase include surgical site healing, acute pain control, edema, and limb volume. Most of these issues center about the stump. While these are all important, there are numerous other considerations in this phase of rehabilitation. Patients with lower extremity amputation, for instance, have a generally increased fall risk. In the acute post-operative phase, pain medication and a lack of familiarity with wheelchair use may contribute to further elevation in fall risk. The patient's recent loss of anatomy and redistributed center of mass adversely impacts balance and movement, creating further complication. This reemphasizes the fact that the entire patient, including their function and societal roles, should be assessed during the evaluation. For example, key areas requiring consideration include comorbidities such as those in the cardiovascular domain as well as mental status, sensation, range of motion and contracture prevention, strength and endurance, balance, bed mobility, transitional movements, and the patient's familiarity and ability with assistive technologies. The evaluation should culminate in collaborative goal setting. As mentioned previously, a visit with a credentialed peer-visitor, peer support group, and a prosthetist may be of value to clarify further what the patient might expect in the future. One other important consideration is whether or not the patient has been fitted with an early or immediate post-operative prosthesis. If so, the physical therapist will work closely with the prosthetist and the surgeon to progress the patient through the pre-determined weight bearing and ambulatory protocol and to assist with stump monitoring.

Pre-Prosthetic Phase (Immediate Post-Acute Hospital)

In the pre-prosthetic phase, the patient's stump is nearly or completely healed. The preparatory prosthesis is now being considered. The patient continues to improve self-care, basic bed mobility and transitional movements without a prosthesis. Rehabilitation in this phase focuses on readiness for prosthetic use including functional mobility, gait training, balance, muscular strength and endurance, range of motion, and conditioning. Contracture prevention continues to be emphasized. In accordance with the patient's goals, the multidisciplinary team determines the patient's functional level and establishes the prosthetic prescription. At times, a prosthetist will meet with the patient in this phase. Some elements of a prosthetic system may also be introduced in this stage. For example, if a patient's prosthetic prescription is to include a gel liner system, it may be appropriate to fit and deliver the liner to the patient in this stage. Doing so offers advantages in determining if there are any adverse skin reactions to the material, and in familiarizing the patient with the process of managing and maintaining an element of the prosthesis. Thus, when the prosthesis is delivered, one aspect of the system is already familiar to the patient.

Prosthetic Phase (Intermediate Recovery)

In this phase, the prosthesis is delivered to the patient. This may be an initial or preparatory prosthesis if this is the patient's first artificial limb. Rehabilitation focuses on the patient's goals. As always, however, in this phase integration of the prosthesis into the patient's function is central. Donning, doffing, hygiene, skin care and monitoring, gait training, and transitional movements including sit to stand and stand to sit are among the areas of emphasis. With regard to gait training, it is important to ensure that the patient is able to walk at multiple speeds over multiple surface types and with varying degrees of distraction. Stair and ramp ascent and descent are also important gait functions to consider. Assuring the patient is able to change footwear and use the prosthesis with different types of footwear is also important. Prosthetic maintenance is a new domain for the patient that must also be addressed. Finally, the therapist should conduct a prosthetic checkout to make sure the device is working properly and to assist the patient in meeting their rehabilitation goals (see Appendix). As mentioned previously, integration of the prosthesis into the patient's function is vital in this phase. However, it is also important to consider the integration of the whole patient, who now uses a prosthesis, back into their societal role(s).

Lifelong Care (Maintenance)

Many factors could result in a patient with amputation seeking physical therapy after lengthy periods of prosthetic use or having lived with an amputation for many years. In this stage, a patient with amputation may have experienced a change in health or functional status or be receiving a new prosthetic component or entirely new prosthesis. It is important to determine specifically what has motivated the patient to seek out therapy through a thorough history and examination so that intervention can be appropriately tailored to the current needs and goals. Some health systems recommend that patients with amputation who use prostheses be seen on at least an annual basis even if things are going well [54].

CASE STUDIES

Example 1

A 72-year-old female with a right transfemoral amputation due to peripheral vascular disease presented to a multidisciplinary rehabilitation clinic and is evaluated by a physical therapist, prosthetist, and physiatrist. The patient's main complaint was that she cannot use her prosthesis to walk independently in her home or to return to some of her pre-amputation community activities, such as weekly bingo and going to church. During the appointment, a family member admits that the patient suffered a fall in the last month, and she only wears her prosthesis for a few hours a day. The physical therapist performed a full physical exam to include observation of transfers, mobility, and gait.

The rehabilitation team also selected several patient-reported outcome measures to administer during the appointment. The ABC, PLUS-M, and SCS were selected to quantify the patient's balance, mobility, and self-rated socket comfort. These instruments were printed and placed on a clipboard, and the patient was allowed time to complete the surveys on her own after the directions were read aloud to her by a clinician. The instruments were collected and scored for immediate interpretation.

On the ABC, the patient scored an average balance confidence of 52%, which is lower than the fall risk cut-off (67%) [44] and suggests that she is at higher risk of falls. On the PLUS-M, she had a T-score of 28, which is well below the 50th percentile T-score for patients with dysvascular transfemoral amputation. Finally, she rates her current SCS with a 4 out of 10, highlighting a level of discomfort in her socket that may be inhibiting her utilization of the prosthesis. This initial physical therapy evaluation was coded 97162 for moderate complexity due to more than two comorbidities (peripheral vascular disease, falls, amputation) and three or more tests and measures (PROMs, physical exam of multiple body structures, activity limitations, and participation restrictions). Her evaluation could have been coded higher given her history and examination, but the therapist should code to the lowest factor. In this case, her clinical presentation is evolving

as opposed to unstable. The PROMs helped to isolate the complications so a treatment plan could be developed.

These results were shared with the patient and a patient-specific treatment plan was generated to include a prosthetic socket evaluation and possible replacement to address the socket discomfort, followed by physical therapy for a balance training program. After the treatment plan was fulfilled, the patient reported back to the multidisciplinary clinic. She was wearing her prosthesis for up to 8 hours a day to walk within her home and had recently started leaving home and attending church regularly. A clinician re-administered the same PROMs and scored them for interpretation. With the new prosthetic socket replacement, the patient reports a SCS of 8 out of 10, which corresponds with her increased prosthesis wear time. The more comfortably fitting socket allowed the patient to fully participate in the balance training program, and subsequently the ABC score at follow-up increased to 72%. The patient's PLUS-M T-score also increased to 45, showing an improvement in her overall mobility. Together the prosthetic socket replacement and physical therapy regimen improved the patient's balance and mobility, allowing her to wear her prosthesis longer and be more independent in her mobility. The entire rehabilitation treatment was patient-centric and guided by PROMs. The benefit of the intervention was readily documented and interpreted with the ABC, PLUS-M and SCS results.

Example 2

A 57-year-old male was admitted to an inpatient rehabilitation unit after a 3-day acute-care hospital stay post right traumatic transtibial amputation. The patient stood only one time since his surgery and was dependent on caregiver support to transfer, toilet, and perform most self-care tasks. He identified a goal of discharging to his home where he lived alone in a two-story home. Upon admission to the rehabilitation unit, the patient was observed and rated with a total FIM score of 82. This score was at the lower end of the range of reported FIM scores upon admission (85.4 ± 16.0) [55], highlighting the need for intensive physical and occupational therapy to prepare the patient to discharge to his desired location. During his first physical therapy session, the AMPnoPRO was administered to identify weaknesses and design a patient-specific physical therapy program that would prepare him to ambulate with a prosthesis once his stump was fully healed. On the AMPnoPRO, he scored a total of 19, and the patient had difficulty or did not attempt many of the ambulatory and standing balance-related tasks. Based on this score, and with knowledge of the patient's desire to discharge to home, the physical therapist focused on increasing balance on the sound side limb and practicing transfers, hopping, and ascending stairs in simulated exercises. Similar to the first case, the initial evaluation was coded 97162 for moderate complexity. The number of personal factors which included discharge to a two-story home; low FIM and AMPnoPRO scores; and the evolving clinical presentation with changing characteristics all led to the classification of this evaluation.

By the time the patient was ready to discharge following his 6-day inpatient rehabilitation stay, he had experienced rapid improvements in his independence and functional mobility. When re-assessed with the FIM, his total score improved to 98, showing a total change of 16 points (2.67 points/day). His performance on the items in the AMPnoPRO improved as well. His AMPnoPRO score at discharge was 27 points, and he improved most notably by demonstrating capacity to hop with a walker and ascend stairs using a handrailing. This patient's AMPnoPRO score is comparable with the reported AMPnoPRO average for patients who are community ambulators (MFCL 3 (K3) Mean = 31.36, SD = 7.38) [19]. During the single limb stance item of the AMPnoPRO, the patient balanced for 30 seconds without holding onto the walker, which presents another strong predictor that he will be successful with a prosthesis.

Following successful primary healing from his transtibial amputation surgery, the patient was cleared for prosthetic fitting and received his preparatory prosthesis. The patient returned for physical therapy outpatient clinic for training with his prosthesis. Intending to evaluate the patient's fall risk, his physical therapist set up and administered a TUG. Finishing the TUG in 17 s, the patient's score was below the fall risk cut-off score (TUG = 19 s), but observing the patient perform the test allowed the physical therapist to identify areas of needed improvement. The patient was reliant on his walker and exhibited a step-to gait pattern with a short prosthetic side step duration. The patient required several steps to make the 180° turn and at the end of the test the patient appeared to be slightly winded. Despite showing great progress, the outpatient evaluation was coded 97162 as moderate complexity due to the continued evolving presentation, personal factors, and the number of elements assessed during the examination.

Within the first 3 weeks of outpatient physical therapy, the patient's balance and gait with the prosthesis had improved. He no longer relied on a walker and instead used a single point cane. When re-attempting the TUG, the patient was able to improve his time to 13 s, demonstrating an improvement in functional ambulation. To continue to challenge the patient and maximize his rehabilitation, his physical therapist selected the 6 min TWT and the SAI as the next two PBOMs to administer. At this stage in his prosthetic rehabilitation, the patient walked 210 m in the 6 min TWT (velocity = 0.58 m/s) and he received a rating of 4 on the SAI, which corresponds to ambulating on stairs "with assistive device, step-to pattern" [40]. Knowing that the type of prosthetic foot has an impact on gait efficiency as well as traversing stairs and other terrain, the patient's

physical therapist worked with the patient's prosthetist to recommend a new type of prosthetic foot for his definitive prosthesis.

The patient received a definitive transtibial prosthesis which included a hydraulic prosthetic ankle and energy storing and returning foot. These components provide hydraulic dampened ankle range of motion as well as increased energetic contribution of the prosthetic foot during the gait cycle. Following specific training by the physical therapist to teach the patient to take advantage of these functional benefits of the new prosthesis on stairs and level ground, the patient was able to walk further and traverse stairs better than before. With his definitive prosthesis, the patient was able to increase his distance walked in the 6 min TWT to 280 m (0.78 m/s) and he received an SAI rating of 10, which corresponds to ambulating on stairs "with rail and assistive device, step-over-step pattern" [40]. These successful prosthetic outcomes and documentation through various instruments show the value of PBOMs and interpretation of scores at all levels of rehabilitation of patients with lower extremity amputation.

SUMMARY

This chapter has presented key tenets of the evaluation of the patient with amputation. It is important that a framework such as the ICF is used to assure that the evaluation is consistent across diagnostic groups and patients and that it is also comprehensive in terms of evaluating issues at the tissue level all the way up to the level of functional integration. The chapter also presented key items to consider for inclusion in the patient evaluation including outcome measures which enable comparison to cut-off scores, normative data, and more. Finally, the CMS evaluation complexity codes were described with examples given to help determine which codes to use.

REFERENCES

[1] Andrus B, Gawenda R. Farewell, 97001: how to use the new PT and OT evaluation codes. WebPT. Accessed January 25, 2017. https://www.webpt.com/blog/post/farewell 97001-how-to-use-the-new-pt-and-ot-evaluation-codes. 2016.

[2] APTA. *APTA Guide to Physical Therapist Practice* 2.0, 2001. American Physical Therapy Association, Alexandria, VA.

[3] Guccione AA. Physical therapy diagnosis and the relationship between impairments and function. *Phys Ther.* 1991;71(7): 499–503.

[4] APTA. *APTA Guide to Physical Therapist Practice* 4.0, 2023. American Physical Therapy Association. Accessed September 2024. https://guide.apta.org.

[5] Escorpizo R, Stucki G, Cieza A, et al. Creating an interface between the International Classification of Functioning, Disability and Health and physical therapist practice. *Phys Ther.* 2010;90(7):1053–1063.

[6] Kohler F, Cieza A, Stucki G, et al. Developing Core Sets for persons following amputation based on the International Classification of Functioning, Disability and Health as a way to specify functioning. *Prosthet Orthot Int.* 2009;33(2):117–129.

[7] Hebert JS, Wolfe DL, Miller WC, et al. Outcome measures in amputation rehabilitation: ICF body functions. *Disabil Rehabil.* 2009;31(19):1541–1554.

[8] Deathe AB, Wolfe DL, Devlin M, et al. Selection of outcome measures in lower extremity amputation rehabilitation: ICF activities. *Disabil Rehabil.* 2009;31(18):1455–1473.

[9] Tucker CA, Cieza A, Riley AW, et al. Concept analysis of the patient reported outcomes measurement information system (PROMIS(®)) and the international classification of functioning, disability and health (ICF). *Qual Life Res.* 2014;23(6):1677–1686.

[10] Magee DJ. *Orthopedic Physical Assessment*, 2006. 4th edition. WB Saunders Publishing, Philadelphia, PA.

[11] Smith DG, Bowker J, Michael J, eds. *Atlas of Amputations and Limb Deficiencies: Surgical, Prosthetic and Rehabilitation Principles*, 2004. 3rd edition. American Academy of Orthopaedic Surgeons, Rosemont, IL.

[12] Robinson C, Fatone S. You've heard about outcome measures, so how do you use them? Integrating clinically relevant outcome measures in orthotic management of stroke. *Prosthet Orthot Int.* 2013;37(1):30–42.

[13] Centers for Medicare & Medicaid Services. *Functional reporting: PT, OT, and SLP services frequently asked questions (FAQs).* Accessed September 23, 2024. https://www.cms.gov/medicare/billing/therapyservices/downloads/functional-reporting-pt-ot-slp-services-faq.pdf.

[14] Centers for Medicare & Medicaid Services. *Medicare Claims Processing Manual.* Accessed September 23, 2024. https://www.cms.gov/regulations-and-guidance/guidance/manuals/downloads/clm104c05.pdf.

[15] Centers for Medicare & Medicaid Services (CMS). *Publication 100-02 Medicare Benefit Policy.* Transmittal 255. Date: January 25, 2019. Change Request 11120. CMS Manual System Department of Health & Human Services (DHHS). Accessed January 30, 2025 at: https://www.cms.gov/Regulations-and-Guidance/Guidance/Transmittals/2019downloads/R255BP.pdf.

[16] Gaunaurd IA, Gailey RS, Raya MA, Roach KE. Exercise prescription protocol based upon the amputee mobility predictor: a case report. In: Proceedings of the 13th IPSO World Congress, Leipzig, Germany. May 14, 2010.

[17] Portney LG, Watkins MP. *Foundations of Clinical Research: Applications to Practice*, 2015. A Davis, Philadelphia, PA.

[18] Fitzpatric R, Davey C, Buxton M, Jones D. Evaluating patient based outcome measures for use in clinical trial. *Health Technol Assess.* 1998;2:1–74.

[19] Gailey RS, Roach KE, Applegate EB, et al. The Amputee Mobility Predictor: an instrument to assess determinants of the lower-limb amputee's ability to ambulate. *Arch Phys Med Rehabil.* 2002;83(5):613–627.

[20] Noridian Healthcare Solutions. Local coverage determination (LCD) for lower limb prostheses (L33787), 2016. American Medical Association, Chicago, IL.

[21] Kaluf B. Evaluation of mobility in persons with limb loss using the Amputee Mobility Predictor and the Prosthesis Evaluation Questionnaire–mobility subscale: a six-month retrospective chart review. *JPO: Journal of Prosthetics and Orthotics.* 2014;26(2):70–76.

[22] Leung EC-C, Rush PJ, Devlin M. Predicting prosthetic rehabilitation outcome in lower limb amputee patients with the functional independence measure. *Arch Phys Med Rehabil.* 1996;77(6):605–608.

[23] Muecke L, Shekar S, Dwyer D, et al. Functional screening of lower-limb amputees: a role in predicting rehabilitation outcome. *Arch Phys Med Rehabil.* 1992;73(9):851–858.

[24] Panesar B, Morrison P, Hunter J. A comparison of three measures of progress in early lower limb amputee rehabilitation. *Clin Rehabil.* 2001;15(2):157–171.

[25] Vellas BJ, Wayne SJ, Romero L, et al. One-leg balance is an important predictor of injurious falls in older persons. *J Am Geriatr Soc.* 1997;45(6):735–738.

[26] Schoppen T, Boonstra A, Groothoff JW, et al. Physical, mental, and social predictors of functional outcome in unilateral lower-limb amputees. *Arch Phys Med Rehabil.* 2003;84(6):803–811.

[27] Hermodsson Y, Ekdahl C, Persson B, Roxendal G. Standing balance in trans-tibial amputees following vascular disease or trauma: a comparative study with healthy subjects. *Prosthet Orthot Int.* 1994;18(3):150–158.

[28] Schoppen T, Boonstra A, Groothoff JW, et al. The Timed "up and go" test: reliability and validity in persons with unilateral lower limb amputation. *Arch Phys Med Rehabil.* 1999;80(7):825–828.

[29] Resnik L, Borgia M. Reliability of outcome measures for people with lower-limb amputations: distinguishing true change from statistical error. *Phys Ther.* 2011;91(4):555–565.

[30] Dite W, Connor HJ, Curtis HC. Clinical identification of multiple fall risk early after unilateral transtibial amputation. *Arch Phys Med Rehabil.* 2007;88(1):109–114.

[31] Bohannon RW. Reference values for the timed up and go test: a descriptive meta-analysis. *J Geriatr Phys Ther.* 2006;29(2):64–68.

[32] Datta D, Ariyaratnam R, Hilton S. Timed walking test—an all-embracing outcome measure for lower-limb amputees? *Clin Rehabil.* 1996;10(3):227–232.

[33] Brooks D, Parsons J, Hunter JP, et al. The 2-minute walk test as a measure of functional improvement in persons with lower limb amputation. *Arch Phys Med Rehabil.* 2001;82(10):1478–1483.

[34] Kark L, McIntosh AS, Simmons A. The use of the 6-min walk test as a proxy for the assessment of energy expenditure during gait in individuals with lower-limb amputation. *Int J of Rehabil Res.* 2011;34(3):227–234.

[35] Lin S-J, Bose NH. Six-minute walk test in persons with transtibial amputation. *Arch Phys Med Rehabil.* 2008;89(12):2354–2359.

[36] Lahiri S, Das PG. Reliability of the six-minute walk test in individuals with transtibial amputation. *Indian Journal of Physiotherapy and Occupational Therapy—An International Journal.* 2012;6(2):100–102.

[37] Major MJ, Fatone S, Roth EJ. Validity and reliability of the Berg Balance Scale for community-dwelling persons with lower-limb amputation. *Arch Phys Med Rehabil.* 2013;94(11):2194–2202.

[38] Wilken JM, Darter BJ, Goffar SL, et al. Physical performance assessment in military service members. *J Am Acad Orthop Surg.* 2012;20:S42–S47.

[39] Highsmith MJ, Kahle JT, Kaluf B, et al. Psychometric evaluation of the Hill Assessment Index (HAI) and Stair Assessment Index (SAI) in high-functioning transfemoral amputees. *Technol Innov.* 2016;18(2–3):193–201.

[40] Hafner BJ, Willingham LL, Buell NC, et al. Evaluation of function, performance, and preference as transfemoral amputees transition from mechanical to microprocessor control of the prosthetic knee. *Arch Phys Med Rehabil.* 2007;88(2):207–217.

[41] Hillman SJ, Donald SC, Herman J, et al. Repeatability of a new observational gait score for unilateral lower limb amputees. *Gait Posture.* 2010;32(1):39–45.

[42] Gaunaurd IA. The Comprehensive High-level Activity Mobility Predictor (CHAMP): a performance-based assessment instrument to quantify high-level mobility in service members with traumatic lower limb loss. Dissertation, University of Miami, 2012.

[43] Miller WC, Deathe AB, Speechley M. Psychometric properties of the Activities-specific Balance Confidence Scale among individuals with a lower-limb amputation. *Arch Phys Med Rehabil.* 2003;84(5):656–661.

[44] Lajoie Y, Gallagher S. Predicting falls within the elderly community: comparison of postural sway, reaction time, the Berg balance scale and the Activities-specific Balance Confidence (ABC) scale for comparing fallers and non-fallers. *Arch Gerontol Geriatr*. 2004;38(1):11–26.

[45] Mandel A, Paul K, Paner R, et al. Balance confidence and activity of community-dwelling patients with transtibial amputation. *J Rehabil Res Dev*. 2016;53(5):551.

[46] Hafner B, Morgan S, Askew R, Salem R. Psychometric properties of self-report outcome measures for prosthetic applications. *J Rehabil Res Dev*. 2016;53(6):797–812.

[47] Hafner BJ, Gaunaurd IA, Morgan SJ, et al. Construct validity of the Prosthetic Limb Users Survey of Mobility (PLUS-M) in adults with lower limb amputation. *Arch Phys Med Rehabil*. 2016;epub.

[48] Prosthetic Limb Users Survey of Mobility (PLUS-M™) Short Forms Users Guide (v1.2). https://plus-m.org/files/PLUS-M_Users_Guide_US_ENGLISH_v1.2.pdf.

[49] Hanspal R, Fisher K, Nieveen R. Prosthetic socket fit comfort score. *Disabil Rehabil*. 2003;25(22):1278–1280.

[50] Heinemann A, Bode R, O'Reilly C. Development and measurement properties of the Orthotics and Prosthetics Users' Survey (OPUS): a comprehensive set of clinical outcome instruments. *Prosthet Orthot Int*. 2003;27(3):191–206.

[51] McAndrew PM, Wilken JM, Dingwell JB. Dynamic stability of human walking in visually and mechanically destabilizing environments. *J Biomech*. 2011;44(4):644–649.

[52] Rabago CA, Dingwell JB, Wilken JM. Reliability and minimum detectable change of temporal-spatial, kinematic, and dynamic stability measures during perturbed gait. *PLOS One*. 2015;10(11):e0142083.

[53] Gailey RS, Clark CR. Physical therapy. In: Smith DG, Michael JW, Bowker JH, eds. *Atlas of Amputations and Limb Deficiencies. Surgical, Prosthetic and Rehabilitation Principles*, 2004. 3rd edition. American Academy of Orthopaedic Surgeons, Rosemont, IL.

[54] U.S. Department of Veterans Affairs, U.S. Department of Defense. *VA/DoD Clinical Practice Guideline ror Rehabilitation of Individuals With Lower Limb Amputation v. 2.0*, 2017. Accessed September 24, 2024. https://www.healthquality.va.gov/guidelines/Rehab/amp/VADoDLLACPG092817.pdf.

[55] Chiong Y, Lim PA. Results from a prospective acute inpatient rehabilitation database: clinical characteristics and functional outcomes using the Functional Independence Measure. *Ann Acad Med Singapore*. 2007;36:3–10.

CHAPTER 7

Lower Extremity Amputee Gait

Leif M. Nelson, M. Jason Highsmith, and Phil M. Stevens

OBJECTIVES

Upon completion of this chapter, the reader will:

1. Understand basic, underlying reasons why gait deviations are common in persons who use lower extremity prostheses.
2. Recall common causes for prevalent gait deviations.
3. Recall common interventions for prevalent gait deviations.

Lower extremity prosthetic technology continues to progress, from the now well-established advancements of carbon fiber energy storage and return (ESAR) prosthetic feet and microprocessor-controlled knees (MPK) into even more biomimetic technologies. Examples include an ankle system permitting dorsiflexion in swing phase or the addition of positive power to mimic concentric muscular contractions [1, 2]. However, challenges remain present for individuals with lower limb amputations and the associated anatomical disadvantages towards achieving a smooth, natural gait. Gait deviations are commonly observed in individuals ambulating with a lower limb prosthesis, resulting from the inherent loss of proprioceptive input, the pseudoarthroses that occur at the limb–socket interface and imbalances in muscle strength and range of motion. These deviations are often both more common and more pronounced at more proximal amputation levels. Whether the individual is just learning to walk following

amputation, or is able to ambulate in a nearly balanced reciprocating manner, minimizing gait deviations should be a core aim of prosthetic rehabilitation. Minimizing gait deviations and promoting symmetric gait, may help preserve the proximal and contralateral joints from onset of pain and/or degeneration [3–5]. Delivering the most appropriate intervention thus involves the process of observing gait deviations, determining the cause utilizing all information from a thorough evaluation, and then focusing the goals, interventions, and plan of care.

Successful physical therapy prescription for a person with lower extremity limb loss is devised through a combination of observational gait analysis and physical evaluation findings. A simple strategy is to observe for symmetry of motion or the lack thereof [8]. While there are a few outlier asymmetrical gait deviations that would historically be considered "normal" for this population [9, 10], access to currently available prosthetic technologies

DOI: 10.4324/9781003526025-8

provides an opportunity for improved gait symmetry [11, 12] particularly for the patient who is both intrinsically motivated and has the proper physical therapy prescription [3].

The process for assessing gait deviations in this chapter relies on the physical therapist diagnostically categorizing the deviation within what would be expected as a typical gait cycle. Placing an asymmetry within the context of the gait cycle can lead to more accurate classification as there are common deviations that will be observed during swing phase, stance phase, and the sub-phases within those gross components of the gait cycle.

Observational findings can lead to specific intervention once they are coupled with a full evaluation of the patient with and without the prosthesis donned. Decreased walking speed, wider base of support, and decreased balance are often common findings for persons with lower extremity limb loss [3, 13–18]. Mitigating causes should be investigated by the clinician. Knee flexion contractures for transtibial amputees and hip flexion and/or abduction contractures for transfemoral amputees are also common, and will cause the patient to ambulate with an asymmetrical gait pattern. Range of motion assessment for the intact lower extremity is also crucial, especially in traumatic etiology, as this can be an overlooked root cause for a gait deviation. Manual muscle testing should also be performed to determine needs for a pre-ambulation therapeutic strengthening program. Subjective feedback from the patient, along with hands-on assessment of socket fit, will help the physical therapist have a complete picture for determining causality of an asymmetrical gait pattern.

During the observational gait analysis, it is absolutely necessary to observe the patient ambulating in both the frontal and sagittal planes. This chapter will cover the most common gait deviations in persons with lower extremity limb loss. Additional comorbidities may lead to additional deviations not considered "common" in this chapter, but should also be evaluated on and individual basis and managed with the appropriate interventions.

STANCE PHASE DEVIATIONS

Foot Slap on Prosthetic Side at Initial Contact

With over 100 prosthetic feet available in the marketplace [19], most of which are non-articulating ESAR feet, popular with users because of their light weight, smooth roll-over, and perceived reductions in energy costs [20], this deviation is less common today. However, research suggests that for the older population with limb loss secondary to vascular disease, an articulating ankle may be indicated to promote a rapid foot flat, thereby improving ipsilateral knee stability [21]. While a rapid foot flat at

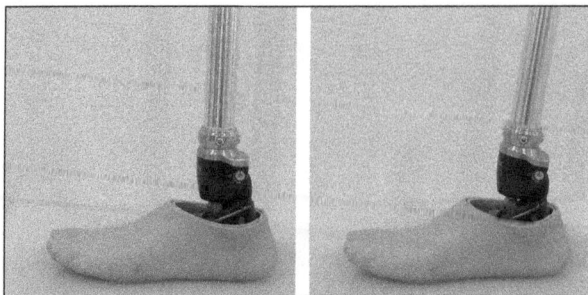

Figure 7.1. Normal foot position at A. heel strike and B. foot slap.

loading response is desirable for transtibial patients with compromised knee extensors and transfemoral patients with weak hip extensors, an abrupt foot slap (Figure 7.1) can be detrimental. For instance, a rapid foot slap can lead to a prematurely extended knee that a patient has to fight to climb over and compromise gait efficiency. An observable foot slap is typically caused by a worn out or missing plantarflexion bumper on an articulating ankle prosthetic foot and is best visualized in the sagittal plane.

Foot Rotation on Prosthetic Side at Heel Strike

Increased wear on the lateral aspect of the heel of proper footwear is typical, suggesting a posterior-lateral heel strike [22]. In the population with lower extremity limb loss, if the prosthetic heel is too firm, this force will cause the foot to pivot externally at initial contact and loading response phases of gait (Figure 7.2). This will lead to excessive toe-out or foot rotation on the prosthetic side.

A more common cause of foot rotation can be a poor socket fit on the residual limb. Rotation of the entire prosthesis can occur if transverse plane movement is not controlled by proper socket fit. Recurrent patient education on assessing and maintaining proper sock ply can address this gait deviation when a loose socket fit is determined. As the day progresses, loss of limb volume is common, and

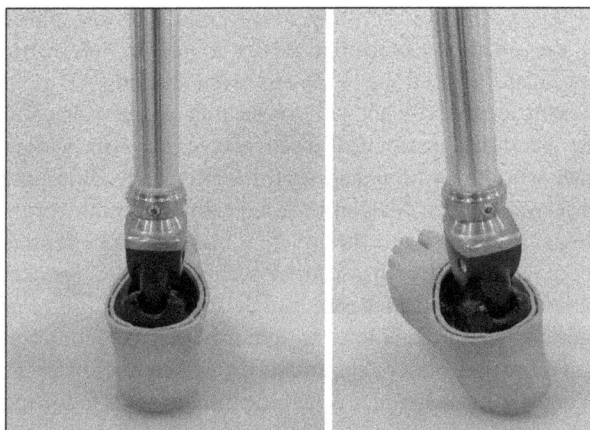

Figure 7.2. Foot maintaining normal transverse position at A. heel strike and B. a foot laterally rotating at heel strike.

thus the addition of residual limb socks can help maintain socket fit and suspension. Alternately, excessive sock ply can also compromise a socket fit. This prevents the residual limb from fully seating itself within the prosthetic socket. As a result, the structural rotation controls built into the socket design and suspension method will not be effective in limiting unwanted rotation.

Weak hip musculature is an additional possible cause of this deviation. This type of weakness creates an inability to control the prosthesis with the residual limb. Due to the hip being the most unstable link in the lower extremity chain at this stage in the gait cycle, dynamic muscular control of the femur is essential to prevent excessive uncontrolled rotation within the acetabulum, leading to observable unwanted lower limb transverse rotation.

Excessive Toe-Out

Unilateral limb loss commonly leads to observable excessive toe-out on the intact limb over time. Although this can be due to a congenital gait pattern, it is disproportionately observed in the population with limb loss compared with the general population. This accommodation allows the patient to compensate for a loss of balance and proprioception due to the limb loss. This compensation aids in maintaining center of gravity within their base of support mediolaterally. Interventions to treat excessive toe-out should focus on improving single limb balance on the prosthetic side and secondarily on the intact side. In addition, the fit of the prosthesis should also be assessed as the user may have donned the prosthesis in an externally rotated position or may have improper sock ply.

If an ESAR prosthetic foot is excessively rotated externally, the patient will not receive the desired energy return from that foot. Thus, for an individual who walks with excessive toe-out on their contralateral sound limb, prosthetic toe-out represents one instance where symmetry may be abandoned for biomechanical efficiency.

Knee Buckling at Initial Contact to Loading Response

When observed on the prosthetic side in the transtibial population, this may result from quadriceps' weakness, a short residual limb length, or prosthetic foot dysfunction. In addition, excessive prosthetic socket flexion or an overly firm heel can create this deviation. Additional prosthesis alignment causes include an excessively dorsiflexed foot or socket placement in an anterior position over the foot.

During loading response, the knee joint is the most unstable point in the weight-bearing lower extremity chain [10]. The implication of this for transfemoral prosthesis users is that the ground-reaction force can shift posterior to the prosthetic knee joint, causing it to buckle. Control of the prosthetic knee after heel strike relies on the intrinsic controls of the prosthetic knee along with the volitional concentric control of the hip extensor muscles. If decreased activation of the gluteus maximus, and/or lack of intrinsic knee control, cannot counteract the knee flexion moment and stabilize the knee [23], buckling may likely occur.

A hip flexion contracture or prosthetic malalignment can also cause this deviation. When the soft tissue is shortened on the anterior aspect of the hip, the gluteus maximus is functionally positioned in a mechanical disadvantage. Further, if this contracture is not accommodated in the prosthetic alignment, it will position the ground-reaction force posterior to the knee, undermining knee joint stability.

An additional prosthetic cause may involve the knee being aligned too far anteriorly, leading to a similar posterior position of the ground-reaction force. Alternately, an alignment of insufficient socket flexion can give rise to inhibited gluteus maximus activation. Prosthetic causes of early knee buckling may be overcome in an individual with strong hip extensors, but guarding in the trunk and ipsilateral hip will be visualized.

Knee Extension/Hyperextension at Initial Contact to Loading Response

Knee flexion of less than the typical 15° to 18° is common for persons with lower extremity amputations of all levels [17, 24, 25]. Individuals with transfemoral amputation have a prosthetic knee joint, thus hyperextension is typically associated with limb loss at the transtibial level. This can be propagated by weak quadriceps at initial contact as the ground-reaction force briefly causes the knee to move into an extended position. Less frequently, the prosthesis can also cause this deviation. Excessive foot plantarflexion, lack of proper socket flexion, or a posterior shifted socket are all alignments that may cause hyperextension at the knee. In addition to alignment, prosthetic componentry including a worn-out or excessively soft heel can lead to this deviation.

For the population with transfemoral limb loss, this gait deviation is commonly caused by prosthetic alignment. In some cases this abnormality may be intentionally created by the prosthetist to prevent falling or to address a fear of falling, but should not be encouraged when a patient is using a prosthesis with a fluid-controlled knee or other component prescribed for an active ambulator.

Wide Base of Support

In an effort to maintain balance, many prosthesis users will ambulate with a wide base of support. Maintaining center of mass within the base of support is necessary to prevent falling in an individual with lower extremity amputation who does not have adequate single limb balance control over the prosthetic limb. Alternately, among transfemoral prosthesis users an abducted prosthetic alignment or volitional hip abduction to reduce medial socket pain are alternate causes. However, decreased balance is the most frequently encountered cause of the wide base of support [3, 13–18].

Trendelenburg or Lateral Trunk Lean

Trendelenburg gait is classically due to gluteus medius weakness on the weight-bearing limb. Visualization of this deviation routinely appears as a slight lateral lean over the weight-bearing limb, and is due to a lack of ability to stabilize the pelvis during stance.

For persons with limb loss, this would typically occur on the prosthetic side, and pure Trendelenburg gait would be due to hip abductor dysfunction [15]. Lateral trunk lean that is not caused by the true Trendelenburg mechanism is frequently observed in transfemoral prosthetic use. The lack of a rigid connection between the residual femur and the external prosthesis compromises the patient's ability to stabilize their pelvis in the coronal plane during single limb stance. Rather, an intentional lateral shift over the prosthesis provides this coronal stability. This is frequently accomplished by a gross shift of the upper torso. With training, this lateral shift can occur at the hips rather than the trunk, restoring a smoother gait.

This deviation can be further exacerbated by a functionally short prosthesis, such as may occur when a patient is not wearing enough sock ply, and thus bottoming out in the socket. For persons with transfemoral amputations, pain in the groin area from medial socket brim impingement will also result in lateral trunk lean as a pain avoidance behavior.

Knee Buckling in Mid Stance

Slight knee flexion from loading response to mid stance of up to 18° is normal. This stance flexion is commonly observed in the general population. Stance flexion serves as a shock absorber which can decrease impact and stress on proximal joints. Knee flexion to the point of buckling will occur if stance flexion cannot be controlled eccentrically by the quadriceps in patients with limb loss at a level distal to the knee joint. In those with an amputation that requires a prosthetic knee, buckling is caused by prosthetic dysfunction from either improper alignment (typically the knee is positioned too far anterior) or improper programming or setting of the knee joint's mechanical

stance control features. A patient with transfemoral limb loss with a hip flexion contracture is more prone to this gait deviation as the hip extensor muscles are in a position of mechanical disadvantage.

Excessive Knee Extension/ Hyperextension (genu recurvatum) in Mid Stance to Late Stance

Genu recurvatum is typically an issue in the population with an intact knee joint on the prosthetic side. As the body moves over the limb, from mid stance to terminal stance, the ground-reaction force shifts anterior to the knee joint center [10]. If this moment is overpowering, excessive knee extension will be observed. Prosthetic causes that lead to this deviation can stem from both the prosthetic foot and the socket alignment. An overly plantarflexed foot, toed-in foot, long toe lever, or hard dorsiflexion bumper or setting (in an articulating foot) can all propagate genu recurvatum. Additionally, lack of appropriate socket flexion or an excessively posterior socket alignment can also give rise to this deviation.

For the population with a transfemoral amputation, many prosthetic knees require full extension in late stance while loaded with the patient's body weight to trigger a shift in knee function from stance to swing mode. However, true hyperextension should be biomechanically impossible unless it is built into the alignment by the prosthetist.

Lack of Hip Extension in Terminal Stance

This is most common in patients with transfemoral amputations and hip flexion contractures. More proximal amputation levels resulting in shorter transfemoral residual limbs may be at more risk of hip flexion contractures. Asymmetry due to decreased hip extension can be limited with early rehabilitation interventions to prevent the contracture.

Once present, a hip flexion contracture must be accommodated in the alignment of the prosthesis to allow functional hip extension. This is done by aligning the prosthesis in exaggerated hip flexion. When these individuals have full hip extension range of motion on their intact limb, the result will be an asymmetrical gait pattern in which patients take a full stride with their prosthesis, but the step length on the sound side is limited by the lack of hip extension on the affected limb. This limitation can also result in compensation at the lumbar spine to maintain an upright posture or need for an assistive mobility aid for ambulation.

Drop Off in Late Stance on the Prosthetic Side

The term "drop off" is an abbreviated name for a premature loss of anterior support. This deviation is observed more frequently in persons with transtibial or more distal limb loss, but maybe present in any level of lower extremity amputation. Drop off is due to an actual or functionally shortened lever arm in the prosthetic foot. The lever arm can be actually shortened due to the foot being the wrong size or stiffness, or can be artificially shortened by having an over-flexed socket, an anteriorly shifted socket, an overly dorsiflexed foot, or a soft/broken dorsiflexion bumper (in an articulating foot). This can be clinically correlated with a physical examination, as full knee extension range of motion and good to excellent knee extensor strength in the residual limb would likely indicate a prosthetic cause of the deviation. If the patient has a knee flexion contracture and/or weak quadriceps, there is a possibility of knee buckling in late stance that may look similar to drop off.

Decreased Push Off in Terminal Stance to Preswing

Due to the replacement of the dynamic contractile tissue of the gastrocnemius-soleus complex across the ankle joint with a simple keel, persons with limb loss have an inevitable loss of power at push off [26]. Extreme instances of this deviation are easily observed as a lack of a crease in the forward third of the shoe on the prosthetic side. If this is observed, the patient is not maximizing the energy return from the prosthetic foot. A commonly expected compensation is increased hip extensor activation [26].

In the less common instance that the individual with limb loss has a powered ankle foot prosthesis that can generate push off, then the user's technique and the program settings of the foot should be evaluated for the lack of push off. A powered ankle foot prosthesis should be able to replicate the missing gastrocnemius-soleus complex in a biomimetic fashion during the late aspects of the gait cycle.

SWING PHASE DEVIATIONS

The ankle is the most unstable joint in the weight-bearing chain at terminal stance. Even though many prosthetic feet are non-articulating at the ankle, creating inherent stability, proper dynamic alignment of the prosthesis is crucial to control the forces that aid in transition from stance phase into swing phase. The energy returned through the keel of the prosthetic foot relies on the position of the prosthetic foot in relation to the shank, the socket, and the ground to determine trajectory as the prosthetic foot leaves the ground. As with stance phase deviations, these asymmetries in the gait cycle may have causes propagated by the prosthesis, or the user and the potential need for proper training.

Excessive Heel Rise During Early Swing

Excessive heel rise in early swing can be considered "normal" for transtibial amputees [10], as this compensation assists in toe clearance as the lower extremity progresses toward mid swing [18]. If heel rise is asymmetrical for the prosthetic side relative to the intact side in a person with unilateral lower extremity limb loss, it should be very slight. In the transfemoral population a slight increase can also be acceptable, and may vary based on the components [25], but in general excessive heel rise may create an unwanted lag in forward progression of the transfemoral prosthesis. Depending upon the knee's mechanical design features, this deviation can often be reduced by the prosthetist by increasing the unit's mechanical resistance to knee flexion or by adding or adjusting the unit's extension assist mechanism.

Lack of Heel Rise During Early Swing

When seen in a person ambulating with a transfemoral prosthesis, the prosthetic cause of decreased heel rise could likely be that the swing flexion resistance is too great, thus limiting heel rise. Knee flexion of less than 60° will also be common in a shuffling gait typical of someone with a step-to gait pattern. This could be a resultant bad habit from forcefully thrusting the prosthesis forward with the hip flexors of the residual limb, or ambulating with a restrictive assistive device such as a standard walker.

Medial Whip

A medial whip is a gait deviation seen in persons with transfemoral limb loss. It is typically caused by malalignment of the prosthetic knee. During initial swing, the proximal segment of the thigh moves into slight abduction as visualized in the frontal plane. The key indicator of this deviation is that the knee points laterally as the heel of the prosthetic foot moves medially during knee flexion

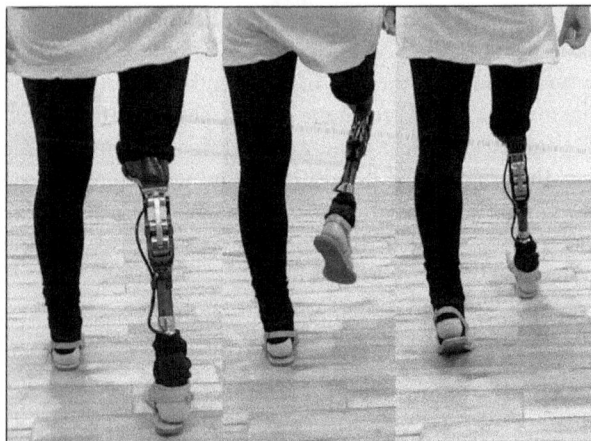

Figure 7.3. In a medial whip, a laterally aligned knee system commonly results in the foot raising medially with knee flexion then traveling laterally during swing phase.

(Figure 7.3). The hip abduction is a compensation for the whip deviation, to prevent the person with amputation from kicking their contralateral limb with the prosthetic foot. If lateral rotation is not present in the static bench knee alignment, other causes may be the result of the user incorrectly donning the prosthesis, or a loose socket that was rotated laterally.

If a medial whip is seen in a transtibial patient, it will typically be less pronounced, and may be from a poorly aligned prosthetic foot. This may also similarly be caused by an incorrectly donned or loose socket. A severe muscle length and/or muscle strength imbalance leading to a functional imbalance propagating this deviation can be ruled out during the physical evaluation.

Lateral Whip

During a lateral whip, the thigh will remain neutrally aligned beneath the pelvis in the frontal plane, the knee will point medially in the transverse plane (Figure 7.4), and the heel of the prosthetic foot whips laterally. This deviation is caused by a medial rotation of the prosthetic

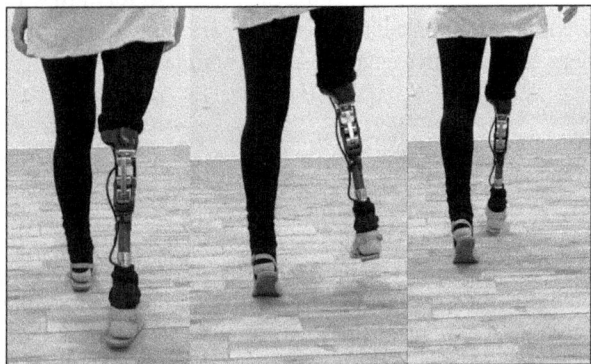

Figure 7.4. In a lateral whip, a medially aligned knee system commonly results in the foot raising laterally with knee flexion then traveling medially during swing phase.

knee, either permanently or due to medial socket rotation from a donning error or loss of suspension.

In the population with transtibial amputation, prosthetic foot alignment or severe muscle strength and/or muscle length imbalance would be the foundation for the presentation of a lateral whip.

Circumduction

Thigh abduction during swing phase is the key aspect of circumduction that differentiates this deviation from lateral whip. This is different from an abducted gait as in circumduction the foot starts at and returns to midline. The knee, whether anatomical or prosthetic, is extended, or very minimally flexed, throughout swing phase. One probable cause of this would be a hip abduction contracture. In the absence of a hip abduction contracture, this would be a compensatory mechanism by the patient to avoid catching the prosthetic foot during swing due to a long prosthesis or an intentional compensation by patients who prefer to keep the knee of their prosthesis extended through swing to ensure sagittal knee stability during stance.

Alternately, excessive length of the prosthesis can be considered. The prosthesis may be functionally long due to loss of suspension, inappropriately donning too many residual limb socks, or an overly plantarflexed foot due to malfunction in an articulating ankle.

In patients with transfemoral limb loss an additional cause could be that the mechanical release into reduced swing phase resistance at the knee is not being triggered by the user. This can be due to lack of weight-bearing into the prosthesis during stance or a shortened step length on the intact side. Physical therapy is essential for training patients with transfemoral limb loss to load the prosthesis during stance phase in order to trigger the knee to transition into swing phase. Alternately, for some MPKs, when the battery of the knee is exhausted, it defaults to permanent stance phase knee resistance throughout the gait cycle, creating an acute occurrence of this deviation.

Vaulting

Vaulting can often accompany circumduction, as this is a sound-side compensation to clear the prosthetic foot during swing [3]. The key observation is plantarflexion during mid stance on the intact limb while the prosthesis is moving through mid swing. This occurs well before appropriate stance plantarflexion that would be visualized as heel rise indicating push off at terminal stance. All causes for circumduction could lead to vaulting. This deviation is typically caused by the prosthesis being too long either functionally or in bench alignment. If this asymmetry is observed in a patient with a properly aligned and suspended prosthesis, the cause is possibly due to a bad habit developed from a previous prosthesis that was too long or simply the patient's desire to ensure swing phase clearance in the absence of active dorsiflexion.

Hip Hiking

This deviation may accompany both vaulting and circumduction due to similar causation. The differentiation is that hip hiking is a lateral elevation of the pelvis on the prosthetic side during swing [17, 24]. This results in side bending of the trunk toward the prosthesis during swing phase. Additionally, this is a necessary deviation for patients with a hip disarticulation or hemipelvectomy with a single axis hip prosthesis.

Long Prosthetic Side Step Length

Common in individuals with unilateral transfemoral limb loss [11, 13, 25, 27, 28], this asymmetrical gait pattern is characterized by a long step length on the prosthetic side (Figure 7.5) and shorter step length on the intact side. Increased stance time on the sound limb in persons with

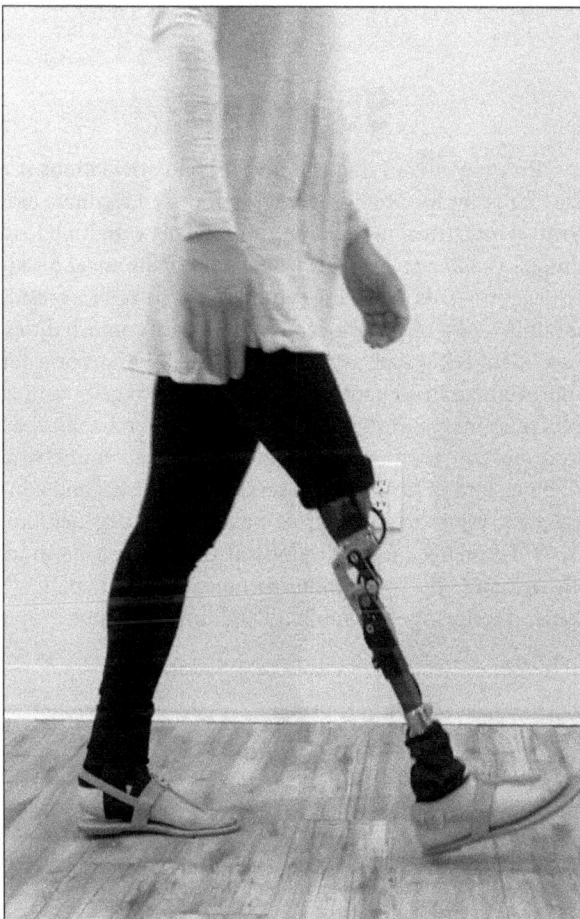

Figure 7.5. Long prosthetic side-step.

unilateral limb loss [15, 24, 28] can be caused by decreased single limb balance or proprioception through the prosthesis, fear of falling, or fear of weight acceptance by the prosthesis. Additional causes include lack of anterior pelvic rotation on the prosthetic side, a hip flexion contracture in the residual limb, or pain caused by impingement of anterior brim of the socket. For long-term prosthesis users, this deviation is sometimes caused by habit from walking on a previous mechanical prosthetic knee that required full extension at heel strike to safely transition into stance phase.

PROXIMAL AND UPPER BODY DEVIATIONS

Gait deviations that occur superior to the residual limb can affect symmetry, efficiency, and overall gait fluidity [13]. Some of the following abnormalities can be targets of direct physical therapy interventions, and others are secondary compensations to other dysfunctions such as decreased balance or pain. While it is initially attractive to focus observational gait analysis and intervention exclusively on the amputated extremity, it is equally vital to view the pelvis, spine, and upper extremities.

Lack of Anterior Pelvic Rotation on Prosthetic Side

Clinically, a lack of prosthetic-side anterior pelvic rotation is common in gait after limb loss, particularly with more proximal amputations. This may be observed as lifting and "kicking" the prosthesis forward using the hip flexors to initiate gait instead of anterior pelvic rotation. As the patient transitions from terminal stance into swing phase, swing initiation should be led by the ipsilateral pelvis transitioning from a maximally posteriorly rotated position toward neutral. At mid swing, this progression should continue until the pelvis reaches maximal anterior rotation at terminal swing of approximately 5°. This is a rarely documented deviation during observational gait analysis but is very common, and must be treated if the patient and physical therapist wish to promote the most symmetric gait possible. If this occurs in early prosthetic use in the new amputee, it could develop into a long-term bad habit. An impinging anterior brim on a transfemoral prosthetic socket, poor balance on the prosthetic limb, and/or fear of falling could also propagate this deviation.

Decreased Trunk Rotation

Moving up the chain to the lumbar and thoracic region, decreased trunk rotation is a potentially symmetrical deviation, which means it must be targeted for observation. The spine and pelvis should rotate fluidly in the transverse plane during ambulation to promote optimal efficiency. This pattern of motion complements arm swing. If this is seen in patients with unilateral lower extremity amputation, who also present with decreased anterior pelvic rotation, asymmetry may be increased as the pelvis and thorax will likely rotate out of phase with each other [13]. Other gait deviations that lead to decreased trunk rotation include a wide base of support and decreased arm swing.

Excess Lumbar Lordosis

Lordosis is the normal curvature of the lumbar spine. However, excess lumbar lordosis is most common in patients with transfemoral limb loss. This is commonly caused by hip flexion contracture, and thus is often seen in patients with short residual limbs. Decreased stability produced by the transversus abdominis and multifidus muscles can also promote this deviation. Other less common causes could be pain avoidance from a high, impinging anterior transfemoral socket brim, or weak gluteus maximus. This can also be caused by a secondary compensation to maintain upright posture when ambulating while trying to maintain an anterior weight line on an unstable knee in stance phase.

Arm Swing Deviations

Patients with extremity loss may present with decreased arm swing, or upper limb guarding as commonly observed in gait of persons with decreased balance. Asymmetrical arm swing typically presents with the upper extremity guarding on the prosthetic side, with potentially excess arm swing on the intact side. Arm swing is regarded as a mechanism to decrease pelvic rotation. Thus, decreased arm swing could be an indicator that the pelvis is not rotating or tilting properly.

COMMUNITY MOBILITY

Successfully navigating community obstacles outside of a controlled physical therapy clinic is a real-life challenge for prosthesis users. Therefore, it is important to train patients to utilize the method best suited for their particular level of mobility. Training on less compliant surfaces such as grass and gravel is an appropriate progression from the flat, level surface commonly found indoors. Transitions between surfaces often provide a challenge for users and can be a source of stumbles and fall.

Ramps, Curbs, and Stairs

Slopes in the community come in varying degrees of incline as naturally occurring slopes are likely inconsistent with Americans with Disabilities Act specifications. Side stepping or step-to gait patterns with the prosthesis maintaining a downhill advantage are starting points for new users and strategies for steep inclines and declines. Step-over-step patterns may be easier to achieve on mild slopes as well as for users with articulating ankles and/or MPKs [29–31].

When traversing curbs and stairs, a similar progression exists. Multiple stairs without handrails may be best overcome in the seated position for new or less ambulatory users. Step-to gait patterns with the prosthesis always being in the trail position when ascending and lead position when descending is the next progression. Step-over-step is the most advanced process and much more easily achieved with the transtibial limb loss population. Foot placement is crucial for descending stairs step-over-step. The prosthetic foot should be placed half to two-thirds beyond the step's front edge to compensate for possible lack of ankle motion and control of the prosthetic foot. This foot placement allows the user to roll over the foot that is less able to dorsiflex at the ankle. Methods other than these described for negotiating community obstacles should be evaluated for user safety and to determine if training and technique modification is needed.

SUMMARY

Properly identifying gait and mobility deviations is a starting point for providing interventions to facilitate efficient, symmetrical mobility for individuals with limb loss. Unique challenges exist in people with anatomical disadvantages towards achieving symmetry, such as short residual limbs, loss of proprioception, or other comorbidities. First identifying gait asymmetries and then striving for improvement in all patients can be a guide to gait training interventions. Both the prosthetic limb and rehabilitation program that are prescribed must facilitate symmetrical mobility, and in turn may preserve the proximal and contralateral joints from onset of pain and/or degeneration [3–7]. Ultimately, focused physical therapy will be more efficient and effective in optimizing each unique patient's gait and restoring their mobility and independence.

REFERENCES

[1] Tacca JR, Colvin ZA, Grabowski AM. Greater than recommended stiffness and power setting of a stance-phase powered leg prosthesis can improve step-to-step transition work and effective foot length ratio during walking in people with transtibial amputation. *Front Bioeng Biotechnol.* 2024 Jul 1;12:1336520.

[2] Kestur S, Zhou S, O'Sullivan G, et al. Comparing the lower limb joint biomechanics of the PowerKnee, C-Leg and Rheo Knee during ramp and stair ambulation. *Biomech.* 2024 Jun;171:112201.

[3] Sjodahl C, Jarnlo G, Soderberg B, et al. Kinematic and kinetic gait analysis in the sagittal plane of trans-femoral amputees before and after special gait re-education. *Prosthet Orthot Int.* 2002;26(2):101–112.

[4] Kulkarni J, Gaine W, Buckley J, et al. Chronic low back pain in traumatic lower limb amputees. *Clin Rehabil.* 2005;19(1):81–86.

[5] Taghipour H, Mohamamzad Y, Mafi A, et al. Quality of life among veterans with war-related unilateral lower extremity amputation: a long-term survey in a prosthesis center in Iran. *J Orthop Trauma.* 2009;23(7):525–530.

[6] Struyf P, van Heugten C, Hitters M, et al. The prevalence of osteoarthritis of the intact hip and knee among traumatic leg amputees. *Arch Phys Med Rehabil.* 2009;90(3):440–446.

[7] Norvell D, Czerniecki J, Reiber G, et al. The prevalence of knee pain and symptomatic knee osteoarthritis among veteran traumatic amputees and nonamputees. *Arch Phys Med Rehabil.* 2005;86(3):487–493.

[8] Hillman S, Donald S, Herman J, et al. Repeatability of a new observational gait score for unilateral lower limb amputees. *Gait Posture.* 2010;32(1):39–45.

[9] Skinner H, Effeney D. Gait analysis in amputees. *Am J Phys Med.* 1985;64(2):82–89.

[10] Perry J. *Gait Analysis: Normal and Pathological Function,* 1992. SLACK Incorporated, Thorofare, NJ.

[11] Graham L, Datta D, Heller B, et al. A comparative study of conventional and energy-storing prosthetic feet in high-functioning transfemoral amputees. *Arch Phys Med Rehabil.* 2007;88(6):801–806.

[12] Kaufman K, Frittoli S, Frigo C. Gait asymmetry of transfemoral amputees using mechanical and microprocessor-controlled prosthetic knees. *Clin Biomech.* 2012;27(5):460–465.

[13] Goujon-Pillet H, Sapin E, Fode P, et al. Three-dimensional motions of trunk and pelvis during transfemoral amputee gait. *Arch Phys Med Rehabil.* 2008;89(1):87–94.

[14] Boonstra A, Schrama J, Fidler V, et al. The gait of unilateral transfemoral amputees. *Scand J Rehabil Med.* 1994;26(4):217–223.

[15] Jaegers S, Arendzen J, de Jongh H. Prosthetic gait of unilateral transfemoral amputees: a kinematic study. *Arch Phys Med Rehabil.* 1995;76(8):736–743.

[16] Lamoth C, Ainsworth E, Polomski W, et al. Variability and stability analysis of walking transfemoral amputees. *Medical Eng Phys.* 2010;32(9):1009–1014.

[17] Su P, Gard S, Lipschutz R, et al. Gait characteristics of persons with bilateral transtibial amputations. *J Rehabil Res Dev.* 2007;44(4):491–501.

[18] Su P, Gard S, Lipschutz R, et al. Differences in gait characteristics between persons with bilateral transtibial amputations, due to peripheral vascular disease and trauma, and able-bodied ambulators. *Arch Phys Med Rehabil.* 2008;(7):1386–1394.

[19] Stark G. How do clinicians select prosthetic feet? *The O&P Edge.* May 2012.

[20] Hofstad C, Linde H, Limbeek J, et al. Prescription of prosthetic ankle-foot mechanisms after lower limb amputation. *Cochrane Database Syst Rev.* 2004;(1):1–42.

[21] Zmitrewicz R, Neptune R, Walden J, et al. The effect of foot and ankle prosthetic components on braking and propulsive impulses during transtibial amputee gait. *Arch Phys Med Rehabil.* 2006;87(10):1334–1339.

[22] *Pedorthic Reference Guide.* Pedorthic Footwear Association, Washington, D.C.

[23] Beyaert C, Grumillier C, Martinet N. Compensatory mechanism involving the knee joint of the intact limb during gait in unilateral below-knee amputees. *Gait Posture.* 2008;28(2):278–284.

[24] Sagawa Y, Turcot K, Armand S, et al. Biomechanics and physiological parameters during gait in lower-limb amputees: a systematic review. *Gait Posture.* 2011;33(4):511–526.

[25] Segal A, Orendurff M, Klute G, et al. Kinematic and kinetic comparisons of transfemoral amputee gait using C-Leg and Mauch SNS prosthetic knees. *J Rehabil Res Dev.* 2006;43(7):857–870.

[26] Yeung L, Leung A, Zhang M, et al. Long-distance walking effects on trans-tibial amputees compensatory gait patterns and implications on prosthetic designs and training. *Gait Posture.* 2012;35(2):328–333.

[27] Maaref K, Martinet N, Grumillier C, et al. Kinematics in the terminal swing phase of unilateral transfemoral amputees: microprocessor-controlled versus swing-phase control prosthetic knees. *Arch Phys Med Rehabil.* 2010;91(6):919–925.

[28] Isakov E, Keren O, Benjuya N. Trans-tibial amputee gait: time-distance parameters and EMG activity. *Prosthet Orthot Int.* 2000;24(3):216–220.

[29] Sawers A, Hafner B. Outcomes associated with the use of microprocessor-controlled prosthetic knees among individuals with unilateral transfemoral limb loss: a systematic review. *J Prosthet Orthot.* 2013;25(4S):P4–P40.

[30] Fradet L, Alimusaj M, Braatz F, et al. Biomechanical analysis of ramp ambulation of transtibial amputees with an adaptive ankle foot system. *Gait Posture.* 2010;32(2):191–198.

[31] Agrawal V, Gailey R, O'Toole I, et al. Influence of gait training and prosthetic foot category on eternal work symmetry during unilateral transtibial amputee gait. *Prosthet Orthot Int.* 2013;37(5):396–403.

CHAPTER 8

Physical Therapy for the Patient with Amputation

Marie Black, Christopher A. Rábago, and M. Jason Highsmith

OBJECTIVES

Upon completion of this chapter, the reader will be able to:
1. Recall the five phases of amputee rehabilitation.
2. Describe key elements of the five phases of rehabilitation.
3. Recall and describe interventions associated with each phase of rehabilitation.

INTRODUCTION

In order to achieve optimal rehabilitation outcomes for individuals with limb loss, an interdisciplinary clinical team must work together with the patient and their family members or caregivers. The clinic team often consists of surgeons, rehabilitation physicians, nurses, prosthetists, case managers, social workers, behavioral health specialists, nutritionists, recreational therapists, occupational therapists, and physical therapists [1]. In this chapter, the entire continuum of care for amputee rehabilitation is considered.

There are five general phases of rehabilitative care for individuals with limb loss: I) Pre-Operative, II) Post-Operative, III) Pre-Prosthetic, IV) Prosthetic, and V) Maintenance & Lifelong Care [1]. A physical therapist's participation in each of these phases depends on the care setting they practice in and a patient's access to care. Ideally, all individuals facing an amputation would progress through each phase with expert guidance from an interdisciplinary clinical team.

PHASE I: PRE-OPERATIVE

Depending on the mechanism that leads to a patient's amputation, a physical therapist may have an opportunity to care for a patient pre-operatively. For example, a patient may be participating in rehabilitation when a choice is made to proceed with a delayed amputation following limb salvage. Additionally, for many individuals with vascular disease, progressive amputation may be inevitable and happen quickly following a recent amputation. Revisions to previous amputations, which may have been traumatic, congenital, or dysvascular in origin, may be needed to control infection, heterotopic ossification, and neuromas. In such cases, clinicians may have the opportunity to provide pre-operative care.

DOI: 10.4324/9781003526025-9

Central to this phase of rehabilitation is patient education, which includes setting expectations and managing the anxiety that often accompanies the unknown. The individual who is soon to have an amputation may desire to know what to expect through their course of care and beyond. Questions a patient facing an amputation may be contemplating can include:

- *What will my limb look and feel like after the amputation?*
- *What does rehabilitation involve?*
- *When will I get my "new" limb?*
- *How long does it take to walk?*
- *Will I be independent or need help from others?*
- *Can I return to work or sports?*
- *How can I prevent further set-backs and the need for more surgeries?*

Some may find it is easier to go through a life changing event such as amputation when they know there is a plan for how to get back to a functional, enjoyable, and thriving lifestyle. Therefore, physical therapists should provide patients with a brief overview of their continuum of care. This patient education should occur pre-operatively and include the patient's family members, loved ones, or caregivers. It should include key milestones the patient may likely experience as they progress through rehabilitation (Table 8.1). Reviewing these milestones helps to manage expectations and provides the opportunity for the patient and their family members to ask questions. While patient education is important in physical therapy, it is not the sole responsibility of the physical therapist. There are questions and concerns that may be out of the scope or experience of the physical therapist. However, beginning this dialogue allows the therapist to determine if the patient may benefit from a consult with another member of the interdisciplinary clinic team. For example, specific questions about the surgical procedures, cost of care, medications, or type of prosthesis may require consults from the surgeon, case manager, and prosthetist. The patient and their family members need to know that every member of the team is there to guide them through this journey and will seek answers to their questions and concerns.

Skin Check

Inspecting the skin of the patient preparing for an amputation and including the patient in this process is important. As clarified in Chapter 3 of this text, many amputation surgeries are the result of vascular issues [2, 3]. Thus, inspecting the sound (or non-operative) limb for any new lesions, changes in skin color, edema, temperature, and pulse can clarify the extent of vascular compromise and the patient's ability to heal. More detail on skin related issues can be found in Chapter 9.

If the therapist is planning to use the inspection as an education intervention, be sure the patient is prepared and equipped to participate in the skin inspection. For example, if they have range of motion limitations, the patient may require a long-handled mirror to inspect the bottom of the feet. Also, make sure the patient has appropriate foot wear. Patients with a dysvascular condition should always wear shoes when the feet are on the floor to prevent further injury or complications. Skin of the involved limb should also be assessed. Stasis dermatitis (i.e. port wine stains) can indicate vascular compromise that may suggest impaired ability to heal, balance, and other issues. If a wound is present, its cleanliness should be noted. This will lead to inquiry regarding who is dressing or otherwise caring for the wound and if the quality and timeliness of the service is adequate. If sub-standard, perhaps further education regarding wound management is indicated. Further assess the skin for any new lesions, changes in skin color, swelling, and temperature.

Range of Motion

Additional areas requiring attention and potential intervention prior to surgery are those associated with setting the patient up for eventual success with a prosthesis. It is generally accepted that greater health and fitness prior to surgery may yield a more favorable post-operative recovery. For basic function, a reasonable range of motion (ROM) is necessary. However, for the patient with lower extremity (LE) amputation there are key joints with a tendency to experience restrictions after surgery. Therefore, it is important to maintain or increase ROM in these joints prior to surgery when possible.

Full hip extension ROM is important, for example. A lack of hip extension prevents a patient from standing up straight and decreases the sound side step length while walking [4]. Another notoriously problematic movement is internal hip rotation. Commonly, when a patient is lying supine in bed after surgery, they tend to keep the hip abducted and externally rotated, potentially limiting functional internal hip rotation.

Patients undergoing transtibial amputation (TTA) benefit from having full knee extension. During mid-stance, normal gait requires near full knee extension on the stance limb in order to clear the contralateral foot during swing without creating deviations. A small knee flexion contracture may be accommodated with prosthetic socket alignment into pre-flexion (Figure 8.1). Conversely, a significant knee flexion contracture can make an otherwise excellent prosthetic candidate struggle with prosthetic gait or prosthetic candidacy all together. To address these ROM deficits, possible interventions may include hip and patella mobilization and manipulation, manual stretching, prone lying on a wedge, or stretches for the hip

TABLE 8.1

Select milestones, goals, and activities that a patient may experience while progressing through each phase of rehabilitation related to limb loss. While not an exhaustive list, this can be used to provide a brief overview of their continuum of care as part of patient education and goal setting.

REHABILITATION PHASE	MILESTONES, GOALS, AND ACTIVITIES
Pre-Operative	• Discuss current status and goals. ◦ Include goals for the procedure and for after the procedure. • Discuss timeline for the rehabilitative process. • Assess current status for future comparison. • Potential meeting with prosthetist, peer visitor, or support group. • Pre-operative functional assessment (i.e. prior level of function).
Post-Operative	• Peer visitor or support group initiated or continued. • Sutures or staples are removed 2 to 3 weeks after surgery. • After suture removal, patients are routinely fit with a shrinker or other volume management device. • Limb healing and volume monitored. • Therapeutic exercises and activities initiated. • Mobility activities initiated.
Pre-Prosthetic Training	• If a prosthesis is being considered, therapeutic exercise, therapeutic activities, and mobility activities are continued in preparation for prosthetic fitting and utilization. • Consultation with prosthetist. • Fit with preliminary prosthetic volume and suspension components as appropriate (i.e. gel liner). • Casted for prosthesis. • Assistive devices considered for prosthetic ambulation based on functional level, balance, and stability.
Prosthetic Training	• Fit with temporary socket. • Prosthetic socket adjusted until properly fit. • Prosthesis fabrication completed, delivered and checked out. (See Appendix.) • Range of motion, strengthening, conditioning, balance, and gait training will continue throughout rehabilitation. Walking on level and uneven surfaces such as stairs, curbs, ramps, and grass.
Maintenance & Lifelong Care	• Patient will follow up with the prosthetic care team as needed for issues such as prosthetic related discomfort, skin issues, prosthetic malalignment or failure, and others. • Some health systems recommend a follow up with the prosthetic care team on an annual basis [1]. • Therapy may be indicated with changes to health, function, or the prosthesis. • Prosthetic changes may be indicated with changes to the patient's health, or function, or if the prosthesis is in disrepair or otherwise failing to meet the patient's goals.

flexors, hamstrings, and quadriceps femoris (Figure 8.2). Home exercise programs (HEPs) are routinely included for patients with joint range restrictions. Compliance with the HEP is necessary and should be assessed; otherwise, ROM gains made in therapy are less likely to be maintained.

Strength

Improving patient function including prosthetic function will likely require strengthening following surgery. Patients with amputation require good general strength,

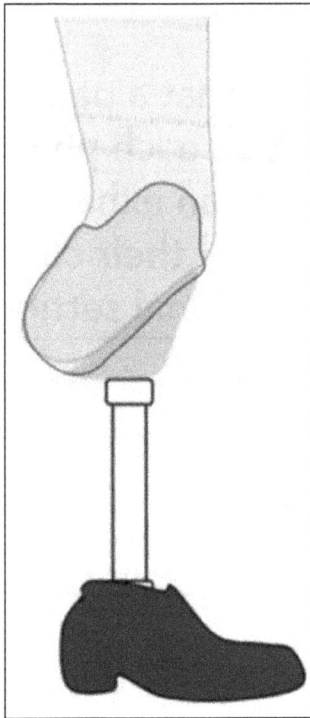

Figure 8.1. The transtibial socket is positioned to enable knee flexion thereby accommodating a knee flexion contracture.

a bolster can be placed beneath the patient's residual limb (RL) or socket. Elastic strengthening bands can be placed around the thighs to add resistance while exercising.

Hip abduction is another movement important in gait. For example, a strong gluteus medius contributes to keeping the pelvis level during single limb stance. This is important for minimizing gait deviations such as lateral trunk bending or toe dragging that could lead to overuse conditions or safety issues. Potential interventions for abductor strengthening may include side lying SLRs, pulley resisted abduction, and balance activities seated on a physio ball.

Strong hip flexion is needed in swing phase particularly for individuals with TFA. The ability to change suddenly from a hip extension to flexion contraction is needed for an individual with TFA. This facilitates control of the prosthetic knee enabling reliable cycling between extension and flexion as the individual walks. The ability to cycle reliably between swing and stance may also have implications for safety and for minimizing gait deviations. Intervention may include prone bridging using a bolster, pulley resisted hip flexion, and supine SLRs. For the individual with TTA, quadriceps femoris and hamstring function are also important. The quadriceps femoris muscle is used through stance phase and the hamstrings are active in swing phase for limb deceleration. Possible interventions for the quadriceps femoris may include isometrics (i.e., quad sets), SLR into hip flexion, varied ranges of concentric knee extension such as short and long arc quadriceps contractions, pulley resisted hip flexion or knee extension, and other progressive resistive hip flexion and knee extension isotonic exercise possibly using ankle weights or elastic resistance bands. Interventions for hamstring strengthening may include body weight only prone knee flexion, resisted knee flexion isotonic exercise (i.e. hamstring curl machine), and squats.

however there are some specific muscle groups requiring particular attention. Hip extension is particularly important at both the transfemoral and transtibial amputation (TFA and TTA, respectively) levels. Strong hip extension is important in sit to stand transfers, maintaining an upright posture, taking a full step length, and ascending stairs. Sample hamstring strengthening exercises include prone straight leg raises (SLRs) (Figure 8.3), bridging (Figure 8.4), and bridging on a physio ball (Figure 8.5). If a patient cannot bear weight through the involved side foot,

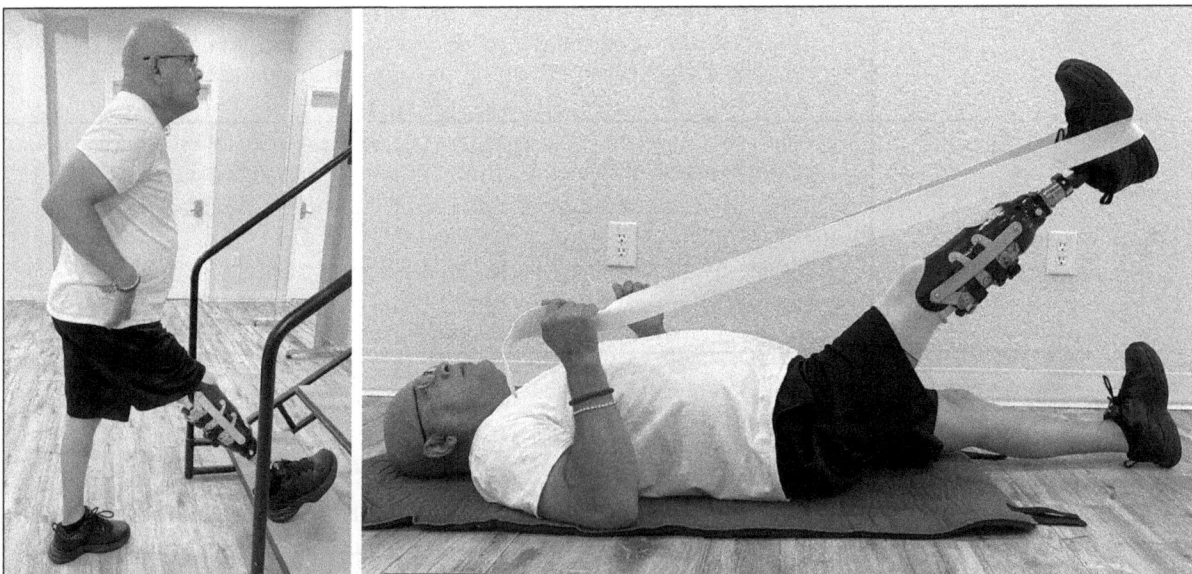

Figure 8.2. Sample stretches for the hamstrings to address knee flexion contracture.

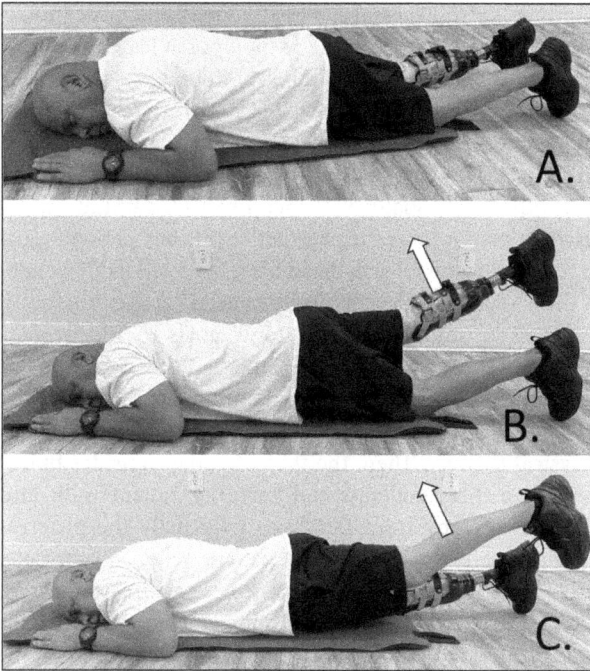

Figure 8.3. Prone straight leg raises. Start prone straight leg raises into extension in prone lying. Upper extremities can be straight out along the sides of the body or flexed as shown here. Both lower extremities are relaxed and in contact with the support surface (A). The participant can begin by raising either side first. Shown here (B), the prosthetic side is raised first. The limb is raised by contracting the extensor muscles (i.e. gluteal muscles and hamstrings) and the knee remains extended. Return to start. Both sides can be worked with this exercise (C).

Finally, core strengthening is universally important for patients with any level of lower extremity amputation. Sufficient core strength may reduce gait deviations such as lateral trunk bending. For the individual with bilateral TFA, adequate core strength may help reduce excessive lumbar lordosis. Core strengthening can begin at a basic level with muscle activation of core muscles such as the transverse abdominis (TrA) (i.e. drawing in the "belly") [5–7]. This can progress to more complex exercises such as maintaining TrA contraction while simultaneously performing a prone plank (Figure 8.6). This can further progress to maintenance of a TrA contraction with more complex dynamic exercise such as large ball roll outs. Core strength plays a role in prosthetic gait and eventually running with the prosthesis if so desired and able to do so. Core strength is also important in preventing low back pain, which is prevalent in the amputee population [8, 9].

Cardiovascular Fitness

Given that prosthetic ambulation requires greater energy than non-amputee gait, cardiovascular fitness must be targeted in rehabilitation [1, 10–12]. Developing and maintaining cardiovascular fitness is an important aspect of rehabilitation throughout the continuum of care for the patient with amputation. Cardiovascular exercise activities may include multiple types of cycle ergometers including an arm bike, recumbent bike, and combined upper

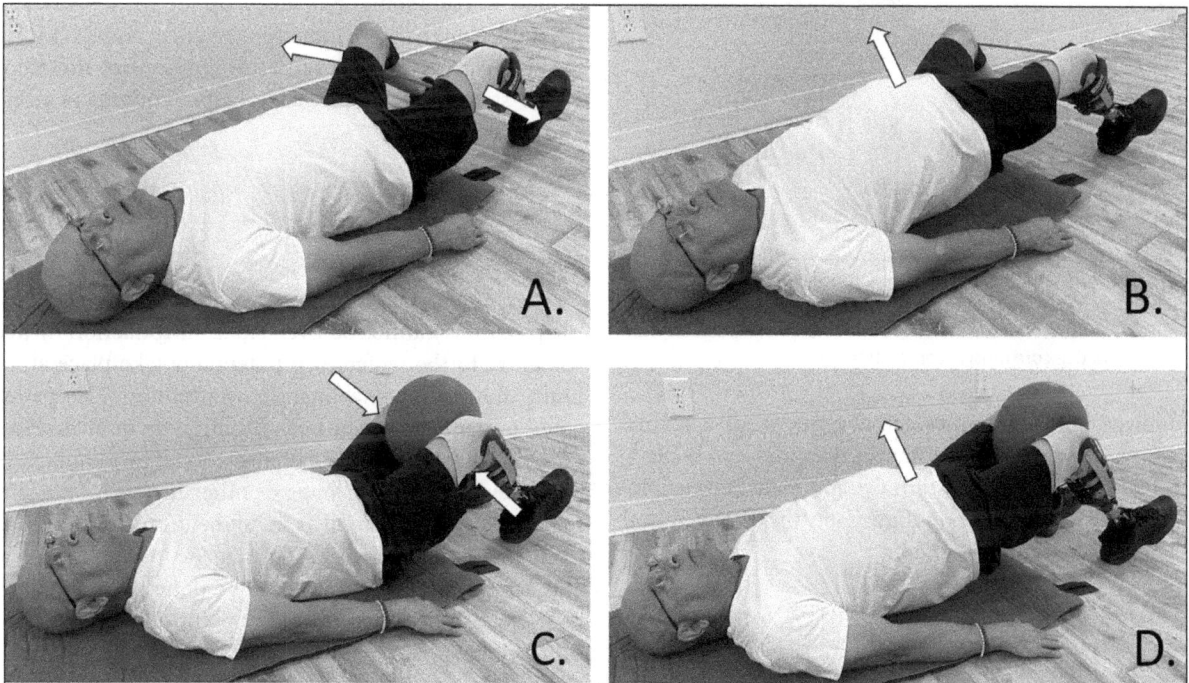

Figure 8.4. Bridging. In supine hook lying (knees flexed and feet on floor), abduct the thighs (A) then bridge upward (B). Return to start. This can be done without external resistance, or as pictured here (A and B) against resistance bands. Another variant of bridging is also in supine hook lying (knees flexed and feet on floor), adduct the thighs against the resistance of a ball (C), then bridge upward (D). Return to start.

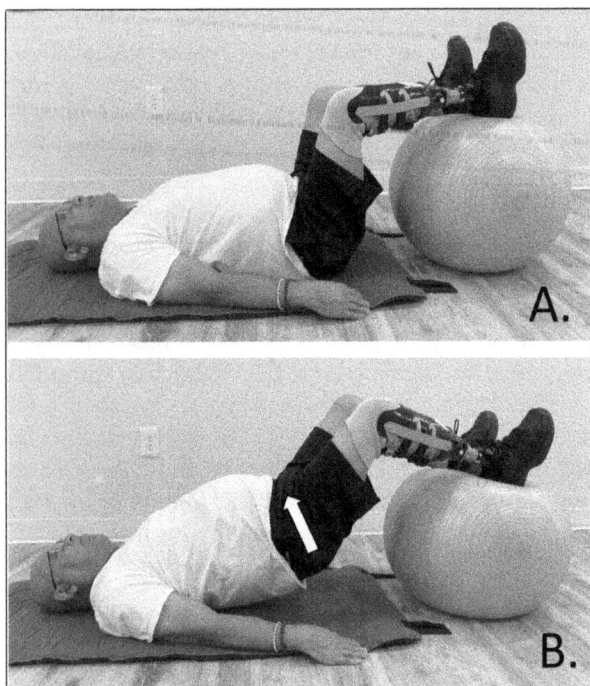

Figure 8.5. Bridging on a physio ball. In supine with heels resting on a physio ball, back is flat and in contact with ground or support surface and hips and knees flexed to approximately 90° (A), bridge up by pressing heels into physio ball and raise buttocks from ground (B). Return to start.

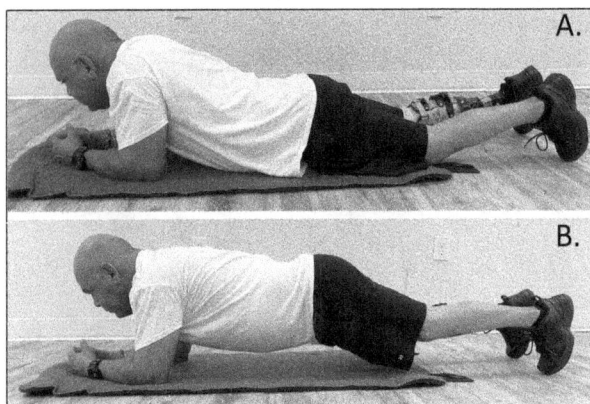

Figure 8.6. Patient with lower extremity prosthesis in prone plank position while contracting the transversus abdominus muscle. Rest position (A). Contracted plank position with active core muscle contraction (B).

and lower body ergometers. Other types of sub-maximal, repetitive exercise may be appropriate and accessible as well including rowing, swimming, and seated or standing elliptical ergometers, depending upon the involved limb and health status of the patient.

Gait, Balance, and Transfers

Pre-operatively, to the extent possible, the patient needs to continue to ambulate. Candidacy for walker or crutch ambulation needs to be determined. Wheelchair training is also necessary to assure safety and basic mobility in times when walking is not possible. However, if walking is feasible, it should be continued pre-operatively and restored as soon as possible post-operatively. Walking maintains a minimal level of cardiovascular conditioning, challenges balance, and facilitates core and extremity strength. Additionally, pre-operative gait training can be used as preparation for prosthetic gait. If a patient's goal is to be a successful prosthesis user, they will likely benefit if they continued to walk prior to receiving the prosthesis. Progressive ambulatory milestones/goals should be outlined and discussed with the patient and their family. For example, if deemed safe, the patient might be encouraged to leave the wheelchair in the waiting room and walk into physical therapy. Then, the therapist may consider building upon that challenge and have the patient walk into physical therapy from their car. Eventually the progression may evolve to having the patient, when appropriate, leave the wheelchair at their home when going to therapy. All of this is training toward reintegration that includes many different domains such as balance, transfer capabilities, functional strength, confidence, and independence. Safety and success are key in this process. Additionally, this sets the tone for ambulatory expectations for the post-operative state.

PHASE II: POST-OPERATIVE

The post-operative phase of amputee rehabilitation is the time period immediately after surgery while the patient is commonly still hospitalized. In this phase of rehabilitation there are numerous issues to address including skin care, ROM as it relates to positioning, functional ROM, strength, transfers, ambulation, equipment needs, and education.

Peer Visitor Programs

The importance of peer visitation and peer visitor programs cannot be overstated. Introduction of peer visitation to the patient can potentially take place at any point along the rehabilitation continuum. The patient could potentially initiate peer visitation themselves. However, it is most likely that patients will not be familiar with advocacy or support groups or other means of engaging this service. Therefore, it is incumbent on the healthcare team to assure peer visitation is made available, offered, and arranged. Again, this could be done pre-operatively, post-operatively, or really at any point during rehabilitation, though post-operatively is a common phase in which this is done.

Benefits of peer visitation are numerous. Creating the opportunity for a patient who has just experienced amputation to meet another person who has successfully learned to manage life with amputation(s), and reintegration following the experience and potentially prosthetic use, can be critically important. The patient can see that it is possible to become independent, to use a prosthesis, and to return to a meaningful quality of life. Additionally, the peer visit can be a place where information imparted to the patient by the healthcare team is reinforced by the peer visitor. New ideas about functional strategies, self-care, and other important topics may be discussed at levels differing from that afforded by providers. Some care should be taken to assure the personalities of the patient and peer visitor do not clash but these engagements are commonly beneficial.

Acute and Inpatient Post-Operative Care

Immediately after surgery, one major concern is keeping the patient free from infection. Preference for post-operative dressing varies by interdisciplinary care team and surgeon preferences; though rigid dressings are demonstrating improved outcomes [13]. There are three types of commonly used post-operative dressings: rigid, semi-rigid, and soft dressings. More technical aspects of post-operative dressings are reviewed in Chapter 4 of this text; however, a brief overview is provided here in the context of therapy. Rigid dressings are applied immediately after the surgery, in the operating room. Rigid dressings provide physical stump protection, and can help prevent contractures, such as a knee flexion contracture in the patient with TTA. They also help with edema management and can facilitate decreased pain. Rigid dressings are typically more expensive than other options and limit ready access for wound inspection.

Semi-rigid dressings are not as stiff as a rigid dressing but they may be more easily removable in some cases. They are more variable in their design, ranging from a simple plaster support splint secured with elastic bandaging to a pre-fabricated removable plastic shell. This latter system affords residual limb protection and edema management while also decreasing the risk of contractures and decreasing pain. Unlike rigid dressings, semi-rigid dressings afford easier access for skin inspection. Semi-rigid dressings are not as protective nor as expensive as rigid dressings.

Finally, soft dressings are not rigid and may use wound dressings such as petroleum impregnated gauze to decrease the risk of a draining wound adhering to the dressing. This may be covered by absorbent elastic bandaging then covered with a final layer of elastic bandaging. This is all commonly covered with and secured by elastic cloth bandaging. Soft dressings are not as protective as rigid and semi-rigid dressings. However, soft dressings are cost effective, afford the ability to provide selective tension, and are widely available.

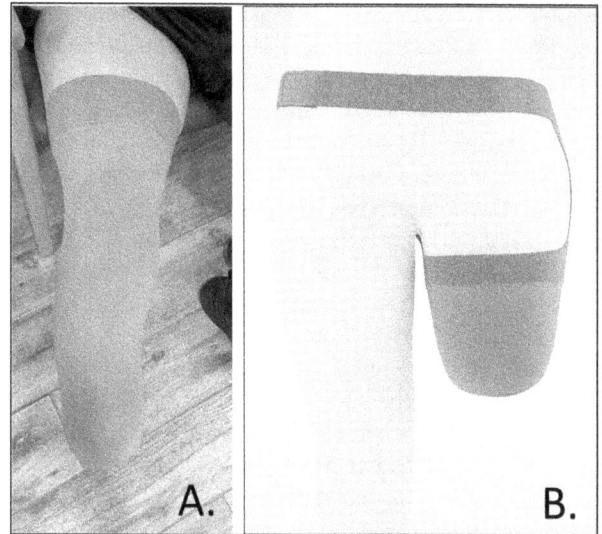

Figure 8.7. Shrinkers donned and displayed. Transtibial shrinker (A). Transfemoral shrinker with waist belt (B).

Sutures or staples are commonly removed 2 to 3 weeks after surgery. Patients are often fit with a shrinker following suture removal (Figure 8.7) Shrinkers are within the soft dressing family of volume management devices but should not be used until the wound is healed sufficiently such that tension on the incision line will not be problematic. They are donned like a sock so distal tension is created in the process which could be problematic for a healing incision. Shrinkers reduce volume and facilitate proper stump shaping. They are regarded as an acceptable volume management device post-healing and throughout many phases of rehabilitation.

Sound limb care should be emphasized in all phases but particularly post-operatively. This is because the patient will rely heavily on the sound limb for mobility. For instance, skin should be inspected daily. If the patient is unable to readily inspect the bottom of their foot, a long-handled mirror may facilitate the inspection. The patient should also be taught to check for any abrasions, scrapes, skin discoloration, or other visual abnormality. They should be encouraged to palpate for texture and skin temperature changes. If the patient has diabetic related or other sensory impairments on the bottom of their foot, they should be instructed not to walk without a shoe (i.e. bare foot). Precautions must be taken to preserve and protect the sound limb.

Range of Motion

Maintaining adequate ROM and preventing contractures is imperative for prosthetic related and general function. Specific joints and associated movements are particularly important to observe due to higher risk of restriction. Hip extension is a movement commonly restricted due to hip flexion contracture. Post-operatively, patients may want to keep the stump elevated to reduce swelling, but this can lead to a flexion contracture. Flexing the hip is commonly reported to be more comfortable post-operatively as well relative to keeping the hip in neutral. However, prolonged rest with the hip flexed will almost certainly result in a hip flexion contracture and limit hip extension.

Another common post-operative rest position that can lead to a hip flexion contracture is sitting in a wheelchair or sitting in general for extended periods of time. If the patient develops a hip flexion contracture, they will quite likely be unable to stand fully upright. The patient may also be unable to take a full-length step with the sound limb. The prosthetist is able to pre-flex the socket alignment to accommodate for some hip flexion contracture, however there is a limit to the benefit of a pre-flexed socket.

Still another hip movement at risk of restriction is internal rotation. In supine lying with knees extended and hips in neutral position, the hips tend to rotate laterally as evident by the toes pointing laterally. Extended bed rest with supine lying can lead to external hip rotation contracture. Towel rolls can be placed in the patient's bed and wheelchair to promote neutral hip rotation and minimize the risk of hip rotational contracture.

Patients need to maintain full knee extension as discussed previously. Patients report more comfort post-operatively with a pillow beneath the knee in supine resulting in knee flexion. However, prolonged rest in this position will likely lead to a knee flexion contracture. If the patient expresses concern about swelling and they insist on elevating their limb, the pillow needs to be placed distally on the limb so that the leg is elevated and the knee is fully extended.

Another common means of developing knee flexion contractures is from prolonged sitting. If the patient is seated for extended time periods during the initial healing phase, a knee flexion contracture can develop. It is important to educate the patient to keep their knee extended. If they are sitting in a wheelchair, a knee extension board can be ordered as part of the wheelchair prescription. When the patient is sitting at home, they must be instructed and disciplined to keep the knee extended as well. Only a modest quantity of knee flexion can be accommodated within a socket, so a lack of full knee extension complicates prosthetic fitting and function.

Knee flexion contractures further complicate the patient's ability to walk and can lead to gait deviations. A lack of knee extension makes it difficult to take a normal length sound-side step resulting in a generally shorter length step. This creates gait asymmetry which contributes to inefficiency, fatigue, and secondary overuse conditions such as pain. Intervention techniques include education in the prevention of joint contractures as well as stretching and ambulating with appropriate joint excursion. If a contracture is present, hip and knee joint as well as patellar mobilization may be useful along with physiological

mobilization such as hip internal rotation, manual stretching, prone lying on a wedge, stretching for the hip flexors, hamstring stretch, and quadriceps femoris. Home exercise should also be included relative to ROM.

Strength

Strength may be addressed in several phases of rehabilitation of the patient with amputation. During a hospital stay, strengthening may include active ROM (AROM) exercises in critical areas including the hip and knee. A common progression is to advance from AROM to AROM using resistive strengthening bands. Important movements that commonly receive focus in terms of strengthening include hip extension, abduction, and flexion. Core muscle strengthening is also important for prosthetic and other general function.

Transfers

Maximizing independence with transfers should be included in this phase of rehabilitation. Key functional transfer situations including bed, toilet, shower, bath tub, couch, recliner, and vehicle scenarios are important to include in assessment and training. It is advisable to begin with level surface transfers, and progress to un-level and compliant surface transfers. It is important to practice transfers such as toilet, shower chair, bathtub bench with bare buttocks, because this is how patients will truly perform them. Considerations include preserving patient modesty as well as opposite gender appropriateness. If the patient is leaving the hospital in a wheelchair, family training should be included regarding ascent and descent of curbs, ramps, and stairs as well as emergent situational preparedness. Vehicle transfers should also be practiced with the actual vehicle the patient and family will use.

Gait

Commonly, patients will ask when they will start walking. Under typical circumstances, ambulation may begin the day after amputation. This often starts with a rolling walker and progresses to crutches. It is important to practice ambulating in this manner over ramps, grass, carpet, up and down curbs and stairs, and any surface the patient is likely to encounter in their living environment. Gait training has many benefits including getting patients out of their wheelchair and minimizes wheelchair reliance, builds endurance, strength, and confidence. If the patient is a prosthesis candidate, walking without the prosthesis in this post-operative and pre-prosthetic period may allow the patient to learn to walk with a prosthesis more rapidly.

Assistive Devices

It is also important in the post-operative phase to consider the equipment the patient may need at hospital discharge. Common items the patient may need are an appropriately selected walking aid, a wheelchair (with leg board for the patient with TTA), and bathroom equipment. Patients with a prognosis favoring rapid return to ambulation with a prosthesis may be best served with a rented wheelchair whereas others may permanently require one. Bathroom equipment may include an elevated toilet seat or 3-in-1 commode, shower chair, or bathtub bench. If the patient has sensory issues, padded bathroom equipment may be indicated.

PHASE III: PRE-PROSTHETIC TRAINING

If healing continues favorably, the patient may be fit with a gel liner. The liner is likely the first prosthetic component the patient receives. Gel liners are one means of suspending a prosthesis and liners also cushion the limb during weight bearing in prosthetic stance. Providing a liner to the patient early pre-prosthetically has several benefits. First, emerging evidence demonstrates that silicone may have beneficial effects on scar tissue [14]. Additionally, if the patient's future prosthesis includes a gel liner, this element of donning, doffing, and maintenance will already be familiar to the patient while learning donning and maintenance of their entire prosthesis. The liner may also provide continuing benefits in terms of stump shaping and volume reduction. It generally takes time, several days in some cases, for the patient and their skin to acclimate to the donning, doffing, and maintenance processes as well as the material.

If it hasn't already happened, the patient will likely be discharged to home. Casting for a prosthetic socket may take place prior to discharge in the institutional setting or in an outpatient setting. Approximately 1 to 2 weeks after casting, the patient is fit with a temporary, or "test" socket. The prosthetist assures the socket is properly fitted. After confirmation that the socket is properly adjusted for the patient, the prosthetist will add the rest of the componentry completing the prosthesis.

Prosthetic gait training begins immediately following delivery of the properly fit prosthesis. Strength training, ROM exercises, cardiovascular conditioning, balance and gait training continue throughout this phase. As before, walking on varied terrains and speeds are included in gait training. Further, acceleration, deceleration, turning maneuvers, walking in complex environments, and walking while distracted are also included in gait training with the prosthesis.

Skin

Continue to emphasize the importance of wound inspection and cleanliness to the patient. The therapist should continue monitoring for signs of infection including erythema, warmth, swelling, discharge, and odor. Sound limb care should continue to be emphasized also, as previously discussed. This emphasis, monitoring, and education are important given the high prevalence of vascular pathology in the amputee population and the risk of losing the second limb within 2 to 3 years. Maintaining skin health and hygiene aims at prosthetic fitting and ambulation as soon as possible as well as sound limb preservation.

Range of Motion

As discussed in prior rehabilitation phases, adequate ROM is imperative to function. The risk of contractures is always present. Thus, monitoring for restriction and education for prevention remain important. Again, the common contractures include hip flexion, abduction, and external rotation, and in the patient with TTA, knee flexion contractures are also a persistent risk. Positioning, stretching, and activity are keys interventions to prevent contractures. Assure the stump is not propped into flexion with pillows while resting in bed and discuss this with the patient. For the patient with TTA, a leg board or knee extension board should be used when sitting in a wheelchair. Other interventions may include joint or other physiologic mobilization and stretching for involved muscles including the hip flexors and hamstrings. A home exercise program including stretching should also be considered. Finally, having the patient ambulate and do so with proper posture plays a role in decreasing contracture risk.

Residual Limb Shaping

As healing continues and the sutures are removed, shaping and shrinking the stump becomes increasingly important to prepare for fitting the prosthetic socket. Common stump shapes routinely observed are bulbous, conical, and cylindrical (refer back to Figure 4.1).

When the stump is bulbous shaped, the distal circumference is greater than the proximal circumference, which is a difficult shape to fit with a prosthesis. The bulbous shape likely occurs as a result of insufficient distal compression and proper or excessive proximal compression. This problematic bulbous shape may be set up with improper pressure gradients initially post-operatively or over the course of subsequent dressing changes through the pre-prosthetic period and up to the prosthetic fitting stage.

Another shape, the hourglass shape, sometimes occurs when there are proximal and distal circumferences greater than the mid portion of the stump. Like the bulbous shape, the hourglass shape can also be created starting post-operatively and across the pre-prosthetic period and up to prosthetic fitting. Commonly, the slender portion with the smallest circumference is around the bony area of the knee joint. The hourglass shape likely develops from applying greater tension to elastic bandaging in the mid-section of the stump with less tension proximally or distally. If the patient is using a shrinker, the proximal suspension band can create high tension leaving less tension proximally and distally also contributing to an hour glass shape.

Another common stump shape is conical. The conical shape occurs when the distal end is smaller in circumference than the proximal end. De-bulking of distal tissue mass during trauma or surgery can contribute to a conical shape. Further, excessively shortening the fibula in surgery can also contribute to a conical shape. Over time, muscle atrophy at the distal end of the stump may also be a factor in a limb that develops a conical shape over time.

The ideal stump shape is cylindrical. In this case the circumferences at various points along the length of the stump are very similar. This shape is most compatible with contemporary prosthetic interface designs and componentry. A cylindrical shape is the goal of stump shaping interventions.

Dog ears are another feature of some post-operative residual limbs. Dog ears are created when the tissue is closed during amputation surgery. The medial and lateral edges of the incision line may tend to not lay flat with the rest of the stump contour, resulting in abnormally shaped expansions. These expansions and abnormal contours are referred to as dog ears.

Common methods used to shape and shrink the stump include post-operative dressings and shrinkers as previously discussed. Rigid dressings are rigid casts placed on the stump immediately after surgery, and then periodically removed and the replaced to accommodate circumferential change.

Semi-rigid dressings afford modest protection and are more easily removable. They may be prefabricated or custom. Often, circumferential change is accommodated by increasing strapping or by adding prosthetic socks.

Elastic bandaging is a form of soft dressing that may be used to shrink and shape a limb. The pressure gradient should be applied such that greater pressure is applied distally with progressively less proximally. A figure of eight style of wrapping prevents a tourniquet effect. The advantage of limb wrapping with elastic bandaging is that shapes are readily accommodated, and pressure can be selectively applied over irregular shapes such as in the presence of dog ears and bulbous presentations. The disadvantages of elastic bandaging include the inability of some patients to re-apply the dressing, uneven pressure gradient leading to poor shaping or volume reduction or even skin breakdown. Further, soft dressings are not protective in the case of events such as falls.

At this phase, shrinkers may be considered provided the incision is healing well and sutures are removed. The advantage is that with reasonable dexterity and hand strength, they are simple to apply. Disadvantages include lack of protection, risk of proximal constriction, and the need to change the shrinker with considerable volume reduction due to their semi-custom sizing

Scar Tissue

After surgery, scar tissue adhesions could develop. This can result in a healed incision that is not mobile. Some clinicians suggest that scar tissue that is depressed below the level of the surrounding skin or scar may be adhered to deeper tissue layers and, consequently, immobile. At times a scar can be so depressed that it can contribute to skin breakdown as the skin folds in on itself becoming invaginated.

Scar mobility should be assessed and mobilized manually in all directions. Ideally, the scar should move easily in all directions. If movement is limited in a certain direction, mobilization in that particular direction is likely indicated.

Scar tissue massage is a method of tissue manipulation that includes, within its indications, mitigating adhesions and weakening scar tissue. Techniques vary; however, straight and circular motions along the incision line are fairly common. Scar tissue massage should only be performed on fully healed scars and should not be performed on an open wound.

Other interventions available to manage problematic scar tissue include Kinesio® taping techniques, use of silicone materials, as well as laser and inter-lesion steroid therapies [14]. More recently, ablative fractional CO_2 lasers are being used to improve stump scars in terms of reducing pain, topographic resurfacing, and improving cosmesis [15]. Adherent, keloid, or hypertrophic scarring can complicate socket fitting. Such problematic scars may be irritated when forces are applied to the tissue during prosthetic ambulation. This can continue to the point of pain and tissue breakdown. Beyond the interventions above, scar tissue massage can be incorporated into therapeutic treatment sessions as well as a home program whereby the patient can manipulate the scar as needed. This could potentially be done several times per day.

Pain

In the amputee population there are multiple types of pain to consider; however, two are somewhat unique— stump pain and phantom limb pain (PLP). Stump pain is commonly reported directly at the actual amputation site. Prescription or over the counter pain medications are commonly considered in the management of localized stump pain.

Conversely, PLP is associated with the limb that no longer exists. Currently, the mechanism of PLP is unknown. Therefore, PLP treatment is elusive. Management of PLP tends to be multi-modal [16]. Management commonly includes prescription medication, massage, transcutaneous electrical nerve stimulation, desensitization, compression, mirror therapy, and virtual reality rehabilitation.

Another type of potential limb discomfort is phantom limb sensation. This is an experience in which the patient senses that the limb is still in place even though it is amputated. This is not a pain experience, but can lead to discomfort or annoyance. For example, a patient may feel that their phantom toes are flexed and need to be straightened, resulting in discomfort but not necessarily pain. It is important to discuss phantom limb sensation and pain with patients because they may be embarrassed or reluctant to talk about it. Patients may feel as if something is wrong with them, because it is seemingly illogical to feel or have pain in a limb that is clearly no longer there. In some individuals, phantom limb pain and sensation may disappear over time. In others, these experiences can remain throughout their lifetime. When evaluating these sensory experiences, it is important to document a description of the sensation and when it occurs as well as its duration and frequency.

Following amputation, patients may develop hypersensitivity of the stump. Hypersensitivity includes magnification of light touch, for example, to the level of pain. One example may be magnification of contact such that a pain response is elicited when a bed sheet contacts the stump. This can be a considerable issue affecting prosthetic function because donning, doffing, wearing, and utilizing a prosthesis could be painful due to hypersensitivity regardless of the quality of the fit. Desensitization techniques are ideal for hypersensitivity. Desensitization may include rubbing a progression of materials such as a cotton ball, cotton T-shirt material, a towel, to eventually massaging the skin lightly and then more aggressively to eventually habituate or normalize the skin to touch. This desensitization can be done during clinic appointments but also as part of a home program.

Strength and Conditioning

Strengthening and conditioning in preparation for prosthetic gait training should address any areas of deficiency, with the hip, knee, and core being common focus areas.

For patients with amputation, adequate hip abduction strength is necessary to keep the pelvis level while walking and to minimize coronal gait deviations. Hip extension is important when rising to stand, ascending and descending stairs, and providing stability during stance phase. Hip flexion strength is important for forward advancement of the swing limb and for stair ascent. If the patient has a TTA, quadriceps femoris strength facilitates shock absorption and knee extension during stance phase and is important for stair ambulation as well as in rising to stand. Further, patients will require knee flexion strength for deceleration during the swing phase.

Core strength and stability is important to facilitate an appropriate upright posture and to decrease trunk contributions to gait deviations. In the post-operative phase, the patient likely performed AROM exercises and progressed to resistance band exercises. Core training may have targeted the transverse abdominis and lumbar stabilization. Now, in the pre-prosthetic phase, the patient should build on that foundation and progress the core training regimen as individually appropriate.

Stance phase in gait is a closed chain activity. It is ideal to strength train in closed chain positions as shear stress at the joint can be reduced and the exercises better simulate real-world function. An example of a closed chain exercise is supine bridging with adduction, which emphasizes hip extension. To perform the exercise, the patient should lie supine with a bolster beneath both lower extremities. The patient should push both thighs into the bolster and raise the buttocks. For patients with more extensor weakness, the bolster may be placed more proximal on the thigh. If the patient has stronger extensor strength and has a longer residuum, the bolster may be placed more distally on the thigh or distal to the knee. The patient should not use their arms to compensate for lack of gluteal and extensor strength. As the patient's strength improves, they can bridge and raise one leg up, approximately four extra inches, by flexing the hip, then eccentrically lower the leg and then raise the other leg with hip extension, then down again finally lowering the buttocks back to the mat. The therapist is advised to monitor for compensatory movements as the patient is exercising. For instance, as the patient alternates leg raising, the hips may rotate transversely or drop due to weakness. Similar bridging exercise can be done in side lying to strengthen hip abduction and prone to strengthen the hip flexors if necessary. As the patient's transverse abdominis is strengthened and increases in endurance, specific core strengthening exercises are suggested such as transverse abdominis drawing in [6, 7, 17]. Basic contraction is the first activity when emphasizing such muscles followed by a progression to contraction while simultaneously performing more advanced bridging exercises such as those previously described. If transversus abdominis drawing in becomes less challenging due to a training effect, other options are available. For instance, selecting other starting positions and moving the extremities in other directions during contraction may be beneficial. The therapist is encouraged to use their imagination to relate the exercise to function and the patient's impairments and goals.

Balance

Another area to address in preparation for prosthetic gait training is balance. Balance training plays a role in gait stability and fall prevention. In order to transfer and walk safely with an assistive device, the patient with lower extremity amputation (LEA) will require sufficient sound limb balance. Balance activities can be performed in short and long sitting, tall kneeling, and standing. Examples of balance activities include sitting on a physio ball and performing resisted rows with a resistance band, long sitting on a large bolster while tossing and catching a weighted ball and using a trampoline as the rebounder, resisted walking in tall kneeling, standing on compliant surfaces, and more (Figure 8.8). These are merely a few examples, however there are many more options to improve balance including gaming platforms, instrumented posturography, and other clinical intervention means.

Transfers

Level and slightly unlevel surface transfers at this stage may be at a modified independent level. Transfers at this stage that many LEA patients may require assistance with are those on unlevel surfaces. Transfers such as wheelchair to floor, couch to floor, and sit to stand tend to be challenging in this patient population. If a patient should fall, the patient needs to know how they can get back up. Falling becomes less frightening if a person knows what to do after the fall. If the patient has limited strength, family training may be indicated to assist the patient in transferring from the floor safely. If the patient has good strength, a couch to floor transfer may be a reasonable starting scenario because usually a couch seat is generally closer to the ground than a wheelchair seat and thus less challenging to transfer up to. For the couch transfer, if the starting point is with the patient seated on the couch, the patient will scoot to the edge of the seat and lower themselves to the floor with the upper extremities. Once on the ground, in order to return to the couch, the patient should move to a hands and knees position facing the couch. The patient should then place one arm at a time on the couch. Then, the patient should push down using their arms and leg and rotate into the seat. If the gap between the floor and the couch is too great, then progression from a shorter, but sturdy surface should be considered as an intermediate step. As the patient gets stronger and more confident, progressing from floor to wheelchair is necessary. In this scenario, similar to the couch scenario, an intermediate, shorter surface may be necessary. Practicing these types of transfers is helpful for function at this stage but may also be foundational in preparing the person to practice floor to stand transfers with their prosthesis. While the ultimate

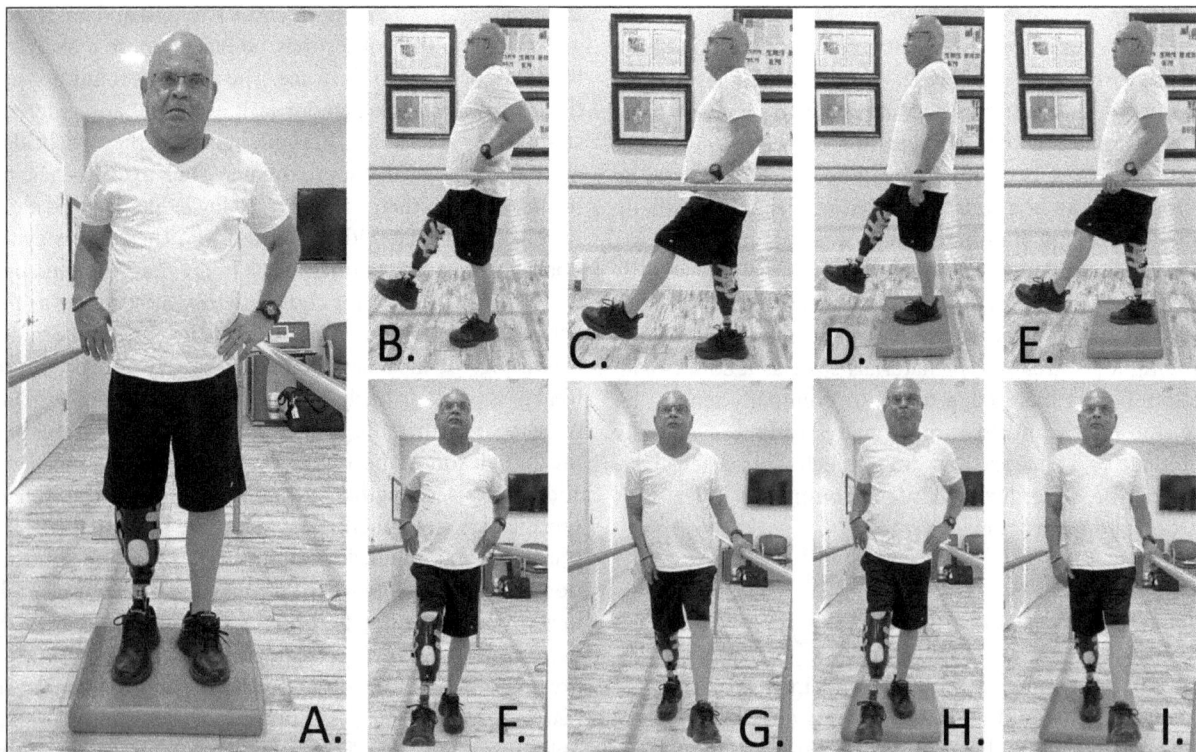

Figure 8.8. Sample balance exercises. Bilateral standing on a compliant surface (A); unilateral sound limb standing, floor support—sagittal view (B); unilateral prosthetic limb standing, floor support—sagittal view (C); unilateral sound limb standing, compliant surface—sagittal view (D); unilateral prosthetic limb standing, compliant surface—sagittal view (E); unilateral sound limb standing, floor support—coronal view (F); unilateral prosthetic limb standing, floor support—coronal view (G); unilateral sound limb standing, compliant surface—coronal view (H); unilateral prosthetic limb standing, compliant surface—coronal view (I).

goal for many LEA patients is to walk, gait may be very limited or not deemed safe. However, the use of a prosthesis for transfers can still lead to greater independence and less reliance on caregivers for mobility.

Gait

Patients who have lost a lower extremity may believe they are not capable of ambulation at this point. Of course, most envision prosthetic ambulation at some point in the future. However, during the time before the person receives a prosthesis, it is important that they build standing tolerance as well as ambulatory strength and endurance. Progressively improving the patient's walking stability and distance may result in reasonably rapid accomplishments such as walking into physical therapy as opposed to coming to therapy in a wheelchair. Gait training and prosthetic mobility at this point are important such that prosthetic ambulation potentially becomes the primary mode of locomotion as opposed to the wheelchair. This includes supervised ambulation over different ground surfaces and environmental obstacles including tile, carpet, curbs, ramps, stairs, rocks, roots, asphalt, slopes, and grass. It is important to practice ambulation on surfaces that the patient will encounter in their daily life. In doing so, the patient will have the best opportunity for success with prosthetic ambulation.

PHASE IV: PROSTHETIC TRAINING

This is commonly a focal point in therapy and tends to be a very exciting time for the patient with amputation. Donning their first prosthetic limb for the first time is commonly a memorable and anticipated milestone within their life. For many this represents a tangible step toward independence or as many describe it, "*getting their life back again.*" Further, this can be a very emotional point for the patient and their family.

Hygiene

When the patient is in therapy with their prosthesis for the first time, it is important to discuss basic prosthesis and residual limb care and hygiene as well as application and care of the gel liner and prosthetic socks if used. The liner is a pliable sleeve, commonly made from gels such as silicone, urethane or others, that directly contacts the skin of the residual limb. The liner should be cleaned daily. Generally, the inside of the liner is cleaned with mild soapy water. It is then rinsed clean and dried on a drying stand. It is routinely advised to clean the liner with the same soap

that is used to clean the skin. For specific cleaning instructions, it is recommended to discuss the process with the prosthetist and to read the manufacturer's instructions for the specific liner. In many but not all systems, prosthetic socks are donned next, upon the liner, to accommodate for circumferential volume loss. Prosthetic socks are ideally hand-washed in mild soapy water, rinsed clean, and air dried. Prosthetic socks may be machine washed and dried but this could also damage and wear the socks prematurely. Prosthetic socks can be washed less frequently than liners as they do not always contact the skin directly. Washing socks weekly may be adequate unless they contact the skin or become soiled. The prosthetic socket can be wiped down with a soapy wash cloth and rinsed with a clean wash cloth. The socket can likely be cleaned weekly unless soiled. Certain cases may require different cleaning instructions. Ultimately, the component manufacturer's cleaning instructions should be followed. Additionally, the prosthetist may be consulted for advice. Maintaining good skin and prosthetic hygiene may help prevent skin irritation or infections that could lead to prosthetic disuse or larger health complications [18–20].

Skin

Prior to beginning, during, and after prosthetic training the skin should be checked. Inspect the skin before donning the prosthesis so the baseline appearance is known. Observe such qualities as the color, presence, location, and quantity of swelling, maceration, abrasions, or other notable findings. Patients with particularly delicate skin, such as burned or grafted skin or scar tissue, may require even more caution and more frequent inspection throughout a treatment session. Assessment during the prosthetic treatment session will provide insight into how the skin is managing the stresses of prosthetic gait training and mobility. It also reveals the quality of the prosthetic fit. The skin should always be inspected again upon completion of the therapy session.

When the patient receives the prosthesis, the person is not to don the prosthesis and wear it all day. This will likely result in skin breakdown. Skin breakdown delays prosthetic gait training as the patient may likely have to disuse the prosthesis until the skin heals. Further, the wound introduces elevated infection risk, and in some cases could potentially lead to more proximal amputation [19]. Therefore, to protect the skin, a prosthetic wearing schedule is advised for patient's receiving their first prosthesis. A wearing schedule informs the rehabilitation team and the patient how long they can wear their prosthesis, and how long they should rest from prosthetic use. An example might be that on the first day, the patient should use the prosthesis for 1 hour on and then rest the limb by being out of the prosthesis for 1 hour. If that was successful, on the second day it may increase to 2 hours of wear time followed by a 1 hour out-of-prosthesis rest period. Eventually, this schedule can progress to the point that the patient is gradually increasing their activity without compromising the skin and is thus integrating into the activities indicated in their goals. Conversely, if the skin begins to look irritated or red or it becomes painful, the wearing time should be decreased until the skin is no longer irritated. With delicate skin, the wearing schedule may start out even shorter than previously described. For instance, 10–30 minutes of wear followed by a 1 hour rest period may be a reasonable starting point. Because there is currently not a widely adopted wearing schedule, each patient's wearing schedule must be individually tailored to the patient's unique attributes.

Donning

There are numerous prosthetic suspension components, methods, and styles. It is recommended to discuss the patient's particular suspension with their prosthetist in advance of the initial therapy session. At the same time, the therapist can discuss the patient's ability to don their prosthesis. Comorbidities can negatively impact a patient's physical and/or cognitive function, limiting their ability to don their prosthesis. Gaining this information proactively allows the therapist to be prepared for the first session to optimize outcomes and assure proper donning and function. This is also in the best interest of safety to mitigate potential prosthetic malfunction, loss of suspension, pistoning (step to step loss of suspension wherein the limb repeatedly moves in and out of the socket), skin trauma, or other issues. Some common suspension systems include sleeve suspension, pin locking, negative pressure, and lanyard systems.

Commonly, when using *sleeve suspension*, the sleeve is doubled over and inside-out on the distal end of the prosthesis to facilitate donning. Donning such a prosthesis then routinely occurs as follows: 1) don the gel liner; 2) don prosthetic socks as needed; 3) place RL into the socket; 4) roll up the sleeve that is on the distal end of the prosthesis so the sleeve covers the liner and the socks and touches skin proximal to the liner (see Figure 8.9). Sleeve suspension is a very common suspension strategy at the TTA level, but is used less frequently at the TFA level. Sleeve suspension is also used as a supplement to another form of suspension to guarantee that the prosthesis stays on, particularly during more strenuous activities such as running.

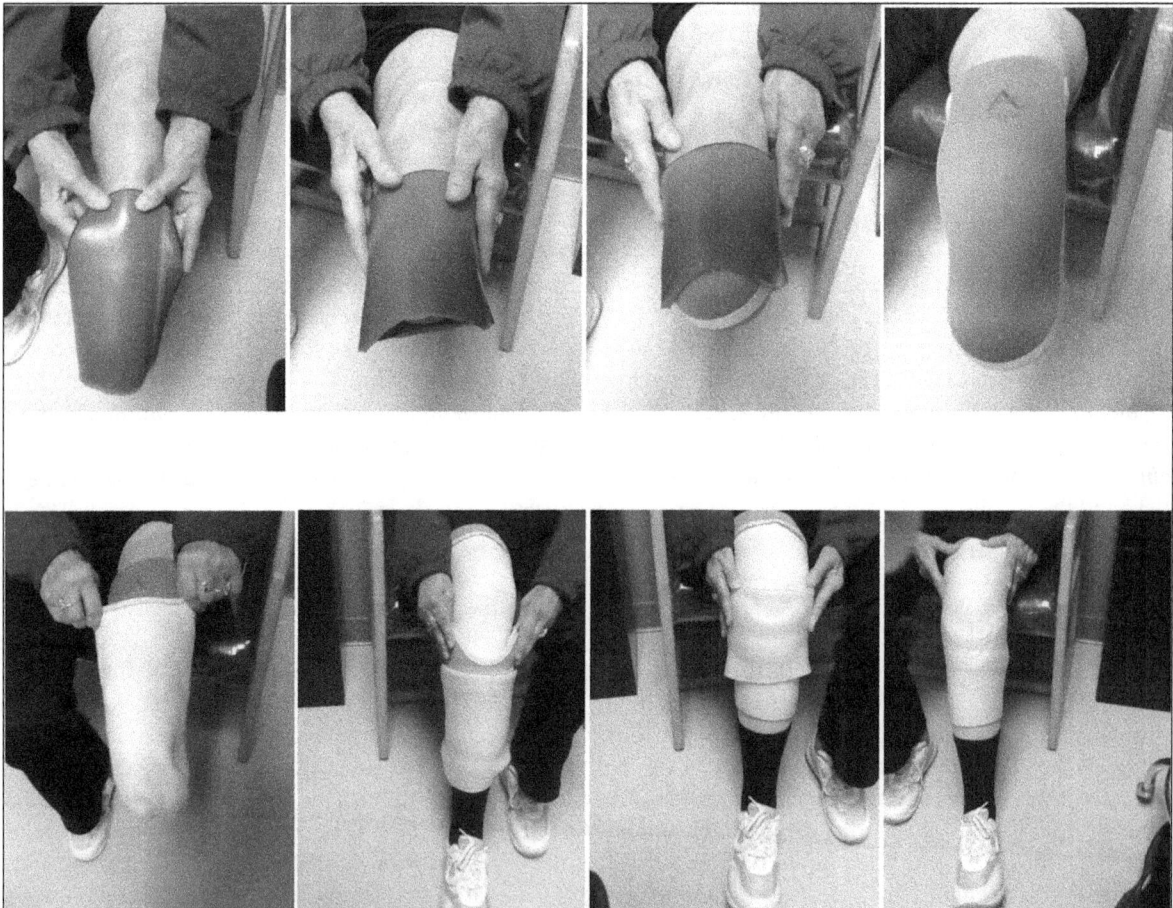

Figure 8.9. Donning a transtibial prosthesis with sleeve suspension and gel liner.
Photo Courtesy of David Hughes of Cornerstone Prosthetics & Orthotics. Everett, WA, U.S.A.

Another common form of suspension is the *pin lock* suspension. In this method of suspension, a pin is attached to the distal end of the liner that will couple into a hole at the distal end of the socket. Donning a pin lock system occurs as follows. 1) The liner is donned by rolling on from distal to proximal. The pin is attached to the distal end of the liner. 2) Prosthetic socks are donned as needed. Prosthetic socks used with pin systems should have a hole at the bottom of the sock to accommodate protrusion of the pin. Prosthetic socks can be ordered by the prosthetist with a hole already in the sock or the hole may need to be cut to avoid fraying and material strands getting caught in the socket lock. 3) The RL is placed into the socket. 4) As the RL goes into the socket, the pin should be lined up with the hole in the socket locking mechanism. Some pin lock systems may produce an audible click (or clicks) to cue the user that the prosthesis is secure. Others may require manipulating the lock on the outer surface of the prosthesis and still others may provide no feedback. It is always recommended that the prosthetist be consulted regarding the type (if any) feedback the particular system provides and means to assure the limb is secure prior to utilizing the prosthesis. Some potential advantages with certain pin lock suspension are audible or palpable feedback indicating a securely donned limb. When provided, this feedback can increase confidence for the user that the prosthesis will not fall off. Further, relative to sleeve suspension, pin lock systems result in less bulk posterior to the knee. This likely improves comfort and knee movement. A potential disadvantage is that pin lock systems commonly produce suction distally on the RL which is uncomfortable or painful to some users. The skin should be assessed regularly for this possibility to avoid complications. Thus, users with grafted skin or focal sensitivity may experience difficulty with pin lock systems, warranting consideration of other suspension options. Persons with TFA may also use this type of suspension.

Negative pressure is still another means of suspending a prosthesis. There are a few means of achieving negative pressure suspension of a prosthesis. Two sub-categories of negative pressure include suction and vacuum. Examples include utilization of external pumps, seals, and one-way suction valving, etc. As previously mentioned, the prosthetist should always be consulted for instruction and education on the particular system utilized. This section will describe the donning process for the seal and one-way valve system which is donned as follows. 1) The liner is donned. Some liners have an integrated rubber seal distally and others have a separate circular rubber seal that is placed on the liner after the liner is donned. If the seal is a separate removable item, place the seal more proximally on the liner or as recommended by the prosthetist. 2) Don prosthetic socks as needed. Prosthetic socks used in suction systems cannot cover the rubber seal as the seal must contact the socket wall. Such prosthetic socks look tubular in that they lack a rounded distal end. 3) Lubricate the

rubber seal. Commonly isopropyl alcohol is used but other lubricants may be used as recommended by the prosthetist. 4) Place the RL into the socket. 4) The person will then slightly piston the RL up and down into the socket and press the release valve of the prosthesis to evacuate air thereby securing the RL into the socket. To check that the RL is all the way into the socket, the valve at the distal end of the socket can be opened. There should not be a gap between the RL and the socket as viewed from the valve opening. Any gapping indicates the RL is not fully in the socket. Inspecting in this manner requires loss of negative pressure. Therefore, negative pressure must be re-established prior to utilization of the limb.

Another form of suspension is the *lanyard* system. In this system there is usually some form of belt or strap attached to the liner. The socket will have a hole for the lanyard to pass through and the lanyard is then secured with some form of locking mechanism, such as a belt buckle, cleat, ratchet system, Velcro®, etc. Donning a lanyard system is accomplished by first donning the liner. Next, if used, prosthetic sock(s) are donned. There will be a hole distally in the sock to permit the strap to pass from the distal liner through the sock. The RL, with liner and socks, is then placed into the socket. The lanyard is then passed through the hole in the socket and secured in the locking mechanism. One benefit of this suspension method, once secured, is that beyond suspension, it limits transverse socket rotation.

Limb Volume

Patients' RLs will likely change in size throughout the course of their rehabilitation and probably throughout the rest of their lives. Acutely post-operatively, the RL is likely to be swollen and edematous. Commonly, near the time of discharge from acute post-operative rehabilitation, the RL is likely to have reduced considerably in size. At some point after the incision area heals, the patient may transition from elastic bandaging to a shrinker sock and volume reduction continues. Eventually, in prosthetic candidates, the temporary prosthesis is fit. Under usual circumstances, the associated use and weight bearing further reduce limb volume. As the socket (temporary or definitive) becomes loose due to volume loss, prosthetic socks are used to accommodate in the reduced RL size. To a certain extent, this restores total contact, the fit, and comfort in many cases.

Most of the time prosthetic socks come in 1, 3, and 5 ply. When a patient dons their prosthesis, the RL should feel snug but not constricting tight. The socket should not be loose allowing aberrant socket translation or rotation about the RL. Pistoning is an example of an aberrant movement due to poor fit that can cause issues with skin, comfort, and function. Therefore, the patient should utilize enough socks to keep tension values appropriate between the residual limb and socket.

For the transtibial amputee, the standard of care is total contact. However, most of the contact pressure is concentrated through the patellar tendon. Toward the anterior distal end of the socket is a protrusion meant to support the limb at the patellar tendon. As the patient's RL shrinks, it sinks deeper into the socket. When this happens, patients may likely begin to feel pressure on the patella, the patellar tendon, or possibly at the distal end of the limb. This can be uncomfortable or even painful. To mitigate this change in limb size, prosthetic socks should generally be added. Adding stump socks increases the diameter of the limb which ideally decreases focal loading at the patella and distal end and equalizes the pressure distribution about the entire limb. Patients sometimes learn very simply that if socks are added, pain is decreased. Other times, too many socks can increase focal pressure causing discomfort in other areas. For instance, the patient may feel pressure on the tibial shaft because the RL becomes too elevated in the socket. In such a case the patient needs to remove socks.

Similarly, for the transfemoral amputee, the RL also needs to be appropriately snug within the socket. As the transfemoral limb shrinks, it moves deeper into the socket. The patient may likely experience pressure from the medial socket wall on the ischiopubic ramus, a very pressure intolerant area. Adding socks restores the pressure gradient and tends to lift the pelvic elements away from the medial socket brim. Patients' learning when to add and subtract prosthetic socks takes time, practice, and experience.

Pressure Relief

There are specific anatomic areas on a RL that tend to be better suited to endure pressure and other areas that are less tolerant. For the TTA, pressure tolerant areas commonly include patellar tendon, medial tibial flare, lateral tibial flare, and the gastro-soleus region. Pressure intolerant areas often include the fibular head, distal end of the fibula, and hamstring tendons. For the TFA, pressure tolerant areas include the ischial tuberosity, medial femoral flare, and lateral femoral flare. Pressure intolerant areas commonly include the pubic ramus, adductor tendon, greater trochanter, and pubic tubercle. In gait training the majority of the pressure for the TTA is borne through the patellar tendon. For the TFA, the majority of the pressure is borne through the ischial tuberosity.

Weight Shifting

An important foundational skill in prosthetic gait training is weight shifting. Efficient and symmetrical gait patterns include optimal weight shifting. Some prosthesis users who achieve ideal weight shifting capabilities may be able to walk with long pants on, and onlookers may be unaware they are an amputee. Therapeutic weight shifting includes a linear shift of the shoulder and hip over the foot. After the amputation surgery and prior to prosthetic gait training, the patient may have been walking using crutches or a rolling walker. Walking in this manner brings the sound limb directly beneath the body. The prosthesis user may then begin incorporating this type of walking as their routine walking pattern. When the amputee receives their prosthesis, it is important to initiate weight shifting activities in front of a mirror. Upon standing up, prosthesis users may perceive bilaterally equal weight bearing but in fact may be asymmetrically shifted to the sound side. The mirror provides visual cueing of their actual position and what a bilaterally symmetric weight shift really looks like. The patient's sound limb needs to be properly positioned beneath the appropriate hip pelvis. The limb should not be outside of the hip or base of support. Weight shifting activities commonly start in parallel bars with a mirror in front. A routine initiating activity is simple side to side weight shifting without moving the feet with both hands supporting on the parallel bars. It is important to focus the patient's attention on the hip being over the foot and shoulder being over the foot. The hip does not shift beyond the foot and, similarly, the shoulder does not shift beyond the hip and foot. Sometimes the patient's attention can be focused on the sound side weight shift so they can realize important points of emphasis for quality weight shifting. Then, the patient can duplicate the weight shift on the amputated side. Weight shifting can be progressed from side to side with feet symmetrically placed to shifting with the sound foot ahead of the involved foot. Shifting back over the rear foot can be incorporated and, finally, shifting toward the forefoot can be important as well. Shifting forward has potential risks in some cases such as those using an above knee prosthesis particularly in the case of knees that flex with toe loading. In such cases, prior to initiating a weight shift forward, the knee mechanism and risks should be discussed. Further, support with the hands on parallel bars should be used in most cases on initial introduction to this task. In addition to safety, proper technique and good form should always be emphasized. Step-ups are one potential activity to progress to after weight shifting. Beginning to progressively remove upper extremity support (i.e. progress from two hand support to one hand to no hand support as appropriate) from the parallel bars are potential next steps in a progression. There are many weight shifting activities that the patient can train with and advance to. Progression to more complex activities should occur following mastery and consistency of performance of prior and current activities.

Balance

Balance is another aspect of prosthetic use and gait training that should routinely be assessed and is often in need of intervention. Regularly, as the patient masters weight shifting, weight shifting and step-up activities begin to rely more on dynamic balance. For example, as the patient is performing weight shifting, balance can be challenged by the addition of throwing and catching a ball in parallel bars. This may be done with the feet both flat on the ground or from a step-up position. An early activity may include tapping a balloon then progressing to catching a ball to eventually to catching a weighted ball. Further progressing to use of a rocker board within parallel bars may assist the patient to determine if they have equal weight on each foot by means of keeping the board level. Keeping the rocker board level while simultaneously performing upper extremity tasks (i.e. shooting baskets, throwing and catching a ball) also challenges dynamic balance. Other balance activities to consider may include walking on a balance beam, standing on compliant surfaces, kicking a ball, stepping over hurdles and others. Challenging the patient to stand on the prosthesis for 30 s without losing balance may be a goal to facilitate a progression toward possible running participation. If the patient has a specific hobby or activity interest, consider linking the patient's therapeutic balance intervention activities with these. If the patient played golf, then consider discussing and working on putting for example. The combination of a thorough patient history coupled with creativity in the selection of intervention commonly reveals a broad selection of possible balance activities.

Motor Coordination

The ability to place the feet in non-traditional places while balancing and walking is one factor in lower extremity coordination. Along with balance, coordination is another aspect of prosthetic gait training that plays a considerable role in efficiency of movement and fall prevention. Cross-over (i.e. braiding) stepping, beginning in the parallel bars and progressing to overground outside the parallel bars, is one potential example of a coordination intervention. Ladder drills such as two step, side stepping, in/out, and zig zag stepping are additional coordination drills to consider. Changes in speed, starting and stopping quickly, are more dynamic and unpredictable and advanced coordination intervention drills to consider. The prosthesis user encounters these scenarios in daily life such as when shopping in the grocery store or mall or when ambulating in crowds such as when attending a sporting event.

Sport and Recreation

As the patient progresses in therapy in terms of strength, balance, coordination and all other domains leading to improved overall functional ability, if they plan on running and returning to sport, agility needs to be part of the intervention plan. For example, teaching patients how to cut and change directions and creating practice opportunities to master these skills is important. Consider beginning by teaching proper form and then increasing speed of movement while maintaining proper form during activity. Implementation of these activities will likely challenge health- (i.e., strength, endurance) and skill- (i.e., balance, agility) related fitness domains.

Gait

It is always impressive to see a prosthesis user ambulate while wearing long pants and noticing that onlookers are seemingly unaware the person walking has an amputation and uses an artificial limb. There are numerous factors that determine the feasibility of such an outcome. Gait training is one potential factor.

Gait is a multidimensional task. A more in-depth discussion about prosthetic gait, gait deviations, and the causes of prosthetic gait deviations—both amputee and prosthetic related—can be found elsewhere in this textbook. The purpose for discussing prosthetic gait in this section is therefore to consider key points of interest for the therapist when applying gait training interventions for the lower extremity prosthetic user. For the TFA for example, it is very important to understand what initiates prosthetic knee flexion, extension, and locking in preparation for ambulation. If the therapist is unfamiliar with how a prosthetic knee functions, they should discuss knee function with the prosthetist. Commonly, there are fewer minute adjustments with mechanical knee users relative to microprocessor prosthetic knee users. Points of interest during gait assessment of the lower extremity prosthetic user include symmetrical weight shift, step length, stance time, upright posture, and reciprocal trunk movement. As the patient begins to walk, typically they will shift more to the sound side and not fully or symmetrically weight shift onto the prosthesis. Mirrors may be used to show the patient visually what a proper weight shift looks like and how they are actually moving during ambulation. The patient may need to be asked or cued to weight shift more to the prosthetic side compared with the sound limb. Depending upon their acuity, progress, and perception, the amputee may report that doing so feels awkward. As previously discussed, it takes time for the body to re-establish a proper body image.

Another point of interest to consider is step length and stance time. Equal or symmetric step length and stance time are commonly desired. Sometimes however, the patient will take a long step with the prosthetic side and a short step on the sound limb. This could be due to the amputee's distrust or discomfort with their prosthesis. Thus, the user likely wishes to minimize prosthetic standing and maximize sound limb standing. Also, for the transfemoral prosthesis user, taking a longer prosthetic step may allow the patient to make sure the prosthetic knee is extended and is therefore less likely to buckle. Perhaps the patient takes a shorter sound side step. This could be for numerous reasons but one is a residual limb hip flexion contracture.

As the prosthesis user ambulates, gait analyses should assess for full upright posture and lateral leaning. The patient may have weak hip abductors, a potential reason for a lateral lean, or there may be socket fitting issues such as an excessively tall medial socket brim. Further, the patient may not wish to shift weight fully onto the socket. Another factor to evaluate is reciprocal trunk movement. In some cases, reciprocal trunk movement is obvious, and the arms are observed to be swinging reciprocally and in the usual manner. Arm swing serves as a means to decelerate pelvic rotation. So if the arms are swinging appropriately and symmetrically, there is a good chance the pelvis is also rotating appropriately and symmetrically. Arm swing may also be asymmetric or of diminished magnitude. Additionally, arm swing may be mistaken for shoulder movement in cases where the pelvis is rotating in a diminished magnitude or asymmetrically. In summary, gait training intervention should be determined as a result of history, goals, and a thorough gait evaluation.

Activities of Daily Living (ADLs)

In addition to considering gait training, it is very important to focus on function and, specifically, function in performing activities of daily living (ADLs). Some examples include the ability to perform transitional movements such as sitting down and standing up. To be able to be independent around the living environment, it is important, for example, to be able to sit for toileting as well as to be able to rise to standing. For males, the ability to stand to urinate is important and requires manipulative hand skills for clothing fasteners, static and dynamic balance, and potentially the ability to manage an assistive device. Staying with the example of sitting and standing, the ability to sit and stand to and from different types of seats and surfaces and at different heights is also important.

Ambulation on different environmental obstacles such as stairs, ramps of different slope, curbs, and others will facilitate enhanced community engagement. Practice with these obstacles should include ascent, descent, and use of different support (i.e. single and double railing, assistive device, etc.). High functioning transtibial prosthesis users may be able to ascend or descend ramps and stairs with either foot leading. However, for most prosthesis users and for those initially learning these skills, it may

be helpful to descend with the prosthesis first and ascend with the sound limb first. If necessary, initial practice may start with a step-to gait pattern on stairs with the intent to progress to a reciprocal climbing pattern if appropriate. When the amputee is descending a step or a curb and the sound limb descends first, it is sometimes helpful if the prosthetic foot is partially off the step or curb as the sound limb descends. Having the toes off the step's leading edge may enable the amputee to roll more smoothly over the prosthetic foot.

For the transfemoral prosthesis user, the type of prosthetic knee is a considerable factor in stair, ramp, and curb ambulation. Generally, transfemoral prosthesis users are initially taught to descend first with the prosthetic side and to ascend first with the sound limb using a step-to gait pattern. However, depending on the type of prosthetic knee it may be possible to descend stairs reciprocally, or to ascend reciprocally [21–25]. As previously mentioned, descent with the toes of the prosthesis over the step's leading edge may ease the ability to transition over the foot and down to the next step [24]. When the therapist is uncertain of the functional capabilities of a prosthetic component, such as knees or feet, it is advised to consult with the collaborating prosthetist to discuss component capabilities, the engagement of the features, and other related issues.

Beyond the previously described tasks, it is important to have the patient ambulate on a variety of terrains such as grass, gravel, sand, hills, and ramps. Consider advancing the ambulatory skills further by completing the tasks at different speeds, turning randomly during the task, or by adding mental distractions such as walking and simultaneously talking or having the patient manipulate their cellular phone. Still additional challenges may include increasing the distance of therapeutic walking sessions, carrying objects during gait, and adding more barriers and variability progressively.

As culminating interventions in gait training, consider taking the patient on functional outings. Examples include shopping at large retail or grocery stores, sharing lunch, or going to a movie. Have the patient practice carry a tray with food and drink, which can be difficult not to imbalance or drop. Have them practice remembering to get a napkin and condiments before sitting. These are all functional scenarios that further enhance community engagement and reintegration.

Advancing to increased levels of activity during prolonged gait training may lead to volume change, thus creating educational opportunities in applied volume management. The prosthesis user may begin to notice the reduced volume and suffer potential discomfort. The therapist should take the opportunity to educate the patient on the optimal volume management strategy for the patient's unique case. Examples include stopping the activity to doff the limb, drying perspiration from the prosthesis and residual limb, and re-applying the limb, donning prosthetic socks or other options as appropriate [20].

Falling

It is important to inform the patient that falling as a prosthesis user is common and that most prosthesis users are at risk of falling several times per month [25]. It is important to teach the patient how to fall safely. It could be the case that the fear of falling, and not knowing how to fall and to get back up from a fall, potentially creates stress and anxiety. Consider beginning fall training with the therapist applying a gait belt around the patient's waist to assist in controlling how quickly the patient will fall. In falling, you want the patient to avoid harming themselves and control the fall to the extent possible. For the transtibial prosthesis user, the individual rises from prone by transitioning from their stomach to on the hands and knees, then to half kneeling, and then to standing. For the transfemoral prosthesis user, the type of prosthetic knee is a considerable factor. In general, however, the patient transitions from the stomach to a hand and knee. Then, the patient straightens the prosthetic leg and finally rises to stand bearing weight predominantly on the sound limb and then shifting weight more symmetrically to include the prosthetic limb. Rising to stand from the floor may initially include the use of stable furniture or an assistive device but should eventually include practice in open floor space without assist in rising to stand.

PHASE V: MAINTENANCE & LIFELONG CARE

Throughout life, it is important to remain as active as possible. The potential level of activity is variable by individual. Individuals may remain active through regular jogging, gym exercise, neighborhood walking, playing sports in the community, and so on. Engaging in the community and participation in activities such as these are elements of the maintenance phase of rehabilitation for persons with amputation, including those who use prostheses.

In the military, if the injured Service Member desires to learn how to run post-injury, running will be taught and the necessary equipment prescribed. Additionally, opportunities for engagement in adaptive sports will be introduced and participation is encouraged after discharge. Similar opportunities may also be available in the civilian population. Participation and training for adaptive sports engagements may not always be an insurance-covered benefit; however, charitable organizations may be of assistance. Examples of adaptive sports engagements may include the U.S. Paralympics, Disabled and Sports U.S.A. Advocacy organizations that may be of assistance with such efforts include the Challenged Athletes Foundation and the Amputee Coalition. Conducting research locally is encouraged to determine what opportunities may be available.

Other functions, activities, and interests merit consideration, discussion, and intervention at differing points in rehabilitation. Among these are intimacy, pregnancy, alternate footwear, and others. Again, while these may emerge in any phase, the maintenance phase may be a phase where some of these topics appear. Practitioners should be equipped to address such topics but should also be aware that peers and support groups may be alternate resources.

Support groups and peer mentoring provide additional means for amputees to network with peers. While clinical providers including therapists, physicians, prosthetists, and others make every attempt to be thorough in preparing the patient with amputation for social and community reintegration, anticipating every life situation and scenario is not possible. Having a support network of other amputees who have gone through similar experiences can be of enormous benefit. Having for instance a peer who has faced similar issues, difficult days, and situations to aid in problem-solving various issues can be exactly what is needed at precisely the right moment and goes beyond clinical care. Whether it is how a peer adapted their home for certain conditions, or their recommendation for a particular organization that provides certain needed service(s), these can be vital pieces of information that can impact quality of life greatly. An analogy to illustrate the impact for the non-amputee may be how a new homeowner asks a neighbor if they have a plumber or air conditioning specialist they've hired and trust, or what church they attend, or restaurant recommendations. The difference of course being the peer to peer interaction with the understanding being from the perspective of issues faced by the persons living with limb loss.

As the amputee continues with prosthetic use and faces issues with their prosthesis throughout the lifespan, they will have a lifetime relationship with the prosthetist. Prosthetic issues may include socket adjustments, the need for new prosthetic socks, liners, or suspension sleeves, alignment adjustments and more. Of course, new prostheses are needed across time so long as the amputee continues prosthetic use.

SPECIAL CONSIDERATIONS FOR PERSONS WITH BILATERAL LOWER EXTREMITY AMPUTATIONS (BLEAs)

Beyond the aforementioned topics, there are areas of special emphasis for the person with bilateral lower extremity amputations (BLEAs). It is important for instance to prevent hip abduction contractures. Persons with BLEAs for example often abduct their legs to prevent them from touching each other while healing. Eventually, however, this can become a habit, which over time can lead to the development of a hip abduction contracture. Functionally, this can contribute to a wider than normal base of support which can decrease walking efficiency and increase the energy needed to walk. Contractures such as these should be monitored in all patients with limb loss but such contractures can be particularly problematic in those with BLEA.

Physical therapy for the patient with BLEA commonly includes lower extremity strengthening. Core strengthening should also be emphasized, which can be particularly important for those with bilateral transfemoral amputation. Additionally, excess lumbar lordosis can result from hip flexion contracture and can be exacerbated by sockets that inadequately accommodate the contractures. A potential prevention and intervention strategy may include core strengthening, hip flexor stretching, and hip extensor strengthening.

Persons with BLEAs are potentially at increased risk of periods of prosthetic disuse [19]. Therefore, these patients need to be skilled in wheelchair use and in many forms of transfers. Among younger, higher functioning patients with bilateral transfemoral amputation (BTFA), for instance, teaching individual, advanced wheelchair-use skills such as curb ascent and decent and the ability to perform a "wheelie" can further enhance mobility options and independence. This can enable the ability to traverse grass and uneven, non-level surfaces more easily. Teaching wheelchair, uneven surface, and floor transfers can further enhance independence and function [26, 27].

Those with BLEA will need a pair of prostheses for prosthetic gait training and for functional ambulation. Some believe that a feasible goal for persons with bilateral transtibial amputation is to walk without visibly obvious gait deviations, even though the ambulatory energy demand is higher than non-amputees and those with unilateral involvement [11].

The ambulatory energy demand for those with BTFA is much higher than those with bilateral transtibial amputation and the goals between these groups are also different. Some believe those with BTFA should consider optimizing the safety and energy efficiency of prosthetic ambulation. Persons with BTFA may start with a pair of shorter than normal prostheses that commonly do not have prosthetic knees. These prostheses are referred to as short non-articulated prostheses or "stubbies." Walking in these prostheses allows the amputee to build strength, endurance, and balance without concern for knee buckling. As the patient improves walking proficiency with stubbies, they may progress to training and ambulation with progressively taller prostheses with articulated knees. Walking in articulated knees is much more complex and difficult in terms of requiring increased dynamic balance,

confidence, ambulatory energy, and more. There are a variety of ways a patient can transition from stubby prostheses to articulated knees. One example includes transitioning through progressively taller stubbies and then to articulating knees. Another example involves starting with an articulating knee on one side and a locking knee on the other and then progressing to bilaterally articulating knees. Still another example includes transitioning from the initial stubbies straight to full-length articulated knee prostheses. Both stubbies and articulated knees play an important role for the ambulatory patient with BTFA. If the patient participates in heavy work, such as clearing land or building fences, use of their stubbies may improve confidence and stability during activity. However, when the patient is participating in social activities that are less functionally intense, such as community outings (i.e., going out to dinner, or to a movie), use of taller articulating knee prostheses may enhance social function and cosmesis. For instance, the latter use of full length, articulating prostheses enables the user to stand taller, take larger steps, and cover more distance with fewer steps.

Transitioning to and from standing is much more difficult for the patient with BLEAs. Thus, aggressive quadriceps and hip extensor strengthening interventions may be needed to improve these capabilities. Practicing moving from sit to stand initially from a higher seating surface, and then progressing to a lower seating surface, is a logical progression. Further, beginning the progression from a chair with arms with the chair being supported against a firm support such as the wall also facilitates success early in the progression. The progression then may include removing the support of the wall against the chair and eventually using a chair without arms. Similar steps of progression should be implemented when practicing the stand to sit transfer.

SUMMARY

This chapter presented common activities and considerations encountered throughout the course of rehabilitation in persons who experience amputation. Phases commonly described in the rehabilitation of persons with amputation include; Pre-Operative, Post-Operative, Pre-Prosthetic Training, Prosthetic Training, and Maintenance & Lifelong Care. It is important to recognize that persons contributing to the rehabilitation and reintegration of these individuals include not only clinical rehabilitation practitioners but may also be contributed to by peers, support groups, and other sources. Further, it must be emphasized that the patient and their goals are central to driving the direction and pace of rehabilitation and that rehabilitation and reintegration is lifelong.

REFERENCES

[1] U.S. Department of Veterans Affairs. U.S. Department of Defense. *VA/DoD Clinical Practice Guideline for Rehabilitation of Individuals with Lower Limb Amputation, v2.0*, 2017. Accessed May 24, 2023. https://www.healthquality.va.gov/guidelines/Rehab/amp/.

[2] Dillingham TR, Pezzin LE, Mackenzie EJ. Limb amputation and limb deficiency: epidemiology and recent trends in the United States. *South Med J.* 2002;95:875–883.

[3] Zeigler-Graham K, Mackenzie EJ, Ephraim PL, et al. Estimating the prevalence of limb loss in the United States: 2005 to 2050. *Arch Phys Med Rehabil.* 2008;89:422–429.

[4] Gaunaurd I, Gailey R, Hafner BJ, et al. Postural asymmetries in transfemoral amputees. *Prosthet Orthot Int.* 2011;35:171–180.

[5] Endleman I, Critchley DJ. Transversus abdominis and obliquus internus activity during pilates exercises: measurement with ultrasound scanning. *Arch Phys Med Rehabil.* 2008;89:2205–2212.

[6] Kim M, Kim Y, Oh S, et al. Abdominal hollowing and bracing strategies increase joint stability in the trunk region during sudden support surface translation but not in the lower extremities. *J Back Musculoskelet Rehabil.* 2016;29:317–325.

[7] Selkow NM, Eck MR, Rivas S. Transversus abdominis activation and timing improves following core stability training: a randomized trial. *Int J Sports Phys Ther.* 2017;12:1048–1056.

[8] Gailey R, Allen K, Castles J, et al. Review of secondary physical conditions associated with lower-limb amputation and long-term prosthesis use. *J Rehabil Res Dev.* 2008;45:15–29.

[9] Highsmith MJ, Goff LM, Lewandowski AL, et al. Low back pain in persons with lower extremity amputation: a systematic review of the literature. *Spine J.* 2019;19:552–563.

[10] Mengelkoch LJ, Kahle JT, Highsmith MJ. Energy costs and performance of transfemoral amputees and non-amputees during walking and running: a pilot study. *Prosthet Orthot Int.* 2017 Oct;41(5):484–491.

[11] Mengelkoch LJ, Kahle JT, Highsmith MJ. Energy costs & performance of transtibial amputees & non-amputees during walking & running. *Int J Sports Med.* 2014;35:1223–1228.

[12] Klenow TD, Mengelkoch LJ, Stevens PM, et al. The role of exercise testing in predicting successful ambulation with a lower extremity prosthesis: a systematic literature review and clinical practice guideline. *J Neuroeng Rehabil.* 2018;15:64.

[13] Highsmith MJ, Kahle JT, Miro RM, et al. Prosthetic interventions for people with transtibial amputation: Systematic review and meta-analysis of high-quality prospective literature and systematic reviews. *J Rehabil Res Dev.* 2016;53(2):157–184.

[14] Del Toro D, Dedhia R, Tollefson TT. Advances in scar management: prevention and management of hypertrophic scars and keloids. *Curr Opin Otolaryngol Head Neck Surg.* 2016;24:322–329.

[15] Aflatooni S, Beekman K, Hennessey K, et al. Dermatologic conditions following limb loss. *Phys Med Rehab Clin of N Am.* 2024 Nov;35(4):739–755.

[16] Urits I, Seifert D, Seats A, et al. Treatment strategies and effective management of phantom limb-associated pain. *Curr Pain Headache Rep.* 2019;23:64.

[17] Park KN, Cynn HS, Kwon OY, et al. Effects of the abdominal drawing-in maneuver on muscle activity, pelvic motions, and knee flexion during active prone knee flexion in patients with lumbar extension rotation syndrome. *Arch Phys Med Rehabil.* 2011;92:1477–1483.

[18] Highsmith JT, Highsmith MJ. Common skin pathology in LE prosthesis users. *JAAPA.* 2007;20:33–36, 47.

[19] Highsmith MJ, Kahle JT, Klenow TD, et al. Interventions to manage residual limb ulceration due to prosthetic use in individuals with lower extremity amputation: a systematic review of the literature. *Technol Innov.* 2016;18:115–123.

[20] Highsmith MJ, Highsmith JT. Skin problems in the amputee. In: Krajbich JI, Pinzur MS, Potter BK, et al., eds. *Atlas of Amputations and Limb Deficiencies Surgical, Prosthetic and Rehabilitation Principles. Volume 2,* 2016. 4th edition, Section 4, Ch. 56.pp. 677–696. American Academy of Orthopaedic Surgeons, Rosemont, IL.

[21] Highsmith MJ, Klenow TD, Kahle JT, et al. Effects of the Genium Microprocessor Knee System on knee moment symmetry during hill walking. *Technol Innov.* 2016;18:151–157.

[22] Highsmith MJ, Kahle JT, Wernke MM, et al. Effects of the Genium Knee System on functional level, stair ambulation, perceptive and economic outcomes in transfemoral amputees. *Technol Innov.* 2016;18:139–150.

[23] Highsmith MJ, Kahle JT, Miro RM, Mengelkoch LJ. Ramp descent performance with the C-Leg and interrater reliability of the Hill Assessment Index. *Prosthet Orthot Int.* 2013;37(5):362–368.

[24] Highsmith MJ, Kahle JT, Lewandowski AL, et al. A method for training step-over-step stair descent gait with stance yielding prosthetic knees. *J Prosthet Orthot.* 2012;24:10–15.

[25] Kahle JT, Highsmith MJ, Hubbard SL. Comparison of non-microprocessor knee mechanism versus C-Leg on Prosthesis Evaluation Questionnaire, stumbles, falls, walking tests, stair descent, and knee preference. *J Rehabil Res Dev.* 2008;45:1–14.

[26] Pauley T, Devlin M, Heslin K. Falls sustained during inpatient rehabilitation after lower limb amputation: prevalence and predictors. *Am J Phys Med Rehabil.* 2006;85:521–532.

[27] Gooday HM, Hunter J. Preventing falls and stump injuries in lower limb amputees during inpatient rehabilitation: completion of the audit cycle. *Clin Rehabil.* 2004;18:379–390.

CHAPTER 9

Dermatoses in Patients who use Prostheses and Orthoses

James T. Highsmith and M. Jason Highsmith

OBJECTIVES

Upon completion of this chapter, the reader will be able to:

1. Describe the prevalence of dermatologic diagnoses in persons who use prostheses and orthoses.
2. Discuss factors, including hygiene, that contribute to dermatoses in persons with amputation(s).
3. Describe prevention, presentation, etiology, and management of dermatologic conditions in persons who use prostheses and orthoses.

INTRODUCTION

Utilizing a prosthesis or orthosis requires care of qualified prosthetists or orthotists to fabricate, fit, align, and maintain the device to maximize function and quality of life. Use of these devices has functional, social, psychological, and economic implications. Interfacing a device with the body introduces stressors beyond those experienced by non-device users. These added stressors create issues that may require evaluation by other healthcare team members. The integumentary system is impacted by prosthetic or orthotic use.

Human skin contains cells that form tissues which function together to form the human body's largest organ. Vital for health and well-being, the skin regulates temperature through multiple mechanisms including glandular secretions, vascular modulation, and contracting dermal erector pili muscles so that hairs on the skin stand, all of which impact conductive and convective heat loss. In addition to covering underlying structures to provide protection, the skin is also vital in fluid homeostasis, insulation, sensation, absorption with selective resistance, production of natural moisturizing factors, solar protection, immunologic surveillance, and more. Interfacing a device with the skin can impair many of these functions. Therefore, occasional collaboration between the prosthetist/orthotist and dermatologist becomes imperative to optimize patient outcomes.

Gross anatomic or functional loss after amputation or injury requires altered loading and adapted movement patterns, generally with a prosthesis or orthosis. With prosthetic use, a socket typically connects the residual limb to artificial joints, limb segments, and ultimately to a terminal device (i.e. hand or foot) to interact with the environment.

DOI: 10.4324/9781003526025-10

Physiologic changes continue occurring after anatomic and functional loss. These changes predispose the limb and body to issues such as volume fluctuation, pain, motor and sensory dysfunction, thermal dysregulation, hygiene problems, infections, cosmetic problems, and scarring.

A prosthetic socket must be intimately fit to the stump or skin problems may occur. Even an excellent prosthetic fit can challenge the skin. For instance, air circulation and heat loss are impeded and perspiration likely increases with little dissipation. Prosthetic use then exposes moist skin to new materials, chemicals, and considerable mechanical forces. This accumulates increased exposure to injury and irritation and provides little opportunity for healing. Often, the situation is confounded by the fact that many amputees are burdened with a number of other health comorbidities such as vascular disease, obesity, multiple limb loss, pain issues, polytrauma including brain injury, and post-traumatic stress [1, 2]. Thus, skin problems in amputees are not solely prosthetically but functionally, economically, medically, socially, and cognitively complex.

EPIDEMIOLOGY

Persons with limb loss who use prostheses can expect increased problems with their skin at rates greater than non-amputees. Where dermatologic issues represent 7% of ambulatory visits in the U.S. [3, 4], 15% to 41% of amputees have a dermatologic issue. This is a 2–6-fold increase in skin problems compared with non-amputees.

A study of 745 prosthesis users reported the following rank order of dermatoses: ulcers (27%), irritation (18%), inclusion cyst (15%), callus (11%), verrucous hyperplasia (9%), blister (7%), fungal infection (5%), cellulitis (2%), and 7% of patients had dermatoses classified as "other" [5]. Rehabilitation providers should therefore be familiar with common skin issues and be prepared to manage them. Knowledge of less common skin issues is also helpful in facilitating prompt referral to a dermatologist when problems are out of the scope of routine prosthetic care. The remainder of the chapter will consider hygiene, cutaneous problems, and classification of cutaneous problems.

HYGIENE

Limb amputation brings adaptation in muscular recruitment which affects strength, balance, energy demand, and also has psychological, social, and other anatomic and physiologic implications. The skin–prosthetic interface environment is occlusive and includes high stress and high friction areas. Some situations are best managed with suction or negative pressure suspension. These factors require increased quality skin hygiene practices.

If a patient did not suffer from skin problems prior to amputation, their pre-amputation skin care practices may be sufficient. If skin problems arise, changes to varied and unusual skin hygiene practices may be in order [6]. Lack of knowledge and training, cognitive or other health comorbidities common to patients with amputations could contribute to suboptimal skin care. Poor skin hygiene contributes to multiple skin issues including odor, intertrigo (skin on skin rubbing inflammation), infection, eczema, auto-eczematization, cysts, and others. Thus, proper instruction for good hygiene is crucial.

Body, stump, and prosthetic interface component cleansing should be a daily routine [7]. Prosthetic components should be dried or permitted to dry and inspected prior to use (Figure 9.1). Bathing in the evening is recommended. This minimizes stump moisture that initiates adherence and friction [8]. Today's increased gel liner use with its associated perspiration is known to be problematic. Moisture (i.e. perspiration) in gel lined interfaces can impair suspension but is somewhat unavoidable. Thus, periodic interface and stump doffing and drying throughout the day should be part of routine hygiene practice with gel lined suspension systems.

Because skin is acidic in nature (i.e. typical pH value near 5), neutral or near-neutral pH cleansers are recommended [8, 9]. This includes washing with neutral or near-neutral soaps (i.e. Dove, Unilever Corporation, London, England) and synthetic detergents, or "syndets" (i.e. Cetaphil, Galderma Laboratories, L.P., Dallas, TX, U.S.A.) using warm water and ensuring all of the cleanser is washed away. Skin cleansing time should be limited to less than 15 minutes and then the skin blotted dry with a towel using a soft touch, pushing motion as opposed to frictional rubbing. This process could be preventative and restorative for many eczematous conditions, xerosis (dry skin), and in facilitating normal cutaneous microbial flora and decreasing pathogenic bacterial colonization (i.e. *Propionibacterium acnes*), which are more commonly seen with most soaps as nearly all soaps have an alkaline pH [10]. Common issues with basic skin care include using hot water, cleansing duration ≥15 minutes, using high alkaline cleansers, leaving some cleanser on the skin, and frictional towel drying. These factors can contribute to inflammation, contact dermatitis, superficial infections, and generally dry skin [11].

CUTANEOUS PROBLEMS

Dermatitis

Dermatitis, or eczema, is skin inflammation. Inflamed skin may be pruritic (itchy), erythematous (red), weeping, crusting, vesicular (multiple fluid-filled blisters), bullous (blood-filled blisters), or have other presentations. There

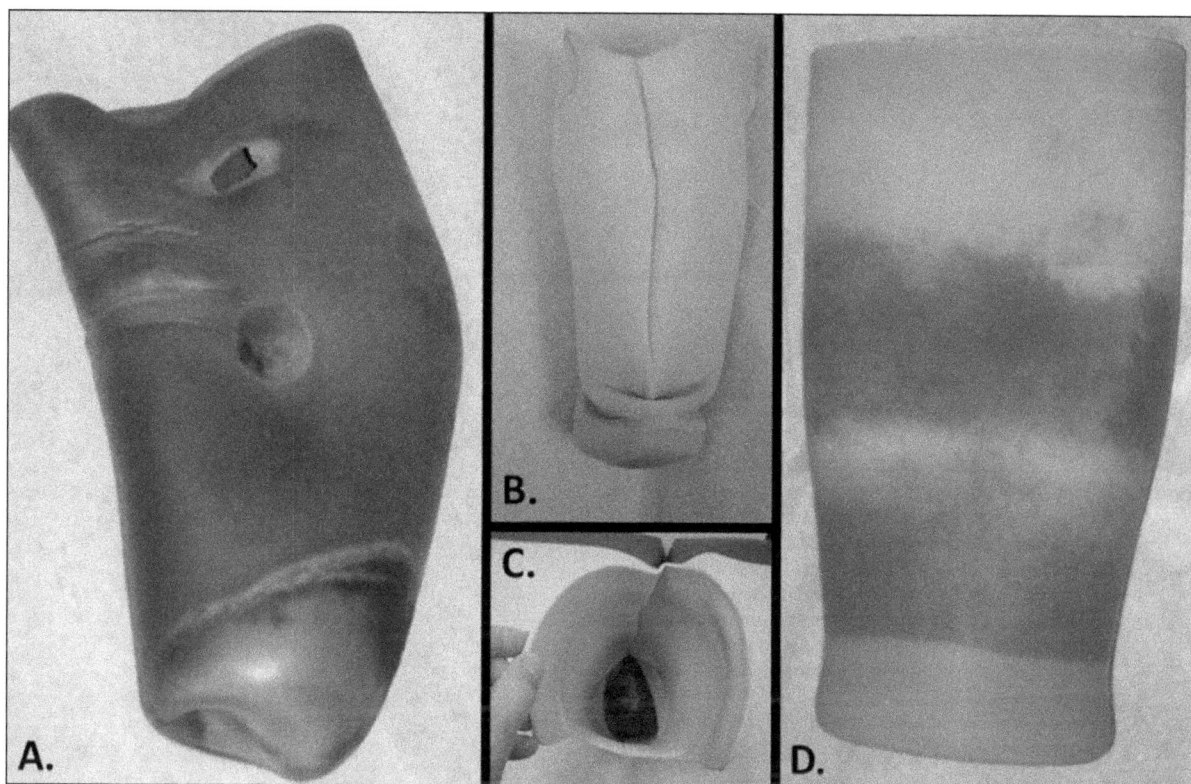

Figure 9.1. Liners that will contribute to dermatoses due to mechanical failure or the presence of irritants. A. Gel liner beyond its useful service life. Note the worn spots where trimlines have worn through the gel proximal to the knee joint and the excess pressure anterior to the knee, at the fibular head, in the popliteal space and distal end. These are all places associated with dermatoses. B. Pelite liner in which the patient is proximally constricted leaving a distal air space. Such gaps lead to verrucose hyperplasia. C. Pelite liner with contaminants accumulated distally. D. Gel liner with mold between the gel and cloth cover.

are multiple causes and types of dermatitis. Selected dermatologic conditions relevant to the care of patients with amputations are discussed here.

Contact dermatitis

Contact dermatitis occurs when a material or chemical contacts skin, resulting in inflammatory signs or symptoms. The two main forms of contact dermatitis are irritant and allergic. *Irritant contact dermatitis (ICD)*, a non-immunologically mediated process, occurs when exposure to a physical agent damages cells and disrupts skin integrity and function. ICD is the most common type of contact dermatitis. ICD results from exposure that could cause a reaction in all human skin equally; for example, a strong acid.

The inflammatory response in ICD is limited to the contact site, which often itches or burns. Among the most common etiologies for ICD include excessive chronic washing with soap and water which can dry and irritate the skin. Chronic excoriation (picking and scratching the skin) and rubbing further exacerbate the problem. Other predisposing factors include age, occlusion, and mechanical irritation. Management primarily includes avoiding contact with the offending agent. Other therapeutic modalities include using a physical barrier (i.e.

Liner-Liner® prosthetic sock. Knit-Rite, Inc., Kansas City, KS, U.S.A.) and topical barrier (e.g. Desitin paste, Johnson & Johnson Consumer Co., Inc., New Brunswick, NJ, U.S.A. and, A&D ointment. Merck & Co., Inc., Whitehouse Station, NJ, U.S.A.), emollients (i.e. Aquaphor, Beiersdorf Inc., Stamford, CT, U.S.A.), and possibly corticosteroids (i.e. hydrocortisone). Frictional ICD (Figure 9.2) is a distinct subtype that results from recurrent low grade friction and can lead to hyperkeratosis and lichenification [9]. However, we will classify the majority of frictional related dermatoses into the 'Volume Changes' section since the associated frictional forces are of a higher magnitude and more directly explain the underlying etiology.

Allergic contact dermatitis or ACD (Figure 9.3) is different from ICD in that agents triggering an allergic response initiate an immunologic hypersensitivity cascade in select persons following repeated allergen exposure. ACD is a delayed hypersensitivity reaction to an allergen developing upon re-exposure. Lesions from ACD are acutely well-defined involving erythema, edema, and, occasionally, vesicles or exudate. Key ACD features include visible reaction upon second but not first exposure. Further, not all persons will react to the offending agent of an ACD in contrast to irritants that can trigger ICD in anyone. Chemicals and materials used in prosthetic fabrication, maintenance, and repair are often suspect in contact dermatitis reactions

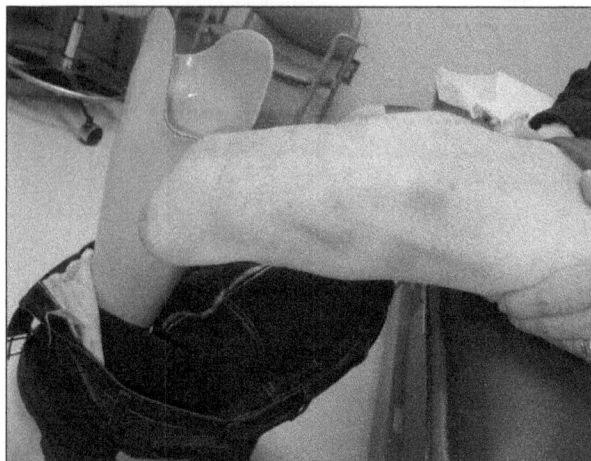

Figure 9.2. Irritant contact dermatitis (frictional). Note the erythematous areas near the fibular head and anterior and posterior aspects of the lateral femoral condyle. Frictional ICD may present in these areas in association with valgus force coupling during stance phase. Alternatively, the socket may be poorly fit or the patient is not properly monitoring and adjusting sock-ply during volume change. If the skin fails to blanch with palpation, then a stage I pressure sore has developed which has begun here only at the most proximal erythematous patch near the anterolateral femoral condyle.

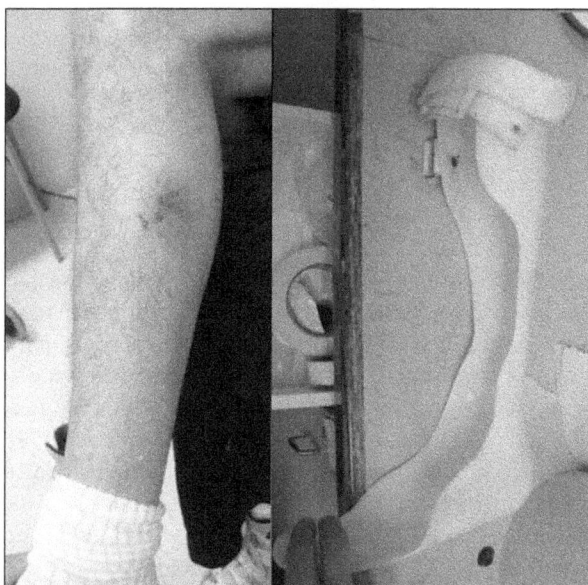

Figure 9.3. Allergic contact dermatitis (nickel). Suspected ACD in a patient using an ankle foot orthosis (AFO) in which the cover has come off the strap rivets thereby permitting metal to directly contact the skin.

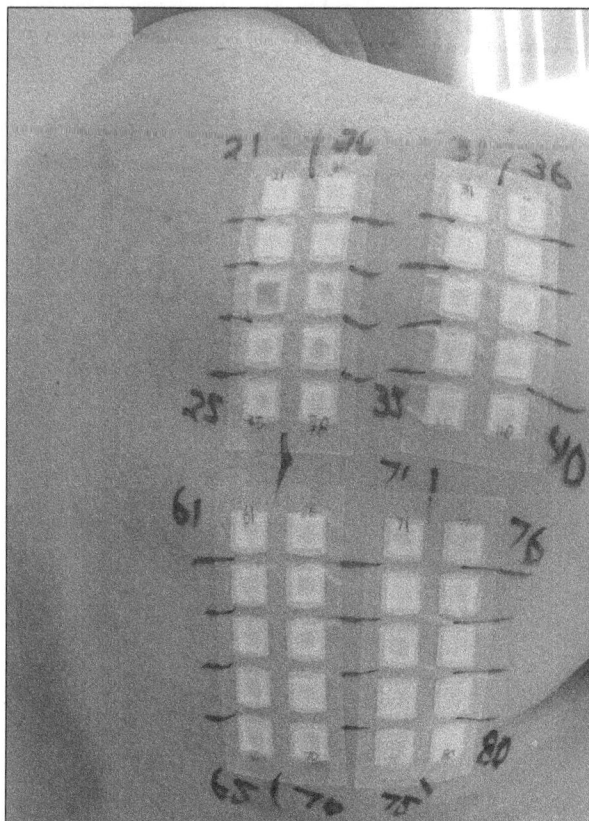

Figure 9.4. Patient undergoing patch testing for possible allergens causing ACD. The back is used due to the broad surface area and to be able to compare site reactions. Patch testing is the gold standard to diagnose ACD but should be supplemented and corroborated with a thorough patient history.

[12]. Varnishes, lacquers, plastics, epoxies, resins, cements, leathers, and others are suspect. Patients with ACD are more likely to have an atopic background including family history of atopic dermatitis, asthma, allergic rhinitis, in addition to the predisposing factors listed for ICD above.

With ACD, conducting a careful history is necessary to determine if a new exposure outside of the prosthesis (i.e. skincare product) is the offending agent as opposed to a prosthetic component. It may not be possible to differentiate ACD and ICD, especially in the chronic phase as the signs and symptoms begin to overlap. Patch testing is the gold standard for determining or excluding an immunologic allergen [9, 13] (Figure 9.4).

If history and patch testing are successful, removal of the inciting antigen is routinely curative for the dermatitis. Otherwise, symptom relief becomes the primary goal, at least temporarily. Beyond avoidance, conservative topical treatment options for symptomatic relief include antipruritics such as Sarna Lotion (Crown Laboratories, Inc., Johnson City, TN, U.S.A.), corticosteroids (i.e. hydrocortisone), and cool compresses [6, 14, 15]. In more aggressive cases or if symptoms are refractory to topical therapy, systemic corticosteroid administration may be considered.

Non-Specific Eczematization (id reaction)

While the dermatitis discussed thus far results in local, contact-site inflammation, it is possible that inflammation appears elsewhere. One example is a dermatophyte fungal infection on a distal extremity resulting in an eczematous patch on the trunk. This is termed a "dermatophytid", or an "id," reaction. Other terms such as auto-eczematization, auto-sensitization, angry skin syndrome, and disseminated eczema have all been used to describe this poorly understood process that does not have to be related to an infection. Although unclear, systemic irritant, allergen, or immune cell (i.e. activated memory T lymphocytes) dissemination plays a key role in inflammation at a distant site from the primary inflammatory source. Id reaction management focuses on recognizing and treating the primary source. Often, emollients and corticosteroids are the most beneficial in treating just the distant eczematous patch(es).

Psoriasis

Psoriasis is a common, chronic immune-mediated systemic inflammatory condition that is characterized by a well-demarcated, red, scaly patch (Figure 9.5). Many sufferers are genetically predisposed, and an external trigger is possible (e.g. infection, hypocalcemia, or medications such as beta blockers). Lesions classically occur on extensor surfaces and are known to occur in friction exposed areas. Injury may lead to a psoriatic plaque directly in the traumatized skin that is often linear, as in a scraped knee, known as the Koebner phenomenon (Figure 9.6). Thus, it

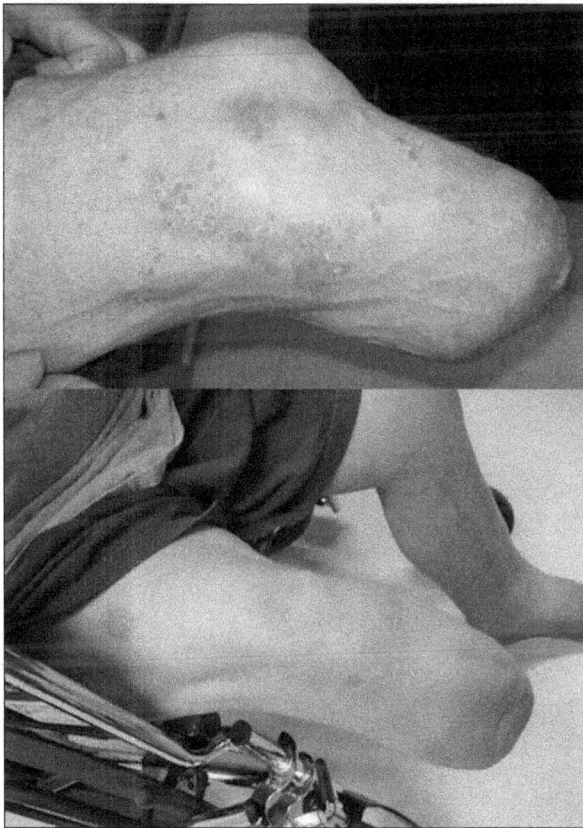

Figure 9.6. Koebner phenomenon. Note the excoriations presenting as linear psoriatic plaques.

is possible for an amputee patient to develop psoriasis on the residual limb. It is recommended to check the elbows, knees, groin, digits, and scalp as well. It is of great service to the patient if the prosthetist can recognize this condition and refer them to their primary care physician or dermatologist. In addition to the skin involvement, about one-third of patients have an associated psoriatic arthritis and an increased risk of diabetes and cardiovascular issues. Most patients are managed with topical prescription medications such as corticosteroids and Vitamin D creams [16]. Topical therapeutics are most beneficial if applied when the prosthesis is not on the body such as during sleep. Collaboration between prosthetist and dermatologist will assure prosthetic use is not undermining dermatologic treatment and vice versa in conditions such as psoriasis. Extensive skin involvement, severe symptoms, or arthritis should be managed with systemic therapies such as ultraviolet phototherapy, biologic agents, chemotherapeutic agents, or systemic retinoids [17].

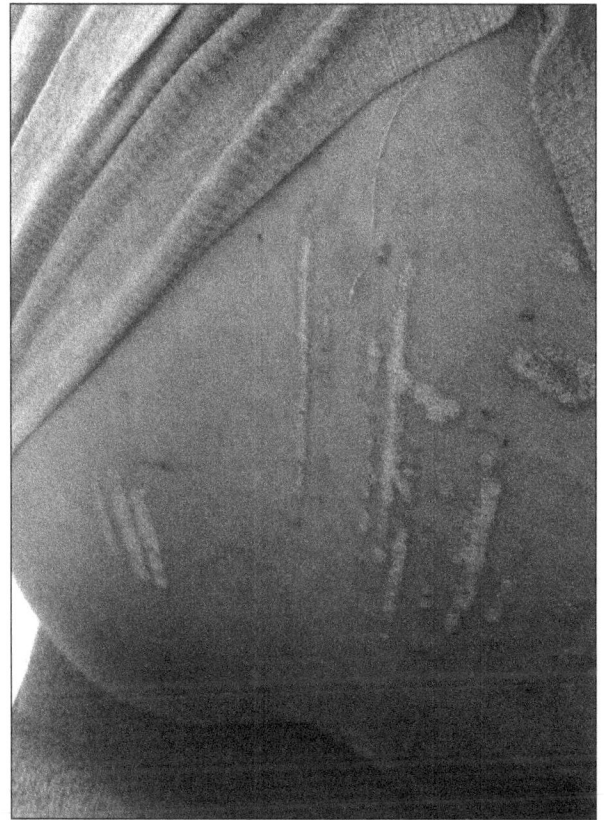

Figure 9.5. Patients presenting psoriatic plaques on their residual limbs. Note the well-demarcated, pruritic, scaling plaques. In the bottom figure, note the psoriatic plaque on the lateral, proximal right thigh. Psoriasis can result in plaques anywhere upon the body but may be additionally burdensome within the socket region for amputees. Note the stasis dermatitis (bottom figure) on the patient's left (non-amputated intact) limb as a result of venous insufficiency.

Intertrigo

Intertrigo is a dermal inflammatory response due to friction between two constantly opposing skin surfaces (Figure 9.7). Commonly involved areas include the axilla, the sub-mammary areas, and inter-gluteal cleft. In obese persons, intertrigo can develop between abdomen or thigh tissue folds and is common on residual limbs in amputee patients. Here, two skin surfaces on either side of an invaginated scar are in constant direct contact while squeezed together inside a prosthetic interface [18]. Inflammation is caused by occlusion, heat, maceration, movement related elevated forces that degrade keratin on the stump's skin. The compromised tissue is subject to further mechanical irritation and secondary infection. Fissures, eczema, pigment alteration, ulceration, or lichenification can result with chronicity. Intertrigo is the non-specific term for dermatitis in contacting surfaces when other pathology is not present. Steps should be taken to identify active infection or specific underlying pathology. A skin biopsy or microbial culture may be necessary to diagnose underlying pathology in a persistent intertriginous lesion. It is therefore prudent to refer the patient with intertrigo who fails to respond to conservative treatment beyond a 2-week time period.

Management recommendations include good hygiene practices along with the application of a topical barrier, emollient, corticosteroid or some combination thereof, depending on the clinical presentation. Furthermore, appropriately selected, fitted, and aligned prosthetic componentry can minimize stress in the invaginated region. Components worn beyond their service life, that are ill-fitting/functioning, or that are contaminated can complicate intertrigo. Once prosthetic components are functioning optimally, care, maintenance, and cleaning are reviewed to optimize stump protection. Finally, if an underlying cause or secondary infection is determined, it should be treated as indicated.

Heat Rash

Obstruction of eccrine sweat ducts may lead to heat rash or miliaria (Figure 9.8). Miliaria has been categorized by the depth of pathology and is ordered here from superficial to deep. Miliaria rubra, or prickly heat, is characterized by occluded sweat that leaks into the lower epidermis or superficial dermis and elicits an inflammatory response with erythematous macules, patches, and papules. Prickly heat rash is commonly seen under the prosthetic device due to the artificial interface with sustained exposure to friction and elevated temperatures. Typically, resolution will occur rapidly if the device is not worn for a single day, usually requiring no further treatment. However, it should be noted that anhydrosis, or a lack of sweating, commonly follows a true heat rash for a week or two as the normal physiologic function returns. Since eccrine sweat glands discharge their contents directly onto the skin surface, they are independent of the hair follicle unlike apocrine and sebaceous glands.

Urticaria

The final type of dermatitis considered here is urticaria, also referred to as hives (Figure 9.9). Urticaria is

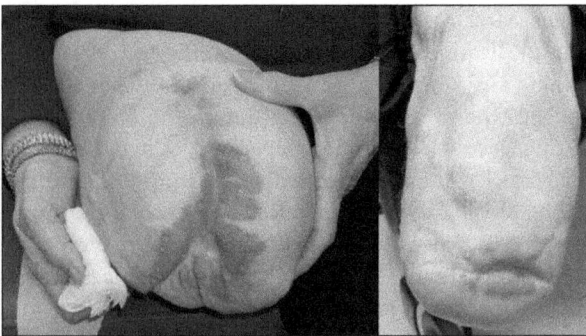

Figure 9.7. Lesions within opposing skin surfaces of invaginated scars which are unfortunately common in amputee residual limbs. These lesions would commonly be referred to as intertrigo. Intertrigo is a non-specific diagnosis and when suspected infections or other diagnoses are present, further testing may be indicated. For instance, the left lesion shown here is well demarcated and beefy red so a competing differential diagnosis may be inverse psoriasis and this patient was referred for biopsy as compared to the mild inflammation seen in typical intertrigo on the right picture.

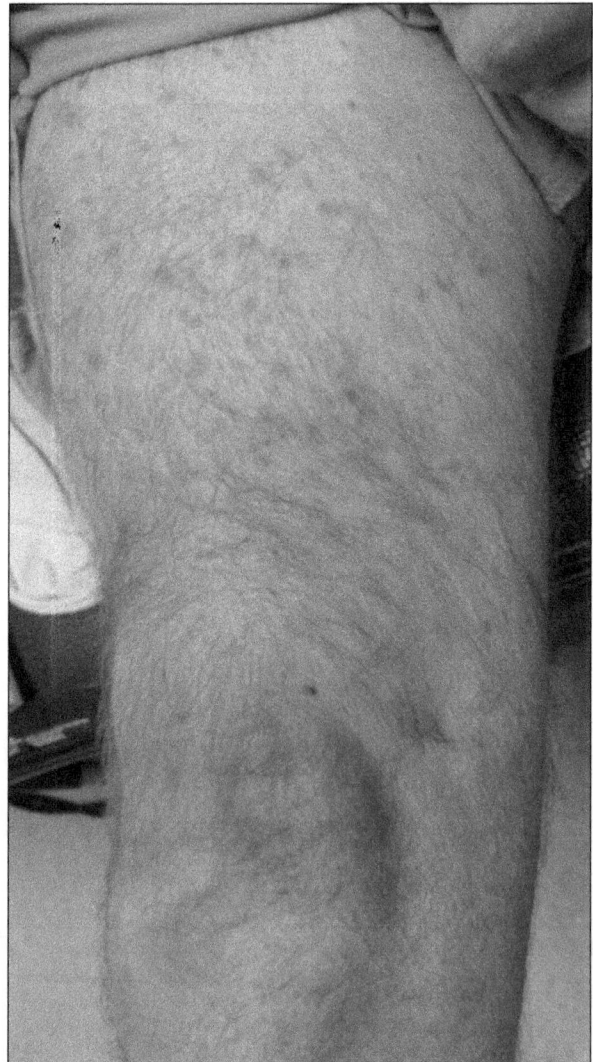

Figure 9.8. Patient presenting miliaria rubra (prickly heat rash) of the distal thigh where the skin contacts gel from his suspension system.

characterized by transient pruritic raised wheals formed from central pale dermal edema and surrounded by redness that blanches with pressure. Individual wheals can resolve rapidly, often within an hour but many persist for an entire day. Wheals that stay in the same location longer than one day should be biopsied to rule out an underlying process, such as urticarial vasculitis or systemic lupus erythematosus. Hives can be acute or chronic. Acute urticaria is defined as lesions that continue to come and go within a 6-week period of time and chronic urticaria occurs beyond 6 weeks. Urticaria can be subcategorized by the underlying etiology. Subtypes of urticarial include physical, cholinergic, cold, heat, pressure, solar, vibratory and others [19]. A careful history should help elucidate if the patient is indeed having hives or physical urticaria. Testing physical urticarias should not be done unless the practitioner is trained and equipped to treat a possible anaphylactic reaction. Treatment of physical urticarias often includes oral antihistamines but topical corticosteroids provide some benefit [19].

Infection

Skin is equipped to prevent infection. Defenses have been divided into the innate and adaptive immune systems. The innate system is non-specific and is known as the first line of defense. It is composed of components such as the intact skin barrier, antimicrobial peptides (e.g. beta defensins, cathelicidins), neutrophils, macrophages, and eosinophils. The adaptive immune system is known as having a delayed but pathogen specific response with memory involving Langerhans' cells, T cell lymphocytes, B cell lymphocytes, and plasma cells. Other barriers to infection include competing normal flora of microbes and the complement system which plays a role in both the innate and adaptive immune systems. The artificial prosthetic interface predisposes the host tissue to elevated temperatures, moisture, and maceration that potentially compromises many of these defenses. As a result,

microbes may invade the skin resulting in an infection. In persons with an amputation, common skin infections include fungi and bacteria. The classic infectious presentation is localized. Systemic infections are possible and should be recognized early by constitutional symptoms as seen with an elevated core temperature, accompanied by fever or chills, to avoid serious and even life-threatening complications [18].

Folliculitis, literally translates to hair follicle inflammation (Figure 9.10). It is an extremely common problem related to microbial infection in amputee patients. Lesions are characterized by a small pustule that is centered on a hair follicle. It is more prevalent in individuals with hyperhidrosis, increased hair, oily skin, obesity, shaving, and friction. Mechanical stress escalates symptoms, particularly in summer months, with higher ambient temperatures, increased perspiration, and is exacerbated by the lack of evaporative cooling under the prosthesis [8, 20]. These infections are typically caused by Staphylococcus aureus but other bacteria or even fungi, such as Malassezia, are common. It is paramount to recommend against shaving and to emphasize keeping the area cool and as free from friction as possible. Other therapies generally include OTC topical antimicrobials (i.e. benzoyl peroxide 2–5%), prescription topical antimicrobials (e.g. Clindamycin solution, Ketoconazole shampoo), and even systemic antibiotics (i.e. Doxycycline), depending on the severity and microbes involved. For recurrent lesions, permanent laser epilation can also be considered.

A deeper dermal infection than folliculitis is termed a furuncle, or more commonly, a boil [21]. If more than one follicle is involved the lesion is termed a carbuncle. A pustule is not visualized in these lesions. Instead, furuncles present as an indurated erythematous nodule often with tenderness or irritation. Furuncles are generally found on areas of mechanical friction and increased sweating [6]. Commonly affected areas include the axilla and groin so it is not surprising to see them on the residual limb of a patient with an amputation. Associated systemic disorders include diabetes, immunosuppression, alcoholism, and malnutrition.

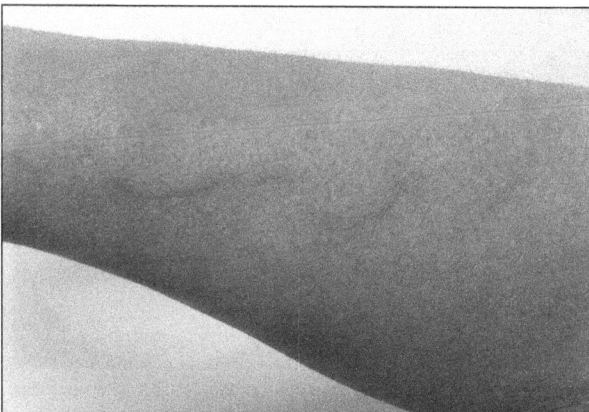

Figure 9.9. Patient presenting with urticaria (hives). Note the elevated lesion with a central, pale dermal area.

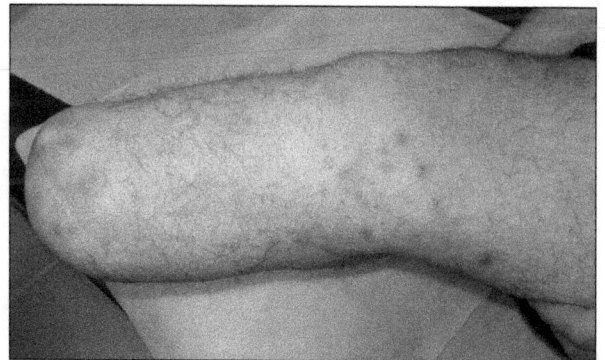

Figure 9.10. Patient presenting with folliculitis on his residual limb. A key feature of folliculitis is inflammation, often one or more pustules, centered about a hair follicle.

Boils are typically caused by Staphylococcus aureus bacteria and may spontaneously resolve. Furuncules are often treated like folliculitis. Recurrent folliculitis or furunculosis may also require antimicrobial soaps or cleansers (i.e. chlorehexidine) several times per week and can be purchased over the counter without prescription though a discussion with a dermatologist is advisable depending upon the previous rate of skin problems and hygiene.

If the infection involves more surrounding and yet deeper tissues, it may result in a fluctuant and very painful abscess. An abscess could result in systemic symptoms and a wound culture should be taken to determine the microbial etiology and susceptibility to antibiotics. Treatment must include incision and drainage of these purulent lesions. Although systemic antibiotics are commonly used they are generally not necessary as long as the lesion is drained appropriately.

Superficial fungal infections (e.g. jock itch, athlete's foot) are also common due to the artificial interface [5]. These dermatophytes produce an erythematous annular patch which is a ring of redness (i.e. ring worm) along with central clearing inside the ring (Figure 9.11). Yeast could also affect the skin and is a distinct fungal infection from the dermatophytes discussed above. A yeast infection is commonly identified as having a beefy red appearance with satellite lesions beyond the primary area of inflammation. Candida albicans is the typical yeast involved and improves best with prescription topical treatment. Topical antifungals are the mainstay of treatment which are available over the counter (e.g. Terbinafine or Clotrimazole) or as a prescription (i.e. Ciclopirox).

Improving hygiene practices may assist to prevent all of the infections presented in this chapter [7]. This is important as the stump's skin may have altered microbial flora compared with sound limbs in the same person. Levy reported that sound hygiene adherence may be curative in patients with recurrent folliculitis [6]. Other general treatment options may include some amount of prosthetic discontinuance [18] and referral to the patient's primary care physician or dermatologist. If the patient is being treated for an abscess, the prosthesis and all of their prosthetic soft goods should be cleaned and evaluated. If the patient is experiencing chronic or severe infections, replacing soft goods (i.e. gel liners, socks, etc.) could prevent recurrent infections, contamination, or further complication [18].

Volume Change

Volume change in patients with amputation is fairly common. Volume mismatching between stump and prosthetic interface is among the most common and significant source of dermatologic maladies and impaired function for the prosthesis user. Several specific forms of volume change and their specific medical diagnoses are discussed below.

Prosthetic use abnormally stresses tissues of the stump. Note for example that typical non-amputee walking generally results in 15°–25° of knee flexion during loading response for shock absorption. When this happens in transtibial gait, the socket rotates about the stump into flexion creating a force couple with the stump in all three planes during movement. The amputee attempts to cease the socket on stump flexion by extending the knee. This causes force coupling as stress increases at the distal anterior tibia and proximal posterior aspect of the socket near the distal hamstring tendon region. Further, during weight bearing, axial loads are applied through the stump resulting in forces acting upon and through tissues that are not anatomically suited to manage them. In contrast, axial loads in the non-amputee are dispersed through the calcaneal fat pad as well as the arched structure of the foot comprised of intrinsic and extrinsic muscles and a complex ligamentous array. When a lower limb is amputated, many of the aforementioned structures are eliminated, requiring structures not designed for load bearing to manage these loads. Consider that the distal cut end of the tibia, fibula, and muscle bellies are now bearing axial load instead of the foot. It is highly conceivable how this can contribute to abnormal forces and ulceration upon the amputated stump.

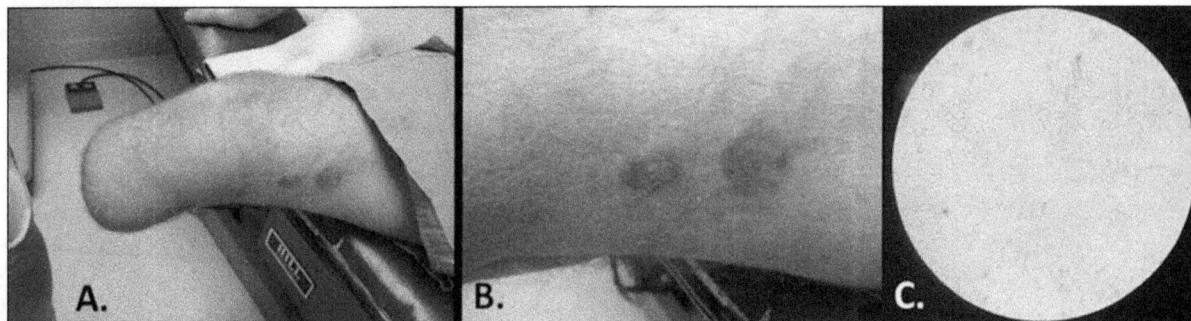

Figure 9.11. A. Patient presenting with two lesions on the distal medial thigh, beneath the liner of his transtibial prosthesis. B. Close-up image of the same patient showing well demarcated borders with central clearing characteristic of fungal infection. Panel C demonstrates a potassium hydroxide (KOH) wet mount microscopic view confirming dermatophyte fungal infection. Note the long, slender hyphae characteristic of dermatophytes fungal infections.

Negative Pressure Hyperemia

One viable prosthetic suspension option includes negative pressure suspension (i.e. suction or vacuum). In negative pressure systems, the prosthesis is held onto the stump during unweighting periods (i.e. swing phase of gait) via suction or vacuum [22]. Any loss of contact between stump and interface with negative pressure suspension will result in a void with lowered resistance to circulation in that area, drawing fluid toward the region of the stump closest to the void. The negative pressure pulls lymphatic and circulating blood into the region creating congestion. If the loss of contact persists, the site will become clearly demarcated, edematous, erythematous, and exquisitely painful (Figure 9.12). The area could begin to weep serosanguinous fluid [18]. Weight gain is a likely contributor but any volume change preventing full and total contact could result in this problem. A period of prosthetic disuse may be recommended due to the pain the suction will cause during unweighting. Total contact must be restored in the interface. Analgesic medication and prosthetic disuse for a short period of time are indicated for pain management from acute symptoms. It is noteworthy however, that one should minimize prosthetic discontinuance in active patients. Temporary padding to restore contact will likely facilitate recovery. However, since the volume change was sufficient to cause this problem in the first place, a cure will likely depend upon the fabrication of a new, better-fitting socket.

Friction (lichenification, blister, callus)

Multiple forces are applied to the stump during prosthetic use. A common suspension type includes the gel liner with pin suspension [7, 18, 23]. When a gel liner is suspending a prosthesis via pin lock, the distal end is firmly attached to the bottom of the socket. A great amount of friction and stress will be applied to the anterior region of the knee with increased knee flexion. Patients using pin systems may complain of knee discomfort if sitting for long periods. This friction will result in changes within the skin. Initially, blisters may form but with time the skin may harden which is termed "lichenification" (Figure 9.13). Clinically, lichenification can be identified easily with exaggerated skin lines secondary to thickening of cutaneous tissue in the affected area. Improving prosthetic fit and teaching pressure relief strategies (i.e. release the pin lock during prolonged sitting, doff the prosthesis) is recommended as first line treatment. Secondary lichenification can be treated with corticosteroids if indicated.

Similarly, excess end-bearing as opposed to proportionally distributed loading through total surface bearing could result in distal stump callusing [24]. Calluses are the skin's protective response to friction and pressure and are generally not problematic. Calluses are caused by an accumulation of terminally differentiated keratinocytes strongly connected by cross-linked proteins in the epidermis [25]. Additionally, calluses can lead to skin ulcers or infection. Problematic calluses can be cultured for infection and treated accordingly. If blisters form, which are commonly filled with leached plasma from cells exposed to shearing near the stratum spinosum, continued prosthetic use commonly ruptures them. Blisters can be filled with blood but can also be infected, so if the fluid is suspect then refer the patient to their physician. However, blisters are initially sterile and should not be lanced or drained. If they rupture, do not remove the skin as this forms a biological dressing to protect the underlying tissues.

Ulceration (volume change; pressure sores and ulceration)

Ulcers can result from bacterial infections, vascular disease, or focused mechanical prosthetic pressure [18, 23, 24, 26]. Concerted efforts to resolve ulcers should be made as long-standing chronic ulcers can become scarred and adherent to deeper tissues which can complicate healing and future prosthetic use. Chronic ulcers can also develop malignant tissue changes and referral for biopsy

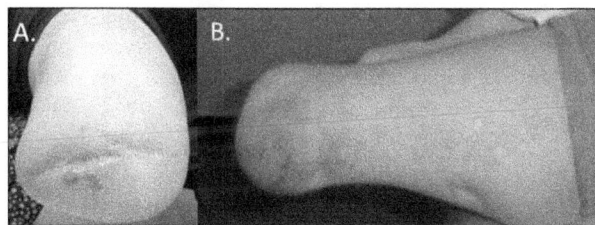

Figure 9.12. A. Residual limb presenting with a blister and distal irritation in conjunction with use of a negative pressure suspension system that resulted in a focal area of suction without total contact. B. Classic negative pressure hyperemia associated with use of a suction suspension prosthesis. Weight gain and an increase in the diameter of the proximal thigh prevents achieving distal contact. Thus, in swing phase there is a constant drawing of fluid to the area of the stump with the least resistance to fluid flow. Fluid congestion, erythema and pain result.

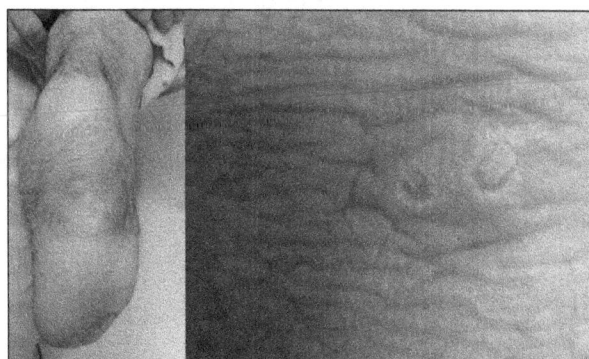

Figure 9.13. Transtibial residual limb presenting with visible lines characteristic of lichenification. Also present are calluses. Both the lichenification and calluses are the result of skin attempting to protect itself from high stress, in this case because of patellar bar pressure.

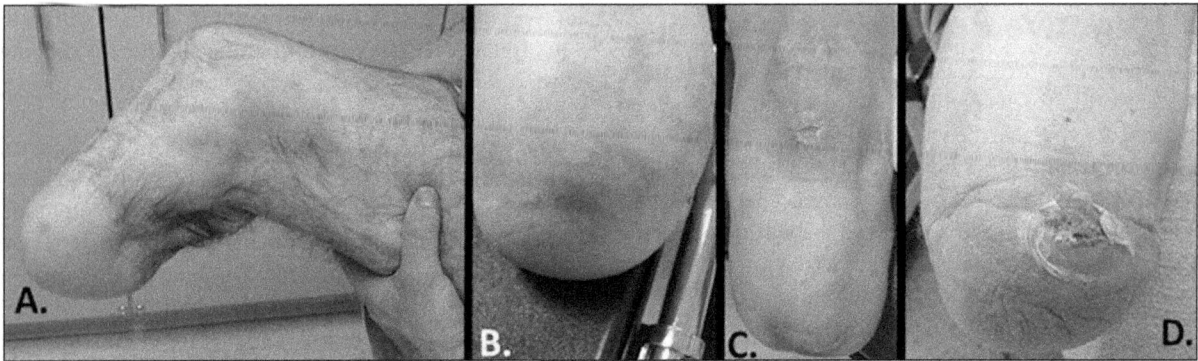

Figure 9.14. A. Classic hot spot (decubitus ulcer, Stage I) over the medial femoral condyle. B. Stage II decubitus characterized by breach of the epidermis. C. Stage III decubitus ulcer characterized by penetration into the subcutaneous tissue layers. D. Stage IV decubitus with purulent discharge that has eroded into muscle tissue.

is indicated. Residual limb ulcerations may result in prosthetic discontinuation until further evaluated.

Decubitus ulcers, or "bed sores," are most commonly seen on the heels and sacrum of supine positioned, bed-bound patients. Decubiti can develop on any skin where mechanical pressure is applied over a bony prominence. A poorly fit or aligned prosthesis creates focal pressure and shear forces over bony prominences referred to as "hot spots" (Figure 14(A)). Irritation and inflammation are introduced to superficial skin layers (Stage I). Continued loading further degrades skin integrity allowing the ulcer to erode deeper into the epidermis or dermis (Stage II), then into the subcutaneous fascial layers (Stage III), and eventually to muscle or bone (Stage IV). Sensory deficits compound this problem and are more commonly seen in patients with diabetes and vascular disease. When protective pain sensation is absent, ambulation continues and the pressure sore is further aggravated (Figures 14(B–D)).

Verrucous Hyperplasia

Verrucous hyperplasia (VH), or lymphostasis papillomatosis, is a warty appearance at the distal end of the stump [8, 27] (Figure 9.15). Human papilloma virus (HPV), which causes cutaneous warts including genital and common warts, as well as lymphatic stasis, has been implicated in the pathogenesis, yet studies fail to isolate any viral particles [28, 29]. The condition is almost exclusively a problem in the distal skin of the amputated residual limb which seems to result from proximal constriction and lack of distal contact or appropriate distal circumferential contact pressures [8, 27, 30]. The differential diagnosis could include HPV infection, squamous cell carcinoma, lymphedema, lymphangioma, venous insufficiency, or lymphangiosarcoma. Nonetheless, the proximal constriction mechanism described above, and treatment of VH are generally agreed upon by using compression, restoring distal contact and optimizing prosthetic fit. A biopsy is indicated if the condition fails to improve or worsens.

VH was possibly more prevalent in previous decades as prosthetic socket designs present at that time minimized distal contact and preferentially loaded proximal

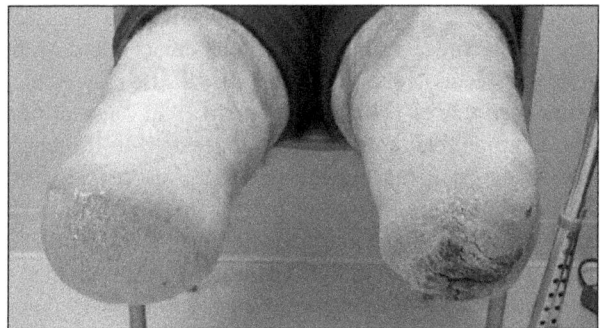

Figure 9.15. Bilaterally amputated patient presenting verrucous hyperplasia secondary to proximal constriction from his prostheses and failure to achieve total contact distally. Medical evaluation to rule out malignancy is indicated in cases this severe. Prosthetic management includes compression when not wearing prostheses and re-fitting prostheses to assure total contact without proximal constriction.

tissues. This constricted fluid exchange and created a space of low resistance at the distal end of the stump [6, 8, 31]. These were the standard of care socket technologies at that time and, consequently, VH was probably more common. Unfortunately, there are no epidemiologic data to corroborate socket type to this pathology. Nonetheless, successful management has been seen with compression and optimizing socket fit.

Contemporary attempts to more uniformly load the stump seem to minimize VH [28, 32]. However, a poorly fit socket or rapid weight gain could create the proximal restriction and distal low-pressure scenario necessary to create VH, so the condition still occurs but with lower frequency. If an acute situation arises that creates a proximal socket constriction and distal contact pressure drop, action should be taken immediately to prevent VH development. Stump compression when out of the socket (i.e. elastic bandage wrapping, stump shrinker) and distal socket padding during prosthetic use are a few recommendations to consider while the bodily situation and new socket are being managed. Chronic or abnormally presenting cases should be cultured for infection and biopsied. It should be noted that VH lesions could be associated with malignancy. For instance, Levy reported a chronic verrucous hyperplasia complicated by extensive ulceration and infection that developed a squamous cell carcinoma in the stump skin and extended into the bone [6, 33].

Tumor

The word *tumor* is of Latin origin which means to swell. The term is often used interchangeably with neoplasia but should not be used synonymously with cancer. Cancer implies a malignant growth into other tissues (local invasion or metastasis) that can alter the function of those structures. Tumors, in contrast, are an abnormal proliferation of cellular growth initiated from an individual cell and may not necessarily invade surrounding structures nor alter their function. Benign tumors typically do not infiltrate into surrounding organs or alter function as opposed to malignant tumors that lead to cancer.

Normally, every cell has a strictly governed growth cycle with suppressive checks and balances. If a cell expresses dysplastic or metaplastic changes, these protective processes (i.e. p53 tumor suppressor) halt cellular growth to initiate repair and are usually successful. In the event of an inability to repair the damage, the cell has a final last chance way to prevent cancer formation through pre-programmed cellular death, termed apoptosis. Apoptosis destroys the abnormal cell for the greater good of the host. However, if the cell evades these cell cycle checks-and-balances, as well as apoptosis, then it can replicate and lead to cancer. A complete discussion of carcinogenesis along with all of the tumors that can affect the skin is beyond the scope of this text. However, a selected few tumors that are common or more prevalent in a patient with amputation will be discussed below.

Benign Tumors

Seborrheic Keratoses

Seborrheic keratoses (SKs) are common skin growths seen on mature adults. SKs are equally prevalent in men and women. SKs typically begin to appear after the fourth decade of life and increase in frequency with age but may occur at a younger age with excessive ultraviolet radiation exposure. A benign clonal proliferation of keratinocytes is the most likely underlying etiology [34]. These common lesions are clinically recognized as a hyperpigmented waxy growth with a "stuck-on" appearance that are generally at least several millimeters in size but can be much larger (Figure 9.16). Although they may have a warty appearance, HPV, which is the virus that causes warts, has very rarely been identified. Reassurance is recommended for most lesions but removal with curettage or cryosurgery is reasonable if the lesion is irritated or inflamed. Differentiating these benign growths from true warts or even malignant melanoma may be difficult so evaluation with a dermatologist is recommended.

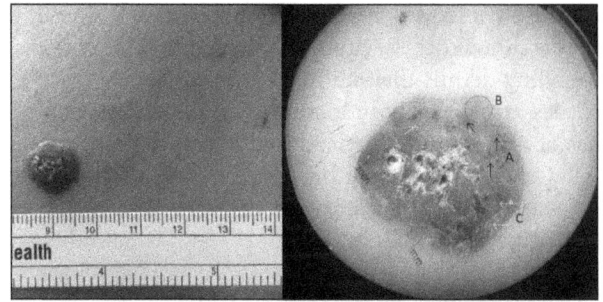

Figure 9.16. Presentation of seborrheic keratoses (SKs). These benign growths are identified as a hyperpigmented waxy growth of several millimeters with a "stuck-on" appearance. The right panel is a dermoscopic picture of the same seborrheic keratosis demonstrating classic findings of comedo-like crypts (arrows labelled A), fingerprint like structure (circle labelled B), and white milia-like cysts (arrows labelled C).

Another benign growth described in patients with amputation is fibroepithelial polyps, also called acrochordons or skin tags. Acrochordons are small, 1–3 mm skin colored to hyperpigmented pedunculated growths that tend to occur on sights of friction and favor the eyelids, axilla, neck, and groin. Friction and weight gain are associated as these lesions may occur within invaginated residual limb scars or a poorly fit prosthesis. Skin tags have been labeled as a marker for diabetes mellitus as well [35]. Treatment is not necessary as they are only of cosmetic significance although snip removal can be done if they become irritated or inflamed.

Neuromas

After amputation of the distal extremity, a potentially painful nerve growth from the distal end of a severed major nerve could develop, termed a neuroma. Neuromas do not appear acutely post-operatively. Most patients use their prosthesis for several months prior to the onset of pain which may suggest a neuroma has formed. While this delay represents the time needed for the neuroma to grow, it also suggests that the extra irritation and inflammation from prosthetic use could be required to initiate symptoms or at least be a significant contributing factor. Conservative management should be attempted to improve fit and offload the tender area. However, an additional surgery may be required to remove the tumor. Following painful neuroma excision, most patients were back into their prosthesis by three months and all patients studied in a large series were satisfied with the surgery and ultimately pain free [36, 37].

Cyst

A true cyst is defined as having an epithelial lining, and epidermoid cysts are the most common type of cutaneous cysts. Patients often present for treatment when the lesions are large, irritated, infected, or purely for cosmetic removal. They range in size from a few millimeters to several centimeters. Epidermal cysts are typically asymptomatic and often have a large dilated keratin-filled pore. However, if the keratinous debris within the cyst ruptures into the surrounding dermis then an intense inflammatory reaction ensues and typically produces a foul odor. Pathogenesis has not been universally accepted as theories range from cellular overgrowth with the adnexal structure to keratin plugs with an inflammatory reaction as well as implanted epidermal cells from trauma. Either way, the infundibular portion of the hair follicle is the suspected site of origin. There are multiple interchangeable labels given to epidermoid cysts including: epidermal cyst, epidermal inclusion cyst, infundibular cyst, and keratin cyst.

In prosthesis users, these cysts have most commonly been reported at locations where trimlines terminate which make trauma with frictional forces more pertinent in this etiology. Commonly affected areas in amputee patients are the hip region in transfemoral patients, proximal adductor thigh, inguinal crease, and ischial region. In the transtibial amputee, skin over the pretibial muscle group has been implicated, possibly associated with contraction of these muscles causing stress between pretibial skin and socket wall during gait. Larger cysts combined with repeated rubbing of the prosthetic interface may lead to pain and may eventually be debilitating in some cases. These can persist and result in infection, abscess formation, ulceration, and scarring, complicating prosthetic use, function, and ambulation [6].

Surgical excision is the preferred treatment intervention [8, 21]. Infections should be treated as previously described. Restoring appropriate interface pressure is necessary to facilitate breaking a chronic repetitive cycle of cyst formations from the aforementioned process. Pressures can be minimized, or more optimally distributed, with appropriately selected interface materials, proper fit and alignment, along with good hygiene practices to optimize care. Other considerations for management include removal of the prosthesis on occasion during prolonged periods of use good and ensuring good hygiene practices to remove keratin and debris from skin that could potentially occlude follicles.

Malignant Tumors
Squamous Cell Carcinoma

Although rare, squamous cell carcinoma (SCC) is the most commonly documented malignant tumor to affect the residual limb of amputees [38] and is the second most common malignant cancer of the skin overall [39]. The relatively flat squamous keratinocytes of the epidermis are the cells of origin. Risk factors for SCC include sun damage, immunosuppression, smoking, HPV infection, prior skin cancers, radiation, arsenic, lymphedema, chronic sores, chronic inflammation, chronic ulceration, or scarring [40–42].

A distinct subset of SCC forms a verrucoid appearance, termed verrucous carcinoma, and has been documented in the residual limb of amputee patients. These lesions are clinically similar to verrucous hyperplasia or viral HPV infections so a biopsy and possibly a skin culture should be done on chronic warty lesions that fail to improve with treatment to exclude malignant potential. HPV has been isolated in verrucous carcinoma and is a predisposing factor. Excision of the affected tissue is the treatment of choice but a residual limb revision leading to a more proximal amputation could be required.

Scar Formation

Scar formation is expected in patients with surgical amputations, but chronic inflammation and chronic ulcerations increase cellular mutations leading to tumorogenesis, termed a Marjolin ulcer. Marjolin ulcers were initially described in burn scars leading to SCC but other less common malignancies have been described to occur in the aforementioned environment and have included basal cell carcinoma, malignant melanoma, and sarcoma [40, 43].

Selected Topics

Having a basic understanding of common skin problems that patients with amputations face is crucial in managing their rehabilitation needs. On occasion however, a patient will present with skin signs or symptoms outside of normal. If unsure of the presentation, referral to a dermatologist is always recommended. As componentry and socket theories have evolved and changed, the principles remain unchanged. Furthermore, these artificial components still predispose the skin to an occlusive artificial environment within a prosthetic socket and this remains a major factor in setting up dermatologic complications. Quality hygiene practices and optimizing fit of the artificial interface remain as the cornerstone of management.

Pruritus

Pruritus is the cutaneous sensation that leads to the desire to itch or scratch and is the most common symptom affecting the skin [11]. The neurological pathways that transmit itch also transmit pain. Therefore, in some cases itch could simply be a misinterpretation of mild pain. Pruritus may present without any visible rash or skin lesions. Typically, there is an associated primary cutaneous condition, although internal systemic conditions involving the kidneys, liver, nervous system, and blood cancers (i.e. leukemia) are possible. The myriad of reasons that cause itching are beyond the scope of this text.

Itching often leads to secondary skin lesions such as excoriations and lichenification. Excoriations can result in pain, cutaneous infections, scars, and a host of additional problems from a compromised skin barrier. Lichenification was previously discussed above with friction, but other selected pruritic etiologies common to persons with limb loss include xerosis and scar formation (discussed in further detail below). It is reasonable to recommend a trial of common anti-pruritic therapies such as a cold compress for 10 to 15 minutes several times per day (note that ice should not come in direct contact with the skin as this could lead to necrosis), emollients, camphor-menthol (i.e. Sarna Lotion, Crown Laboratories, Inc., Johnson City, TN, U.S.A.), pramoxine hydrochloride (i.e. Sarna Sensitive Lotion, Stiefel Co., Research Triangle Park, NC, U.S.A.), or systemic antihistamines as directed by the package insert, over the counter. It is imperative to search for and treat the underlying cause of pruritus as first line management. If the patient fails to improve within 2 weeks of conservative treatment, if the severity of symptoms awaken the patient during sleep, or if systemic symptoms are present, then a referral for systemic evaluation to a physician is indicated.

Dry Skin

Dry skin, or xerosis, is extremely common and is typically associated with pruritus. In the general population, xerosis affects approximately three out of four people over the age of 64 [11, 44, 45]. Xerosis was also the most common skin condition observed in a report of 261 outpatient lower limb prosthetic visits but was rarely the primary reason for scheduling a visit with the prosthetist or other provider [18]. Xerosis is identified by dry, scaly, rough, and possibly itchy skin. Xerosis affects the limbs more than the trunk and is more prevalent in the winter. Xerosis is routinely managed with good hygiene practices and skin moisturizers, such as emollients (e.g. Aquaphor, Vaseline, Unilever, NJ, U.S.A.) orhumectants (e.g. LacHydrin, Ranbaxy, Jacksonville, FL, U.S.A.). A common inciting example would be a prolonged hot bath. Long hot tub baths provide short-term symptom relief but heat exacerbates itch and actually pulls further moisture from the skin and increases desquamation [11]. Drag drying also removes potentially protective, superficial epidermal cells and increases friction and dermatitis.

Moisturizers are available over the counter and should be applied as instructed on the product label as most help to retard transepidermal water loss. Specifically, a technique referred to as the "*soak and smear*" method is recommended [46]. With dry skin, a slightly longer duration (20 minutes) lukewarm bath, using a mild fragrance-free soap or syndet if dirty, is recommended. Immediately after, patting dry with a towel, intentionally leaving a slight amount of moisture that is locked in with the moisturizer at bedtime, preferably in an ointment base such as petrolatum (e.g. Aquaphor, Vaseline) is also recommended. Similar length and temperature showering, or shorter baths, have not shown the same benefit. Additionally, chlorinated water soaks as in sitting in a pool or hot tub lead to increased irritation [46]. Unless otherwise instructed, a moisturizing lotion should not be applied to

open lesions. In prosthetic management, applying a moisturizer on the stump immediately prior to donning a gel liner is not recommended. In such cases, liners with integrated emollients or moisturizers would be preferable but could become a potential chemical irritant. Introduction of new components or chemicals requires skin monitoring for reaction. Another helpful management strategy is to use an air humidifier in bedrooms. Management of xerosis commonly has a seasonal element and is generally a matter of modification of hygiene practices. Patients should be reminded to seek medical advice if symptoms fail to improve or become worse.

Scar

Scars can be a common source of symptoms affecting the residual limb and are an inherent complication of surgery. After the initial amputation, the inflammatory stage of wound healing ensues almost immediately (Figure 9.17). Platelets are the primary player initially and are responsible for platelet derived growth factor (PDGFs), transforming growth factors (TGFs), and fibronectin to serve as a provisional matrix. Chemoattractants increase vascular permeability and attract white blood cells to the area. Neutrophils and macrophages then migrate to and clean the wound and reduce the risk of infection. After about 5 days, the proliferative or granulation stage of healing begins and the focus switches to keratinocytes as the primary cell of significance. These cells of the epidermis begin to fill in the wound laterally as well as from deeper hair follicles. Fibroblasts begin producing type III collagen and myofibroblasts act on the wound to decrease its area with maximal contraction occurring around day 15. Revascularization and angiogenesis occur during this time as well. After nearly 3 weeks, the wound begins maturation and the focus switches to fibroblasts to produce ground substance and more collagen. As time progresses, mature type I collagen replaces type III, and the strength of the scar improves. After 1 year, the scar is fully mature with a peak strength that is about 75% of the pre-wounding strength; it will never attain the strength of normal skin [47].

Following primary healing, consultation with a physical therapist for scar desensitization and myofascial manipulation may be of benefit to optimize scar strength and healing [48]. Itching, irritation, and pain are common complaints related to scar tissue even when the scar is ideal in appearance. If possible, surgical scars are planned to be parallel to Langer's cleavage lines as underlying muscles generally run perpendicular and collagen orientation is primarily parallel to these natural skin creases. These tension lines are more apparent with age, smoking, and sun exposure. Cutting parallel to these lines generally results in a more aesthetically appealing fine scar and scars widen when these lines are violated. It is also important to note that many surgical procedures are done urgently or even

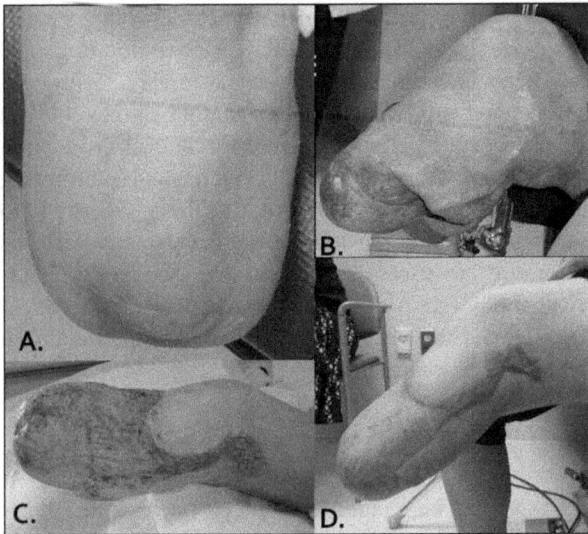

Figure 9.17. A. Well-healed, minimally noticeable scar. It is positioned anterior-distal on this transtibial residual limb, characteristic of a typical transtibial amputation with long-posterior flap closure. B. Residual limb with mottled, dry distal tissue and excess skin flaps with invaginated scarring (beneath). This limb will be prone to intertriginous lesions in the posterior skin folds and scar area. C. Acute, post-operative skin graft covering a residual limb. D. The same residual limb presenting sub-acute scarring.

emergently to prevent mortality. Underlying comorbidities, smoking, nutritional status, suture selection, undermining, and many other technical aspects of closure have all been known to affect the final outcome of healing and scar formation. Healing will hopefully end with a normal, flat, asymptomatic scar. However, the end result may ultimately be an atrophic scar, hypertrophic scar, or keloid. Scars can also break down, ulcerate, or harbor chronic inflammation and even tumor formation (see Tumor above). Thin or atrophic scars generally have a white or nearly transparent look with a flat epidermis and very thin dermis to the point where visualization of underlying blood vessels could be possible. Hypertrophic scars are typically elevated above the skin but not beyond the borders of the inciting trauma, whereas keloids have abnormally enlarged collagen bundles and extend beyond the initial site of injury. Hypertrophic scars and keloids are responsible for the majority of mature scar-related symptoms and treatment is often disappointing. Over the counter silicone has shown to be beneficial in several studies. However, intralesional corticosteroids have proven to be most effective in the authors' experience. Laser treatments are effective in some scars. For example, erythematous scars, which are typically younger, improve with laser treatments using wavelengths near 585 nm. Scar revisions are beyond the scope of this text but serve as another management option. However, improvement would not be expected if there was not a significant improvement in the underlying or associated comorbidities previously described. Scar-free

healing in humans occurs naturally in utero but does not normally occur otherwise. Nevertheless, this exciting possibility is the focus of intense study and several researchers have documented scar-free healing by altering the chemical wound environment in murine models by decreasing growth factors (e.g. PDGF), neutralizing proteins (e.g. TGFbeta1 or TGFbeta2), adding exogenous TGFbeta3, or using mesenchymal stem cells [49, 50].

Sweating
Hyperhidrosis (abnormal increased sweating)

Hyperhidrosis is a condition characterized by an abnormal increase in perspiration beyond the typical quantity required for thermoregulation. It can be associated with burden to quality of life from multiple perspectives including emotional and social domains [51]. Sweat glands tend to be highly concentrated in the areas of the hands, feet, axilla, and groin. These locations are where the majority of people tend to have most of their perspiration take place. Primary (or focal) hyperhidrosis occurs with localized sweating, for instance from the scalp, the hands, or the feet. This tends to begin in adolescence and has a familial or genetic component. Alternatively, secondary (or generalized) hyperhidrosis occurs with total body involvement. Secondary hyperhidrosis can start at any point in life, is less likely to be strongly inherited, and could be the consequence of another systemic condition (e.g. diabetes, thyroid disorders, menopause). The cause of hyperhidrosis may remain elusive but sympathetic over-activity is involved and the condition is generally worse in persons who tend to be anxious. Nutrition and food supplements have been found to play a role (i.e. stimulants) as can other sensory stimuli (i.e. noises, smells) [8, 52].

Heat loss in normally intact skin occurs by radiation, conduction, convection, and evaporation. Radiation is the transfer of heat from one object to another without contact. At room temperature with normal humidity, 60–65% of heat removed from the body is removed via radiation. Ambient temperature is however a major factor in influencing vasomotor responses influencing radiation whereby colder temperatures cause vasoconstriction and heat is conserved. Contact with a prosthesis impairs radiation heat loss. Similarly, convection requires moving air to remove heat and thus prosthesis to skin contact prohibits air movement and convection. The process of conduction exchanges heat between two contacting surfaces [8]. This is clearly functioning in prosthesis users as interface materials warm up to body temperature, and likely maintain it along with any additional temperature elevations resulting from added forces associated with movement. Evaporation of perspiration from skin is another heat transfer pathway that is impaired during prosthetic use.

Reflex sweating is total body sweating that occurs when any single body part is exposed to the threshold temperature that triggers sweat production. It is a condition associated more commonly with spinal cord injury but has been discussed in association with amputation [8, 53]. Reflex sweating induces perspiration in other places of the body even if all other body parts are below the threshold for sweat production. For instance, due to conduction and impairment of all other heat exchange pathways, stump skin temperatures can indicate perspiration is necessary but the amputee's sound limb, hands, and head are at a comfortable sub-sweat production temperature and thus may begin perspiring [8]. Simply donning a prosthesis at rest could increase stump skin temperature by a perceptible 0.5–1.0°C [20]. Walking can therefore easily increase stump skin temperatures into the perspiration range. Following walking, a 2.0°C reduction or more in temperature is required for amputees to begin to perceive cooling, although they could detect a mere 0.5°C temperature increase as previously mentioned. In summary, amputees who use prostheses are likely to feel warmer and experience total-body, reflex sweating at rates higher than non-amputees.

First line treatment using over the counter topical anti-perspirants, not deodorants, containing aluminum ions (e.g. aluminum zirconium, aluminum chloride, aluminum hydroxybromide) provides relief in many patients by temporarily occluding sweat gland pores. This is generally initiated with once-daily application at night due to the relative inactivity of sweat glands at this time. After around 2 weeks, the patient slowly increases the number of nights between applications to maintain symptom control, ideally once per week [52]. Mild associated irritation or dermatitis is treated with sporadic use of over the counter hydrocortisone as needed. The skin should be dry before application because moisture could lead to the formation of irritating hydrochloric acid; therefore, washing just before application should be avoided.

Prescription strength aluminum chloride may be necessary or switching to other topical preparations such as anticholinergics, boric acid, 2–5% tannic acid solutions, resorcinol, or potassium permanganate, but each substance has its own drawbacks. In some patients, systemic anti-cholinergics (i.e. glycopyrrolate) are effective but are associated with the following adverse events: blurry vision, dry mouth, difficulty with micturition, and constipation. Although potentially costly and painful due to the necessity of multiple injection sites, some patients have been treated with neuromodulating toxins, such as Botox® [54–57], though minor muscle weakness secondary to diffusion can occur [58]. Furthermore, laser epilation has been recently used as a successful treatment option in axillary hyperhidrosis. Therefore, we postulate that improvement would also be seen on the residual limb, so it would be reasonable to treat the area under the artificial interface with a 1064 to 1320 nm Nd:YAG laser [59–61].

Odor

Apocrine sweat is secreted as an odorless and sterile substance. Nonetheless, certain bacteria (e.g. Micrococcus spp.) modify the secretion into a sweaty or rancid smell, termed bromhidrosis [9]. Eccrine secretions are also odorless but can soften the skin allowing bacteria to breakdown keratin, also leading to an unpleasant odor. Eccrine bromhidrosis has also been described secondary to ingestion of medications (e.g. bromides), foods (e.g. garlic), or other metabolic abnormalities. When assisting the amputee patient in assessing and managing complaints of odor, the most important aspect is to ensure high quality hygiene as described previously. A thorough diet and medication history is also encouraged to minimize ingestion of known provocative substances. Topical antimicrobial cleansers (e.g. Dial antimicrobial soap, chlorhexidine), prescription antibiotics (e.g. Clindamycin solution), or a novel glycine–soja sterocomplex agent have demonstrated improvement in some cases [62]. Finally, odor could emanate from places in the prosthesis not subject to daily hygiene. In cases where odor is a persistent problem, elements of the prosthesis not included in daily cleansing should be investigated by the prosthetist. Such places include between the flexible interface and rigid frame and between the foot shell and foot structure. These components should be inspected and cleaned thoroughly to optimize management.

CLASSIFICATION SYSTEMS

Classification of skin problems is important for multiple reasons. In order to classify, proper recognition and identification are first necessary. These are early steps in proper management of skin problems. Beyond this, classification is also necessary to facilitate interprofessional dialogue and research. A lack of uniform classification of skin problems is cited as a reason why aggregating epidemiologic data from multiple studies is difficult [63]. This is a valid point. Some studies refer to skin problems by either their diagnosis [13] or by some description of the presenting problem or a combination of both [24]. A classification system has been proposed to either use morphology or etiology of the amputees' presenting skin problem(s) [63]. Both have merit and either may have application depending upon the specific question, clinical or research, to be answered. However, the etiology of problems may be difficult or impossible at times to determine. Therefore, we consider the morphological approach to be superior and more useful to both clinical and research teams. The morphological classification previously recommended is reasonable however, it may lend some confusion. For instance, infections are listed as both a morphological type as well as in the larger problem list. As difficult a task it is to create a classification schema, it is necessary. Using the outline from this chapter, we propose in Table 9.1 a descriptive classification be considered for future inter-professional dialogue and research.

TABLE 9.1

Diagnostic Summary of Dermatoses in Amputees

PRIMARY	SECONDARY	TERTIARY
1. Dermatitis	a. Contact Dermatitis	
		i. Irritant
		ii. Allergic
		iii. Non-Specific Ecsematization
	b. Psoriasis	i. Koebnerization (lichen planus)
		ii. Bacteria
		iii. Fungi
	c. Intertrigo	
	d. Urticaria	i. Pressure urticaria (physical)
2. Infection (pyodermas)		
3. Volume Changes		
	a. Negative Pressure Hyperemia	
	b. Friction	i. Blister
		ii. Callus
	c. Ulceration	i. Pressure Sores (Decubiti)
	d. Verrucous Hyperplasia	
4. Tumor	a. Benign	i. Epidermoid (inclusion) Cyst
		ii. Bursa
	b. Malignant	
5. Specific Signs & Symptoms	a. Pruritus (in addition to dermatitises previously listed)	i. Lichenification
	b. Xerosis	
	c. Scarring	i. Atrophic
		ii. Keloid
		iii. Hypertrophic
	d. Perspiration	i. Bromhidrosis
		ii. Hyperhidrosis

SUMMARY

This chapter presented common dermatoses in persons who use prostheses and orthoses. It is clear that use of an assistive device such as prostheses and orthoses can increase the likelihood of skin issues. Because use of these devices increases skin problems [64], prosthetists, orthotists, and other rehabilitation practitioners must first be able to help patients prevent them as much as possible. When not possible, they must be able to recognize and manage skin problems that occur frequently. Finally, when skin problems are refractory to routine management or are clearly beyond the scope of the rehabilitation team, a referral to the primary care physician or dermatologist must be made. When a referral is made for assistance with skin problems, it is vital to include as much information as possible. This information should include exposures to materials and cleaners as well as interventions that have been tried, any changes that have been made and how long the problem has persisted. At times, disuse of the prosthesis or orthosis may be part of the management plan. Interdisciplinary communication and collaboration will ultimately optimize care in such cases.

The chapter further presented a number of commonly occurring dermatoses along with their etiology, morphology, and management to facilitate improvements in care and referrals. Finally, classification systems were considered and introduced. Until tissue and limb regeneration is a reality, exoprostheses and orthoses will continue as the standard of care. As long as exoprosthetic sockets and orthoses interface with skin, there will be problems with the skin. Those providing care for persons with limb loss who use prostheses, and those who use orthoses, require fundamental knowledge of how to care for all facets of these unique patients' lives including their skin.

REFERENCES

[1] Ziegler-Graham K, MacKenzie EJ, et al. Estimating the prevalence of limb loss in the United States: 2005 to 2050. *Arch Phys Med Rehab.* 2008;89(3):422–429.

[2] Curran T, Zhang JQ, Lo RC, et al. Risk factors and indications for readmission after lower extremity amputation in the American College of Surgeons National Surgical Quality Improvement Program. *J Vasc Sur.* 2014;60(6):1315–1324.

[3] Stern RS, Nelson C. The diminishing role of the dermatologist in the office-based care of cutaneous diseases. *J Am Acad Dermatol.* 1993;29(5 Pt 1):773–777.

[4] Bickers DR, Lim HW, Margolis D, et al. The burden of skin diseases: 2004 a joint project of the American Academy of Dermatology Association and the Society for Investigative Dermatology. *J Am Acad Dermatol.* 2006;55(3):490–500.

[5] Dudek NL, Marks MB, Marshall SC, Chardon JP. Dermatologic conditions associated with use of a lower-extremity prosthesis. *Arch Phys Med Rehab.* 2005;86(4):659–663.

[6] Levy SW. Skin problems of the leg amputee. *Prosthet Orthot Int.* 1980;4(1):37–44.

[7] Hachisuka K, Nakamura T, Ohmine S, et al. Hygiene problems of residual limb and silicone liners in transtibial amputees wearing the total surface bearing socket. *Arch Phys Med Rehab.* 2001;82(9):1286–1290.

[8] Levy SW, ed. *Skin Problems of the Amputee*, 1983. Warren H. Green, St. Louis, MO.

[9] Bolognia JL, Jorizzo JL, Schaffer JV, eds. *Dermatology*, 2012. 3rd edition, No. 1. Saunders/Elsevier, China.

[10] Tyebkhan G. A study on the pH of commonly used soaps/cleansers available in the Indian market. *Indian J Dermatol Venereol Leprol.* 2001;67(6):290–291.

[11] Norman RA. Xerosis and pruritus in the elderly: recognition and management. *Dermatol Ther.* 2003;16(3):254–259.

[12] Munoz CA, Gaspari A, Goldner R. Contact dermatitis from a prosthesis. *Dermitis.* 2008;19(2):109–111.

[13] Lyon CC, Kulkarni J, Zimerson E, et al. Skin disorders in amputees. *J Am Acad Dermatol.* 2000;42(3):501–507.

[14] Hoare C, Li Wan Po A, Williams H. Systematic review of treatments for atopic eczema. *Health Technol Assess.* 2000;4(37):1–191.

[15] Green C, Colquitt JL, Kirby J, et al. Clinical and cost-effectiveness of once-daily versus more frequent use of same potency topical corticosteroids for atopic eczema: a systematic review and economic evaluation. *Health Technol Assess.* 2004;8(47):iii,iv, 1–120.

[16] James WD, Berger TG, Elston DM, eds. *Andrews' Diseases of the Skin. Clinical Dermatology*, 2011. 11th edition. Saunders/Elsevier, China.

[17] Parisi R, Symmons DP, Griffiths CE, Ashcroft DM. Global epidemiology of psoriasis: a systematic review of incidence and prevalence. *J Invest Dermatol.* 2013;133(2):377–385.

[18] Highsmith JT, Highsmith MJ. Common skin pathology in LE prosthesis users. *JAAPA.* 2007;20(11):33–36, 47.

[19] Lang DM, Hsieh FH, Bernstein JA. Contemporary approaches to the diagnosis and management of physical urticaria. *Ann Allergy Asthma Immunol.* 2013;111(4):235–241.

[20] Peery JT, Ledoux WR, Klute GK. Residual-limb skin temperature in transtibial sockets. *J Rehab Res Dev.* 2005;42(2):147–154.

[21] Atanaskova N, Tomecki KJ. Innovative management of recurrent furunculosis. *Dermatol Clin.* 2010;28(3):479–487.

[22] Kahle JT, Highsmith MJ. Transfemoral interfaces with vacuum assisted suspension comparison of gait, balance, and subjective analysis: ischial containment versus brimless. *Gait Posture.* 2014;40(2):315–320.

[23] Bruno TR, Kirby RL. Improper use of a transtibial prosthesis silicone liner causing pressure ulceration. *Am J Phys Med Rehabil.* 2009;88(4):264–266.

[24] Dudek NL, Marks MB, Marshall SC. Skin problems in an amputee clinic. *Am J Phys Med Rehabil.* 2006;85(5):424–429.

[25] Freeman DB. Corns and calluses resulting from mechanical hyperkeratosis. *Am Fam Physician.* 2002;65(11):2277–2280.

[26] Salawu A, Middleton C, Gilbertson A, et al. Stump ulcers and continued prosthetic limb use. *Prosthet Orthot Int.* 2006;30(3):279–285.

[27] Scheinfeld N, Yu T, Lee J. Verrucous hyperplasia of the great toe: a case and a review of the literature. *Dermatol Surg.* 2004;30(2 Pt 1):215–217.

[28] Chang JH, Moon HB, Kim CJ, et al. Intractable verrucoushyperplasia: a surgically corrected case. *PM R.* 2015 Mar;7(3):322–325.

[29] Sbano P, Miracco C, Risulo M, Fimiani M. Acroangiodermatitis (pseudo-Kaposi sarcoma) associated with verrucous hyperplasia induced by suction-socket lower limb prosthesis. *J Cutan Pathol.* 2005;32:429–432.

[30] Kelishadi SS, Wirth GA, Evans GR. Recalcitrant verrucous lesion: verrucous hyperplasia or epithelioma cuniculatum (verrucous carcinoma). *J Am Podiatr Med Assoc.* 2006;96(2):148–153.

[31] Levy SW, Allende MF, Barnes GH. Skin problems of the leg amputee. *Arch Dermatol.* 1962;85:65–81.

[32] Aflatooni S, Beekman K, Hennessey K, et al. Dermatologic conditions following limb loss. *Phys Med Rehabil Clin of N Am.* 2024;35(4):739–755.

[33] Lillis PJ, Zuehlke RL. Cutaneous metastatic carcinoma and elephantiasis symptomatica. *Arch Dermatol.* 1979;115(1):83–84.

[34] Nakamura H, Hirota S, Adachi S, et al. Clonal nature of seborrheic keratosis demonstrated by using the polymorphism of the human androgen receptor locus as a marker. *J Invest Dermatol.* 2001;116(4):506–510.

[35] Kahana M, Grossman E, Feinstein A, et al. Skin tags: a cutaneous marker for diabetes mellitus. *Acta Derm-Venereol.* 1987;67(2):175–177.

[36] Paysant J, Andre JM, Martinet N, et al. Transcranial magnetic stimulation for diagnosis of residual limb neuromas. *Arch Phys Med Rehabil.* 2004;85(5):737–742.

[37] Sehirlioglu A, Ozturk C, Yazicioglu K, et al. Painful neuroma requiring surgical excision after lower limb amputation caused by landmine explosions. *Int Orthop.* 2009;33(2):533–536.

[38] Sarma D, Hansen T, Adickes E. Carcinoma arising in the leg amputation stump. *Int J Dermatol.* 2005;4(1).

[39] American Academy of Dermatology. Accessed July 23, 2024. https://www.aad.org/public/diseases/skin-cancer/types/common#:~:text=Basal%20cell%20carcinoma%20(BCC),a%20pinkish%20patch%20of%20skin.

[40] Furukawa H, Yamamoto Y, Minakawa H, Sugihara T. Squamous cell carcinoma in chronic lymphedema: case report and review of the literature. *Dermatol Surg.* 2002;28(10):951–953.

[41] American Cancer Society. What are the risk factors for basal and squamous cell skin cancers? 2014. Accessed August 1, 2014. https://www.cancer.org/cancer/types/basal-and-squamous-cell-skin-cancer/causes-risks-prevention/risk-factors.html.

[42] Skin Cancer Foundation. Squamous cell carcinoma—causes and risk factors. 2014. Accessed August 1, 2014. https://www.skincancer.org/skin-cancer-information/squamous-cell-carcinoma/scc-causes-and-risk-factors/.

[43] Kowal-Vern A, Criswell BK. Burn scar neoplasms: a literature review and statistical analysis. *Burns.* 2005;31(4):403–413.

[44] Freedberg IM, Eisen AZ, Wolff K, eds. *Fitzpatrick's Dermatology in General Medicine*, 1999. 5th edition, No. 1. McGraw-Hill, New York.

[45] Amin R, Völzer B, El Genedy-Kalyoncu M, et al. The prevalence and severity of dry skin and related skin care in older adult residents in institutional long-term care: a cross-sectional study. *Geriatr Nurs.* 2023;54:P331–P340.

[46] Gutman AB, Kligman AM, Sciacca J, James WD. Soak and smear: a standard technique revisited. *Arch Dermatol.* 2005;141(12):1556–1559.

[47] Cantu RI, Grodin AJ. *Myofascial Manipulation. Theory and Clinical Application*, 2001. 2nd edition. Aspen, Gaithersburg, MD.

[48] Mensch G, Ellis PM. *Physical Therapy Management of Lower Extremity Amputations*, 1986. Aspen, Rockville, MD.

[49] Ferguson MW, O'Kane S. Scar-free healing: from embryonic mechanisms to adult therapeutic intervention. *Philos Trans R Soc Lond B Biol Sci.* 2004;359(1445):839–850.

[50] Sabapathy V, Sundaram B, Sreelakshmi VM, et al. Human Wharton's Jelly Mesenchymal Stem Cells plasticity augments scar-free skin wound healing with hair growth. *PLOS One.* 2014;9(4):e93726.

[51] Kang CW, Choi SY, Moon SW, et al. Short-term and intermediate-term results after unclipping: what happened to primary hyperhidrosis and truncal reflex sweating after unclipping in patients who underwent endoscopic thoracic sympathetic clamping? *Surg Laparosc Endosc Percutan Tech.* 2008;18(5):469–473.

[52] Vorkamp T, Foo FJ, Khan S, Schmitto JD, Wilson P. Hyperhidrosis: evolving concepts and a comprehensive review. *Surgeon.* 2010;8(5):287–292.

[53] Fast A. Reflex sweating in patients with spinal cord injury: a review. *Arch Phys Med Rehabil.* 1977;58(10):435–437.

[54] Kern U, Martin C, Scheicher S, Muller H. Does botulinum toxin A make prosthesis use easier for amputees? *J Rehabil Med.* 2004;36(5):238–239.

[55] Garcia-Morales I, Perez-Bernal A, Camacho F. Letter: stump hyperhidrosis in a leg amputee: treatment with botulinum toxin A. *Dermatol Surg.* 2007;33(11):1401–1402.

[56] Charrow A, DiFazio M, Foster L, et al. Intradermal botulinum toxin type A injection effectively reduces residual limb hyperhidrosis in amputees: a case series. *Arch Phys Med Rehabil.* 2008;89(7):1407–1409.

[57] Kern U, Kohl M, Seifert U, Schlereth T. Botulinum toxin type B in the treatment of residual limb hyperhidrosis for lower limb amputees: a pilot study. *Am J Phys Med Rehabil.* 2011;90(4):321–329.

[58] Schnider P, Binder M, Auff E, et al. Double-blind trial of botulinum A toxin for the treatment of focal hyperhidrosis of the palms. *Br J Dermatol.* 1997;136(4):548–552.

[59] Goldman A, Wollina U. Subdermal Nd-YAG laser for axillary hyperhidrosis. *Dermatol Surg.* 2008;34(6):756–762.

[60] Kotlus BS. Treatment of refractory axillary hyperhidrosis with a 1320-nm Nd:YAG laser. *J Cosmet Laser Ther.* 2011;13(4):193–195.

[61] Letada PR, Landers JT, Uebelhoer NS, Shumaker PR. Treatment of focal axillary hyperhidrosis using a long-pulsed Nd:YAG 1064 nm laser at hair reduction settings. *J Drugs Dermatol.* 2012;11(1):59–63.

[62] Gregoriou S, Rigopoulos D, Chiolou Z, et al. Treatment of bromhidrosis with a glycine-soja sterocomplex topical product. *J Cosmet Dermatol.* 2011;10(1):74–77.

[63] Bui KM, Raugi GJ, Nguyen VQ, Reiber GE. Skin problems in individuals with lower-limb loss: literature review and proposed classification system. *J Rehabil Res Dev.* 2009;46(9):1085–1090.

[64] Visscher MO, Robinson M, Fugit B, et al. Amputee skin condition: occlusion, stratum corneum hydration and free amino acid levels. *Arch Dermatol Res.* 2011;303(2):117–124.

CHAPTER 10

Upper Extremity Prosthetic Rehabilitation

Christopher Fantini and Phil M. Stevens

OBJECTIVES

Upon completion of this chapter, the reader will:
1. Recall epidemiologic data regarding upper extremity amputation.
2. Be familiar with types of pain reported by persons with upper extremity amputation.
3. Recall prosthetic options.
4. Understand intervention options and functional implications associated with differing levels of upper extremity amputation.
5. Be introduced to emerging management options for patients with upper extremity amputation.

INTRODUCTION

Upper limb prosthetic rehabilitation is a challenging endeavor in which patients benefit greatly from multidisciplinary care. Taking into account the individual patient presentation, including amputation level and etiology, vocation, interests, funding resources, and preferences, a core team consisting of the prescribing physician, the treating prosthetist, and a dedicated therapist work with the patient to optimize their function following limb loss or in association with congenital limb deficiencies. This chapter will present general demographics and observations associated with this patient population, introduce general categories of upper limb prosthetic design, discuss amputation level specific prosthetic considerations, treat the concept of successful rehabilitation following upper limb amputation, and address current areas of developing technologies.

GENERAL DEMOGRAPHICS AND OBSERVATIONS

Demographics

The demographics associated with upper limb absence are distinct from those associated with the more

DOI: 10.4324/9781003526025-11

commonly encountered presentation of lower limb amputation. While the latter population is largely characterized by elderly individuals with dysvascular disease and associated comorbidities, amputations of the upper limb are predominantly experienced by younger males with amputations due to traumatic etiologies [1]. Additionally, congenital upper limb deficiencies and acquired amputations secondary to cancer constitute less common causes of upper limb absence. There are nearly ten times as many acquired "minor" upper limb amputations (i.e., fingers and hands) compared with "major" upper extremity amputations (transradial and transhumeral) [1]. The best available estimates, from 2005, indicate that of the 1.6 million individuals living with limb loss, only 41,000 (8%) were living with major upper limb amputation [1].

Pain

The pain experienced by those with upper limb absence is more universal, frequent, and intense than that experienced by their lower limb counterparts [2]. Almost all individuals with upper limb loss experience some type of chronic pain [3]. Both painful and non-painful phantom sensations can be anticipated among those with acquired upper limb loss, followed in prevalence by residual limb pain and pain in the sound side limb, back, or neck due to overuse injury [3]. While phantom limb pain is a frequent source of discomfort, it has been observed to cause less interference with daily activities than other types of pain [3].

For example, the majority of those living with acquired upper limb amputation describe their phantom pain as "discomforting" and "distressing" rather than "horrible" or "excruciating," and quantify the associated lifestyle interference of their phantom pain as "not at all," or "a little bit" [4]. While less common, overuse syndromes appear to be the most disruptive pain sources, with the greatest reported interference with daily activities [3]. Observations suggest that these musculoskeletal overuse pains may have a more deleterious effect on an individual's perceived general and mental health than the absence of the limb itself [5].

In their early work on this topic, Jones and Davidson reported the following overuse diagnoses among a cohort of individuals with upper limb absence: epicondylitis, shoulder impingement, tenosynovitis, osteoarthritis, reflex sympathetic dystrophy type symptoms, carpal tunnel syndrome, and trigger finger [6]. The high prevalence rates of various musculoskeletal overuse pains are of particular interest in this text as therapists are frequently called upon to treat these overuse syndromes within this patient population. The reported prevalence rates of overuse symptoms by location among individuals with upper limb absence are summarized in Table 10.1.

Anxiety and Depression

In contrast to individuals with lower extremity amputation, where prosthetic solutions are both concealable and reasonably functional, upper limb absence

TABLE 10.1

Prevalence rates of overuse symptoms by location among individuals with upper limb absence

PAIN LOCATION	POSTEMA ET AL., 2016	BURGER AND VIDMAR, 2015	OSTLIE, FRANKLIN ET AL., 2011	HANLEY ET AL., 2009	DATTA ET AL., 2004	RANGE
Neck Pain	46%	29%	57%	43%	45%	29–57%
Back Pain	27%	N/R	45%	52%	40%	27–52%
Sound-Side Limb Pain	46%	N/R	57%	33%	N/R	33–57%
Sound-Side Shoulder Pain	33%	40%	59%	N/R	45%	33–59%
Sound-Side Elbow Pain	14%	20%	29%	N/R	28%	14–29%
Sound-Side Wrist Pain	16%	43%	27%	N/R	28%	16–43%
Sound-Side Hand Pain	24%	N/R	26%	N/R	23%	23–26%

is distinctly visible to the outside world. Despite recent technological advances in upper limb prostheses, they only partially replicate some of the physiologic functions and dexterity of the lost extremity. In addition, upper limb amputation is often associated with memories of an acute traumatic event that often precipitates a change in vocation. Collectively, these factors and demographics may explain why up to one-third of those with upper extremity amputation exhibit symptoms of clinical depression [8, 11]. As a result, both life satisfaction and health-related quality of life are understandably reduced relative to the general population for those with both acquired upper limb amputation [12] and congenital limb deficiency [13].

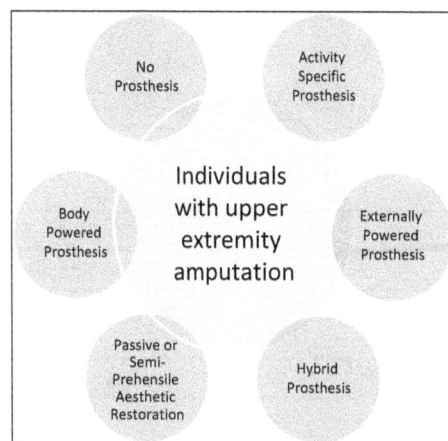

Figure 10.1. General prosthetic options to address upper extremity amputation.

Upper Limb Prosthetic Options

The absence of significant portions of the upper extremity limits the functional capacity of the limb and can significantly impact the individual's ability to perform daily functions with independence and efficiency. Individuals with upper limb absence, and their rehabilitative healthcare teams, should become fully educated about all available options pertinent to clinical and functional needs. Realistic expectations of the benefits and limitations associated with prosthetic use need to be formulated as both can be exaggerated from lack of accurate information. Having accurate and comprehensive knowledge of available solutions empowers the individual with absence of an upper extremity to be the primary driver in the decision-making process while working with the amputee healthcare team. This maximizes the potential for a positive outcome.

Though no individual prosthetic device can restore all the function of a missing anatomical hand or arm, there

are numerous options available which can act to minimize the physical and psychological impact on the individual with absence of an upper limb. The following six general options (Figure 10.1), relating to prosthetic devices, are available for consideration (including combinations thereof):

When appropriate, multiple prostheses may be considered to address strategically diverse needs for variable activities or social/vocational goals. It is important to emphasize that *all* of these design options, including the option of not wearing a prosthesis, provide functional solutions to the individual, based on their given needs or goals. A brief description of each option follows, along with Tables 10.2 through 10.7 which list many of their advantages and disadvantages.

No Prosthesis

Whether the decision is to reject the option of a prosthesis altogether, or to exercise a situational preference of

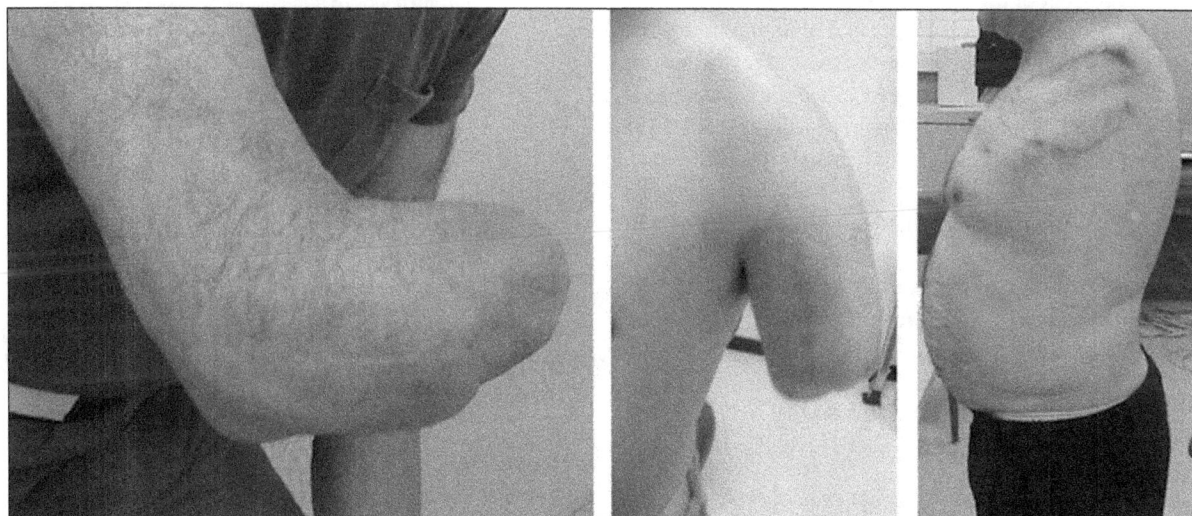

Figure 10.2. Examples of residual limbs at various amputation levels. A. transradial (TR), B. transhumeral (TH), and C. scapulothoracic (ST) (aka forequarter).

TABLE 10.2

Advantages and disadvantages of the no prosthesis option

NO PROSTHESIS	
Advantages	**Disadvantages**
Very simple.	Poor aesthetics.
Comfortable—nothing to don.	No added function.
Full sensory feedback with external environment. (Residuum is not encapsulated by a socket.)	Necessitates either functioning as "one-handed" or with no hands in the case of bilaterals.
Improved mobility—less encumbering to movement.	Reduced or absent ability for bimanual tasks.

when to use one, there are multiple reasons a person with upper extremity amputation may decide not to wear a prosthesis. These include, but are not limited to:

- Perceived negative impact to body image;
- Functional efficiency in the use of the remaining limb(s);
- Comfort;
- Lack of access to clinical expertise/training;
- Unawareness of the available options;
- Prior negative experience with a prosthesis;
- Financial limitations.

In situations where the decision is voluntary rather than imposed by the healthcare system, the choice of no prosthesis may be considered a functional choice, allowing the individual to take advantage of some of the benefits listed in Table 10.2.

Recommended Training: Physical rehabilitation for all individuals with upper limb amputation, regardless of whether they choose to use a prosthesis, should focus on strength, flexibility, and endurance of the remaining musculature, with particular attention to the individual's core muscle groups. Early emphasis should also be placed on skin care and management of the residual limb (Figure 10.2), including techniques to deal with edema and phantom limb pain. Progress should then be made toward teaching alternate one arm or no-arm techniques to perform self-care, activities of daily living (ADLs), and vocational tasks if applicable. The rehabilitation and training should include patient education on adaptive equipment, tools, and utensils to allow the individual to function more efficiently with maximum independence. This provides a foundation of physical well-being and will help minimize overuse syndromes from compensatory body movements during activities.

Passive or Semi-Prehensile Aesthetic Restoration

While there are some disadvantages, this option provides many advantages (Table 10.3) including body image symmetry (Figure 10.3) and practical function. It is often used with amputation at the digit level but can be used for any amputation level. Materials such as acrylic, latex, polyvinyl

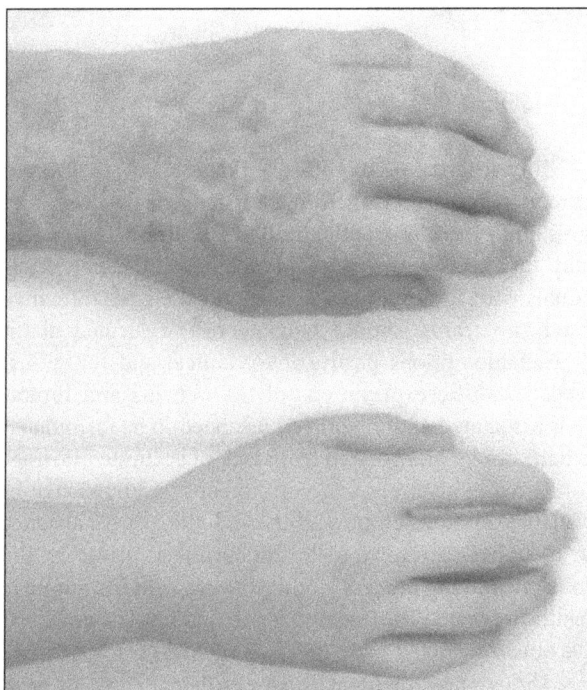

Figure 10.3. Example of aesthetic restoration design. The hand pictured at the top is a custom silicone glove. The bottom hand is a non-customized (aka "off the shelf") hi-definition, semi-prehensile silicone hand.

chloride (PVC), micro coated vinyl (MCV), and silicone are often used to improve cosmesis. These prostheses, especially at the transradial (TR), partial hand, and digit levels (Figure 10.4), can provide functional frictional resistance which can facilitate bimanual tasks such as carrying large objects, or embracing a loved one. When prosthetic hands with semi-prehensile fingers are incorporated into the restoration, the fingers can be prepositioned for specific activities, such as typing on a keyboard or cell phone, grabbing the handle of a bag, or holding small object and tools, such as kitchen utensils. These devices are often made to be self-suspending on the residual limb, without need for a harness.

Recommended Training: In addition to following the same recommendations mentioned for "no prosthesis," rehabilitation should focus on the donning/doffing and appropriate oppositional use of the prosthesis in doing simple tasks as mentioned above.

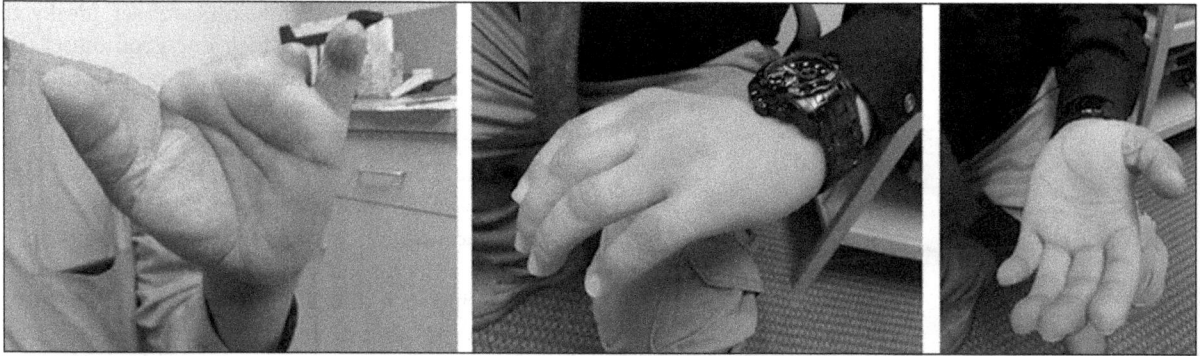

Figure 10.4. Left traumatic partial hand amputation without and with a passive custom silicone restoration (palm up and palm down).

TABLE 10.3 Advantages and disadvantages of the passive or semi-prehensile aesthetic restoration option	
PASSIVE OR SEMI-PREHENSILE AESTHETIC RESTORATION	
Advantages	**Disadvantages**
Relatively lightweight.	No active finger control (i.e., they must be positioned and manipulated by external forces).
No harnessing necessary for transradial level. Only minimal harnessing may be needed for higher levels of amputation.	Custom silicone devices are expensive.
Cosmetic appearance—can be made very lifelike with silicone.	Less expensive PVC products (a type of material used to make non-custom cosmetic gloves) stain easily.
Can have semi-prehensile, flexible fingers which can be prepositioned for specific functions.	Lack of durability.
Can accommodate any level of amputation without causing a length discrepancy with the sound limb.	May require topical agents for donning and suspension.
Restores lost limb length to facilitate a degree of bimanual function.	Exact color matching of the patient's skin tone is uncommon and may frustrate some users.

Externally Powered Prostheses

Externally powered prostheses (Figure 10.5, Table 10.4) are an ideal option for cases where harnessing is to be minimized and active function in reasonable environments is the primary goal. These prostheses feature one or more battery powered, motorized joints actuated by the amputee using one or more control inputs. They could include an interchangeable electric hand and/or hook. Hooks, though less anthropomorphic than prosthetic hands, do provide the advantage of a wider field of view with respect to grasping objects. The number and combination of control inputs used and how they are programmed, constitute the control strategy for the prosthesis. The most common input mechanism is the electromyography (EMG) sensor. The EMG sensor is a non-invasive, surface electrode which acts as an antenna, picking up myoelectric signals from the contracting muscles beneath it. Prostheses that utilize EMG electrodes are commonly referred to as "myoelectric" prostheses. The signals picked up by the EMG sensors are filtered, amplified, and converted by a microprocessor into commands for an assigned motorized function, such as opening or closing an electric hand. The signals may be programmed to be utilized as individual inputs, or used collectively with pattern recognition software, increasing the number of potential input signals. The development of EMG pattern recognition in the prosthetics industry has helped to make control of more complex, externally powered prosthetic devices more intuitive for the user and is discussed in more detail later in this chapter.

There are other control input options for externally powered prostheses, such as linear transducers, force sensitive resistors (FSRs), rocker switches, and inertial measurement units (IMUs), to name a few. These control inputs can take the place of EMG signals when adequate myoelectric signals are not available, or they can be used to complement EMG inputs to provide simultaneous control of two or more functions, or to broaden the number of functions controlled with external power [14].

Externally powered devices are typically heavier, more costly, and require more maintenance relative to other design options. As such, these devices should only

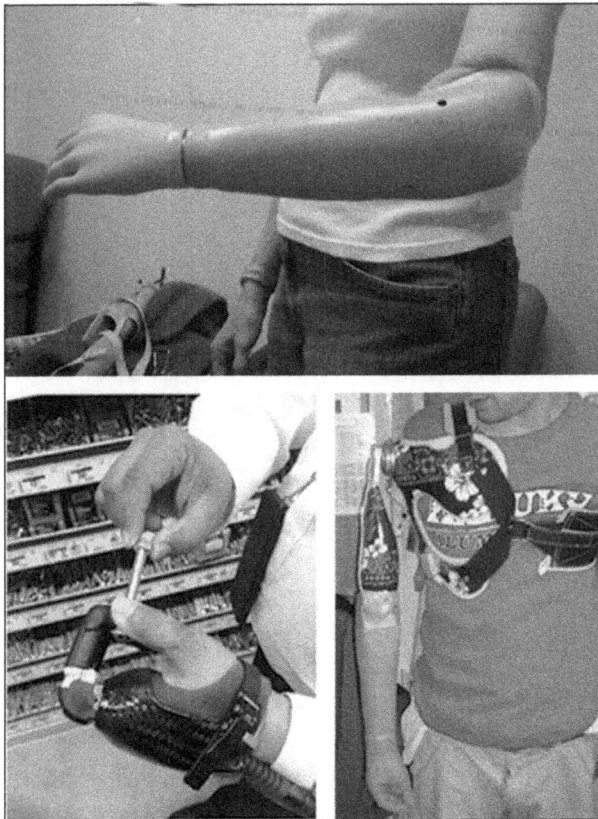

Figure 10.5. Examples of externally powered prostheses at the A. transradial, B. partial hand, and C. shoulder disarticulation level.

be considered if the following factors are met. Ideally, the potential user should have at least one good muscle signal, from their residuum, that they can be trained to use for operating an externally powered device. Other inputs, such as force sensitive resistors or linear transducers, can be considered, but the patient must have sufficient range of motion (ROM) and strength to operate the selected input(s) successfully. Another factor that needs to be considered is the patient's accessibility to an experienced team in fitting such devices. The team should include an experienced prosthetist and therapist who are comfortable with upper extremity prosthetics and rehabilitation. In addition, insurance coverage, or other available funding sources, need to be considered since these devices, as stated earlier, are expensive and will require routine maintenance costs, as well as replacement every few years.

Recommended Training: In addition to the universal training principles, it is very important that the patient be clearly educated as to the functional potential and limitations of externally powered prostheses as many externally powered components can be damaged in extreme usage environments. Training involving an externally powered prosthesis may include collaborative exploration, with the treating prosthetist, of multiple control strategies to select the most advantageous to the user. Whenever possible, the utilization of a trial or preparatory prosthesis should be attempted to verify candidacy. Unfortunately, insurance coverage for such trial fittings is often limited and, in the

TABLE 10.4	
Advantages and disadvantages of the externally powered option	
EXTERNALLY POWERED DESIGN	
Advantages	**Disadvantages**
Minimizes, and may eliminate, the need for harnessing.	More expensive than non-powered options.
	Require more maintenance due to increased susceptibility to damage from moisture, vibration, and impact than other options.
Terminal devices have increased grip force (vs. body powered options).	Some dexterous components are intended for light duty activities only.
More natural control through use of residual muscle contractions, especially for proportional control.	Lack of proprioception in relation to terminal device (TD) position and grip status as compared to harness design.
Increased functional envelope due to an increased ability to use device in all planes of arm movement (reduced harness requirements).	Increased weight relative to non-motorized options.
Easier wrist control as compared to body powered designs is possible.	Battery must be charged on a regular basis.
Improved aesthetics as compared to body powered design.	Consistency of functional performance when using myoelectrodes may be negatively affected by residual limb volume fluctuations, or excessive sweating.
Some powered hands allow for variable grip pattern selection.	

absence of alternate funding sources, externally powered trial prostheses may not be an economically viable option.

When financial conditions support use of a trial prosthesis, training should focus on identifying the most appropriate myosite locations, as well as any other alternate input options, under weight-bearing conditions that mimic those of an actual prosthesis. This approach allows for adjustability in the prosthesis, prior to the final design. Similarly, if available, training the individual in the use of virtual components (i.e., hand, wrist, and/or elbow), via computer software, can also help select appropriate control strategies [15]. Utilizing these training techniques will better improve the individual's development of realistic expectations, ensure formulation of an appropriate definitive clinical prescription, and limit potential rejection of the prosthesis.

Body Powered Prostheses

Body powered devices (Figure 10.6, Table 10.5) require a harness and cable(s) that allow the user to translate gross body motions into control of their prosthesis. While cable-driven hooks are the most common terminal device in such systems, interchangeable cable-driven hands and specialty terminal devices are available. Though prosthetic hands are more cosmetic in appearance, hooks provide several functional advantages over body powered prosthetic hands: they do not obstruct the user's view as much; they allow finer prehension patterns; they require less force to operate; and they have passive function due to their shape, such as carrying a bag.

Body powered systems are most effective when starting from ideal posture. As posture degrades (i.e., a forward head position and rounded shoulder posture), less excursion is available to operate the cable system, resulting in diminished function.

Recommended Training: A postural education and conditioning program should be especially emphasized and incorporated into the rehabilitation of an individual with upper limb loss using a body powered prosthesis.

Hybrid Prostheses

Hybrid prostheses (Figure 10.7, Table 10.6) are most used with more proximal amputation levels, more

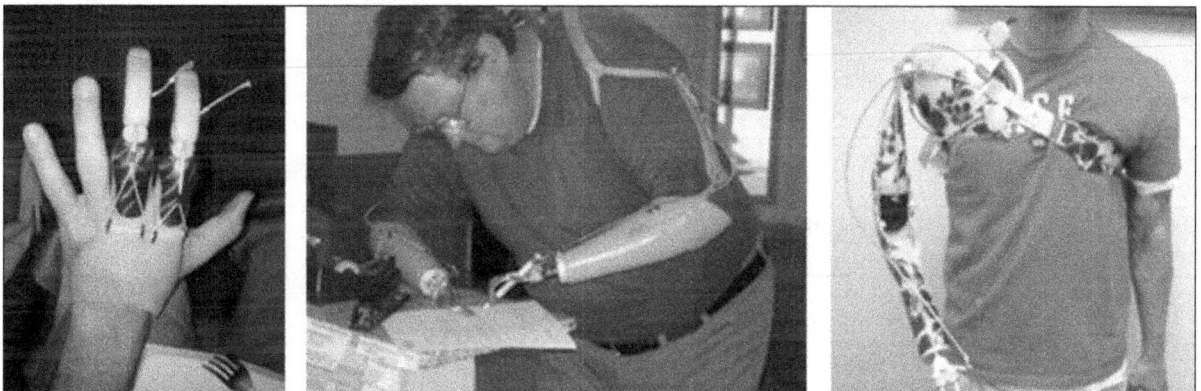

Figure 10.6. Examples of partial finger (A), transradial (B), and shoulder disarticulation (C) body powered prostheses.

TABLE 10.5
Advantages and disadvantages of the body powered option

BODY POWERED DESIGN	
Advantages	**Disadvantages**
Typically, easier to repair than externally powered prostheses.	Requires harnessing which can compromise comfort and restrict movement.
More durable than other options, suitable for use in heavy duty activities and harsh environments (water, dirt etc.).	Requires a certain level of strength, limb length, and ROM in the residuum to operate the prosthesis.
Provides proprioceptive feedback through the harness and socket with regard to joint position and grip status.	Decreased grip force as compared with externally powered terminal devices.
Faster response than externally powered devices.	Less cosmetic compared with semi-prehensile or powered devices.
Less expensive than externally powered devices.	Potential of nerve entrapment syndrome from axillary pressure through the harness over time.
Lower maintenance costs.	

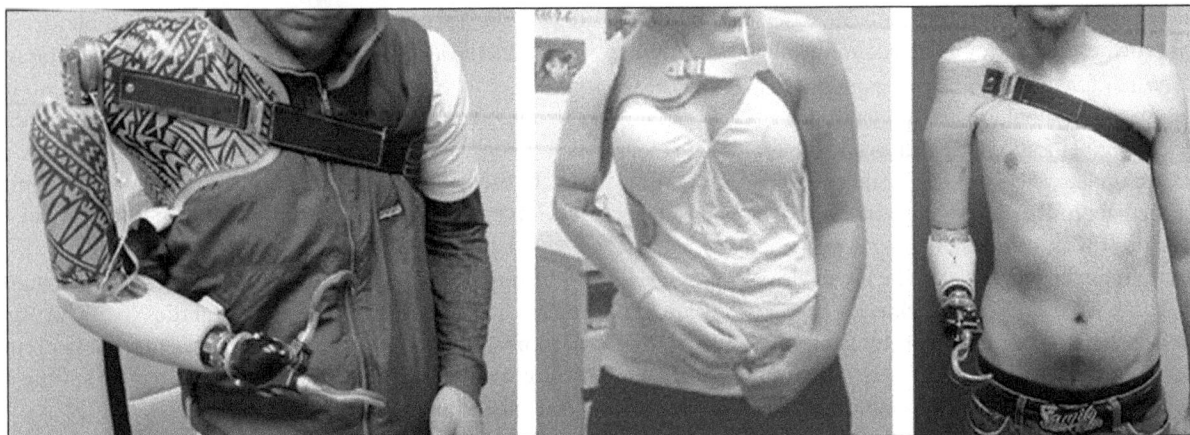

Figure 10.7. Examples of A. shoulder disarticulation, B. interscapular thoracic, and C. transhumeral hybrid prostheses with externally powered terminal devices and passively positioned elbow and shoulder mechanisms.

TABLE 10.6

Advantages and disadvantages of the hybrid option

HYBRID DESIGN

Advantages	Disadvantages
Larger functional envelope than body powered systems.	Harness may be needed for body powered function (usually elbow control).
Less expensive than externally powered devices.	Requires gross body motions to control non-powered components.
Lower weight than externally powered systems.	
Stronger grip force available as compared with body powered devices.	
Simplified control with less need for iterative "mode" switching between components.	More maintenance than non-externally powered options.
Better battery life (due to fewer powered components) than externally powered options.	

specifically with individuals who exhibit sufficient strength and ROM to operate a body powered elbow but lack the additional strength and cable excursion necessary to operate a terminal device efficiently. Though several hybrid set-ups are possible, most hybrid set-ups involve a body powered elbow with an externally powered elbow lock mechanism, combined with a myoelectric controlled terminal device. In some instances, an electric wrist rotator may also be employed.

Though hybrid designs do require a certain level of strength and ROM in the residuum to operate the body powered functions involved, they do provide many of the functional benefits of the externally powered functions. A list of the commonly associated advantages and disadvantages of this design are given in Table 10.6.

Recommended Training: The same training principles that apply to the previously discussed options should be incorporated with the hybrid prosthesis, as this option employs features of both body powered and external powered designs.

Activity Specific Design

Activity specific prostheses (Figure 10.8, Table 10.7) are considered when an individual with upper extremity limb loss wishes to continue, or begin, an activity or hobby that cannot be adequately accommodated with the previously described options. These devices are generally made for life enhancing recreational/sporting activities such as swimming, cycling, weightlifting, golf, playing a musical instrument, etc. They can also be made for facilitating specific vocational tasks, such as holding tools, when more traditional terminal devices are ill-suited for the task.

Recommended Training: Given the variable nature that these devices encompass, specific training should include practicing the specific activity under the supervision of a qualified therapist and subject matter expert. As an example, if a specialty device was made for rock climbing, it is ideal to include a rock-climbing expert or coach in the trial and training of the activity specific prosthesis. This is not only beneficial to the individual with upper limb absence, as it provides a safe and secure environment for evaluating

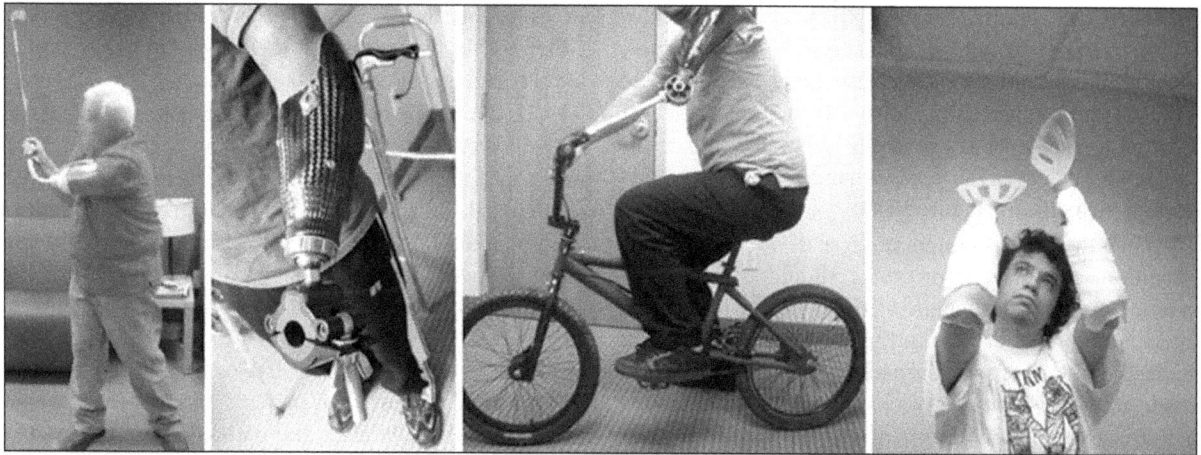

Figure 10.8. Examples of activity specific upper limb prostheses designed for A. golf, B. weightlifting, C. cycling, and D. basketball.

TABLE 10.7	
Advantages and disadvantages of the activity specific option	
ACTIVITY SPECIFIC DESIGN	
Advantages	**Disadvantages**
Customized for a specific function/task.	
Can empower the individual to return to participating in the same recreational activities as before the amputation.	Limited function outside of its intended purpose.

the effectiveness of the device, but better informs the prosthetist and therapist as to the specific and nuanced demands of the activity on the prosthesis. This ensures that appropriate design modifications can be made, if needed, for maximum safety and function.

AMPUTATION LEVEL SPECIFIC CONSIDERATIONS

Partial Finger/Partial Hand

The terms "partial finger" and "partial hand" should be viewed as umbrella diagnoses that encompass a range of potential patient presentations. Partial finger amputations encompass limb deficiencies with absence of one or more digits distal to the MCP (metacarpal phalangeal) level. Partial hand amputations suggest limb deficiencies at or proximal to the MCP joints.

For many years, the prosthetic options at these levels were extremely limited, confined to passive silicone restorations, oppositional posts, and, in the case of carpal level absences, a small selection of transcarpal hands. The introduction of additional components suitable for partial finger and partial hand amputations, in the past decade, have created a broader selection of possible prosthetic solutions.

The advantage of such deficiencies is that the wrist joint and some level of hand anatomy and function are preserved. Further, the residual limb segments are generally sensate. Cumulatively these advantages allow a level of dexterity and function without a prosthesis that often exceeds that obtained with a prosthesis at more proximal amputation levels. Their disadvantage is the lack of anatomic space available for prosthetic restorations and a historic lack of fitting options.

Available solutions at these amputation levels include the choice of no prosthesis, aesthetic silicone restorations, opposition posts, body powered digits, and externally powered digit systems. Patient needs, preferences, and funding resources have a marked effect on which type of prosthesis is most appropriate. Because of the tremendous variability in patient presentations, solutions at these amputation levels are often extremely customized.

For patients whose primary interests are in restoring the cosmesis of a whole hand, silicone restorations can be pursued. Through detailed molding and color matching efforts, these devices can be manufactured to match closely the appearance of the deficient hand or fingers (Figure 10.4). However, as skin tones are transient and affected by several variables, including temperature, diet, and the time of year, a perfect match is difficult to obtain. Practically speaking, patients should be advised that such restorations may fool others at a distance but may draw additional attention up close.

When the residual finger segment approximates or is distal to the proximal interphalangeal (PIP) joint, individual digit restorations can be suspended from the base of the residual finger using suction principles. Absences proximal to this level are generally integrated into a silicone glove worn over the residual hand segment to ensure adequate suspension (Figure 10.4).

While the primary intent of these devices is aesthetic restoration, their functional value should not be overlooked. Restoring the length of the deficient hands and fingers addresses the "hole in the hand" phenomenon in which objects fall through the back of the hand during prehensile activities. However, such devices are not intended for use in extreme environments and have suspect durability. In addition, while guidewires can provide a limited ability to preposition the fingers in relative flexion, they are largely confined to a single alignment.

An alternative to silicone restorations could be found in more durable, but less cosmetic opposition posts. Historically, such posts were fabricated in an ideal alignment that lacked subsequent adjustability. Recent years have seen the commercial availability of full and partial prosthetic digits of robust titanium construction that allow patients to passively position the flexion angle on a task specific basis (Figure 10.9). While body powered and externally powered systems will be discussed shortly, for those individuals who retain active control over proximal digit segments or remaining digits, the grip strength provided by such positionable digits constitutes the strongest, most durable grip option.

Until recently, body powered prosthetic options at these amputation levels were confined to the "handi-hook" approach, in which terminal devices conventionally used in more proximal prosthetic solutions were mounted either within the palm or at the distal end of the residual hand segment (Figure 10.10).

Recent years have seen the appearance of several body powered systems designed for these more proximal applications. These systems are generally driven by mechanical linkage designs or cable driven mechanisms (Figure 10.6A). In both cases, flexion at a more proximal joint segment drives flexion at distal prosthetic joints. Commercial body powered solutions are available for amputation levels at or proximal to the PIP joint. While these mechanisms provide active control of joint position and finger alignment, their prehension is generally weak—a limitation that clinicians and patients should be aware of before pursuing this solution.

External powered prosthetic options are currently confined to those individuals with amputations approximating or proximal to the MCP level. These systems feature powered digits that mount distal to the residual hand segments. Due to spatial limitations, the controllers and batteries for such systems are generally positioned at the wrist (Figure 10.11). Control input is frequently obtained through myoelectrodes positioned over the dorsal interossei, thenar or hypothenar eminance. Alternately, for those individuals with active control over a residual joint segment, FSRs can be used as a source of control input. While such systems provide active control of joint position and alignment and give a stronger grip than that associated with body powered solutions, they are still viewed as light to moderate duty solutions that are ill-suited for extreme usage environments or extreme loading conditions.

Wrist Disarticulation (WD)/ Transradial (TR)

Amputations at or proximal to the wrist are often referred to as major upper limb amputations as the entirety of the hand is now absent. Compared with short TR amputations, wrist disarticulations (WDs) and long

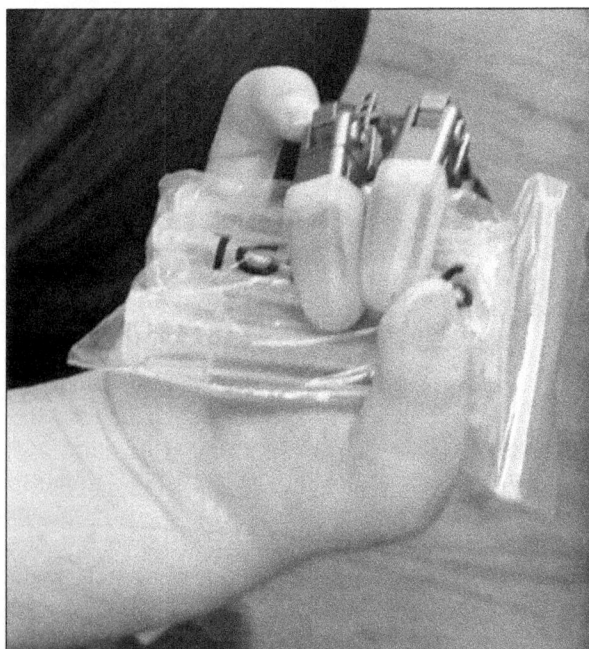

Figure 10.9. Example of an oppositional, positionable partial digit prosthesis.

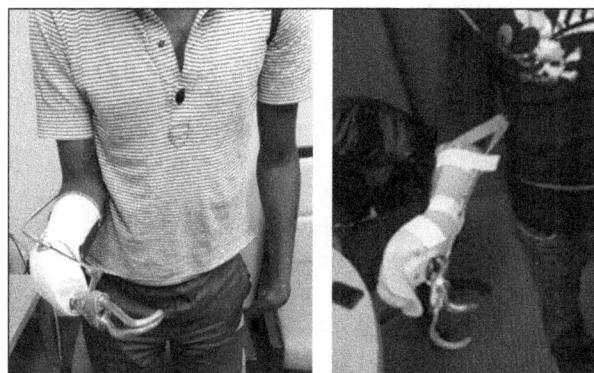

Figure 10.10. Examples of "handi-hook" prostheses with the hook mounted A. distal to the residual hand and B. in the palm of the residual hand.

TR amputations may provide several advantages to the amputee. These include preservation of most, or all, anatomical pronation/supination; increased forearm leverage; and maximized functional ROM at the elbow due to lower prosthesis trimlines.

In contrast, shorter TR amputations result in the elimination of all anatomical wrist function including

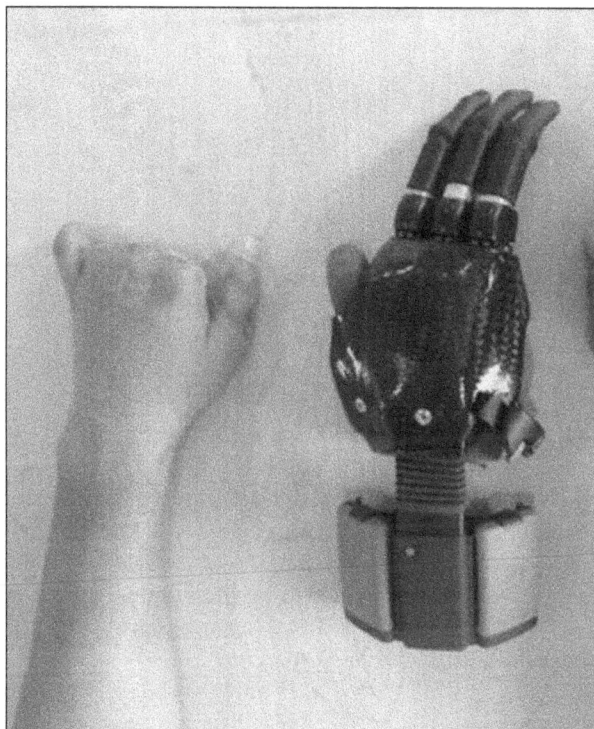

Figure 10.11. Example of an externally powered partial hand prosthesis.

pronation/supination. However, the more proximal amputation level creates additional space that can accommodate the wide variety of prosthetic components that are available to allow the amputee to regain a level of wrist motion.

The disadvantages, relating to fitting of prostheses for the long TR or WD amputee, include the limited selection of functional components. While appropriate for shorter TR levels, wrist units that provide features such as flexion/extension, radial/ulnar deviation, quick disconnect, and/or powered rotation are not practical for longer residual limbs due to the added length of the prosthesis and resulting asymmetry with the individual's body. Table 10.8 lists some of the common wrist units and features used for prosthetic devices.

If the individual's main goal is that of aesthetic appeal, then a self-suspending, semi-prehensile, cosmetic prosthesis should be considered, including the option of a custom silicone hand.

If the individual would like something that is cosmetically appealing with a broader range of function than that of the semi-prehensile design, then a myoelectric device may be considered (Figure 10.5A). Externally powered hands, if used, may also receive custom silicone gloves for enhanced cosmetic appeal.

Body powered designs, utilizing harness suspension, will feature some form of elbow hinges. In general, elbow hinges can be either flexible (made of webbing material, leather, or wire) (Figure 10.6B) or rigid (single axis). Flexible hinges are indicated for long TR, WD, and bilateral TR amputees as they preserve as much of the existing pronation/supination as possible. Flexible hinges are also indicated for children with TR amputations so as not to limit development potential by restricting movement.

TABLE 10.8

Common prosthetic wrist options

COMMON PROSTHETIC WRIST OPTIONS

Type of Wrist Unit	Features
Standard friction wrists	Provide passive wrist rotation; uses friction to control rotation.
Quick disconnect, locking wrists	Allows quick changing of terminal devices (TDs) and locks in the position of the TD during grasping and lifting. These devices are not used with wrist disarticulation amputations or very long transradial levels due to the resulting length discrepancies with the sound limb.
Wrist flexion units	Allows up to three locking positions in flexion and extension for positioning of the TD.
Multiflex wrist unit	Provides resisted flexion/extension and radial/ulnar deviation when unlocked with the additional option of a lock for one of the two axes.
Ball and socket wrists	Allows passive, multidirectional wrist movement with adjustable friction control. These wrists often only resist unwanted movement with light loads.
Quick disconnect for externally powered TDs	Provides a connection between a battery, control input(s), and an electric terminal device. Wrist rotation is possible through manual positioning of the TD.
Electric wrist rotator	Allows quick disconnect of the powered TD and provides the capability for powered wrist rotation. The motor and control for wrist rotation adds significant length to the wrist unit. This is not used with wrist disarticulation cases and may often be impractical for long transradial cases.

Prosthetic designs for the short TR residual limb must address medial/lateral and rotary stability about the elbow and limb. This can be achieved using rigid external hinges in the body powered prosthesis design, particularly if it is intended for heavy duty use.

Lighter duty prostheses, such as semi-prehensile and externally powered designs can be suspended on the limb using aggressive interface designs which extend over epicondyles and olecranon, eliminating the need for a harness (Figure 10.5A). Locking roll-on liners and suction sleeves may also be utilized, either on their own, or combined with a supracondylar interface design (Figure 10.12).

In addition to the array of prosthetic options described above, a forearm cuff, with or without a quick disconnect adapter, should be considered for all individuals with long residual forearms, as they are inexpensive, lightweight, durable, and easy to utilize (Figure 10.13). They can be ordered pre-made or can be custom made from various materials such as leather, plastic, or metal. Forearm cuffs provide a functional alternative in instances when the individual doesn't feel like wearing a complete prosthesis but still requires added functional capacity to the option of "no prosthesis."

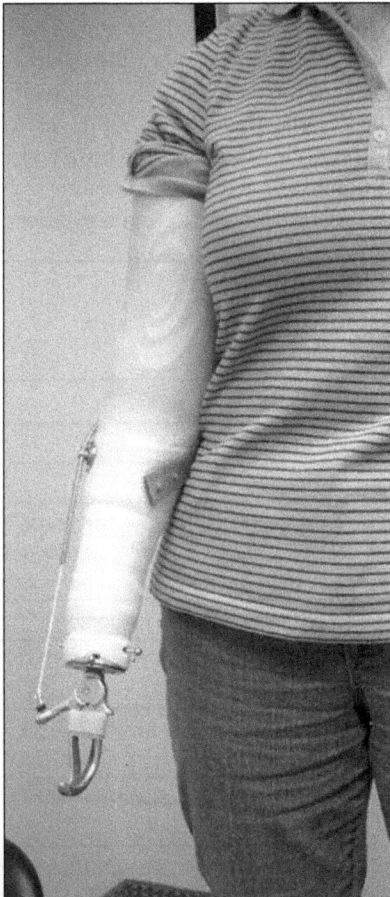

Figure 10.13. Example of a forearm cuff as an alternate functional device to a prosthesis.

Photo courtesy of TRS.

Elbow Disarticulation (ED)/ Tranhumeral (TH)

Amputations at or proximal to the elbow represent another dramatic transition with regard to prosthetic rehabilitation and potential. Lacking an anatomic elbow joint, the patient's ability to preposition the terminal device in space is compromised and functional dexterity with the prosthesis is further undermined.

Elbow Disarticulation

Elbow disarticulations (EDs) provide advantages for suspension and active humeral rotation of the prosthesis due to the preservation of the humeral epicondyles. This is particularly beneficial for bilateral amputees as the ability to actively control humeral rotation with their prostheses results in greater functional control of the device and improved function. Options, however, for prosthetic design are limited. Due to the length of the limb, there isn't enough room to use either a normal or externally powered, prosthetic elbow unit. External locking elbow hinges are usually utilized in the design of a prosthesis made for this level of amputation (Figure 10.14).

External locking hinges add weight as well as bulk to the prosthesis. The extra width resulting from the hinges can limit clothing options for the wearer as tight-fitting sleeves may not fit over the device.

Operation of the elbow is achieved through a dual control harness system. The term "dual control" refers to the two control cables controlled with the harness: 1) the elbow lock control cable, via the anterior elbow lock control strap and 2) the posterior control cable which either functions to enable flexion/extension of the elbow (when the elbow is unlocked) or operation of the TD (when the elbow is locked).

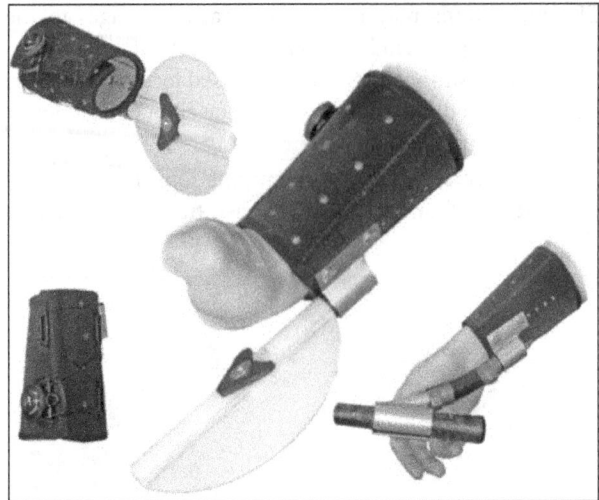

Figure 10.12. Example of a wrist disarticulation prosthesis suspended by a suction suspension sleeve.

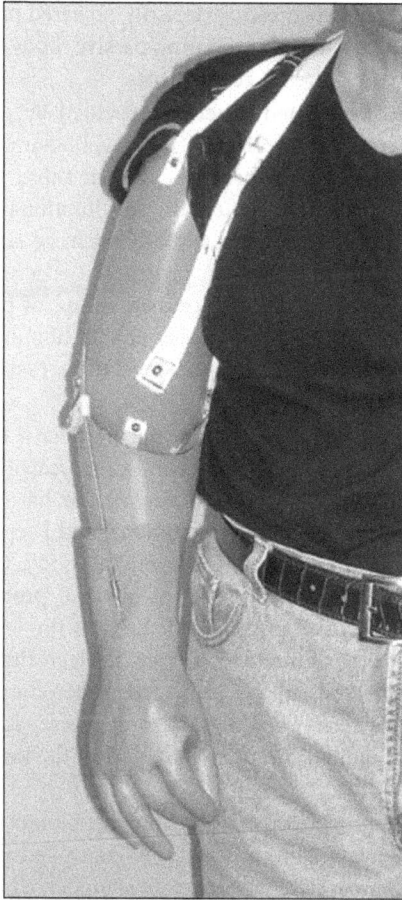

Figure 10.14. Example of body powered elbow disarticulation prosthesis with external locking hinges.

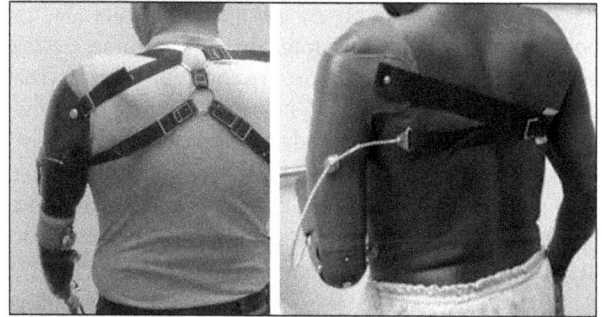

Figure 10.15. Examples of A. figure of eight and B. chest strap harnessing of body powered transhumeral prostheses.

The body motions required for operating a dual control harness are:

- Elbow lock control—simultaneous humeral abduction, extension, and depression.
- Elbow flexion—glenohumeral flexion, abduction, and biscapular abduction. The elbow must be unlocked to control elbow flexion/extension.
- Operation of the TD—same motions as that for elbow flexion control, however the elbow must be locked to control the TD.

Externally powered elbows are usually not used with EDs due to the resulting length asymmetry, so external power, if used, is integrated into a hybrid design in which the elbow would be controlled using body motions, as described above, while the wrist and/or terminal device can be operated with myoelectric control. The amputee can utilize various strategies to switch between wrist and hand control.

Transhumeral Level

Transhumeral (TH) interface designs (Figure 10.15) are usually harness-suspended but they can be self-suspended with the use of suction, elevated vacuum, or with a roll-on liner system. The harness-system can be that of the TH figure of eight design or a shoulder saddle and chest strap (Figure 10.15), however both include an anterior control strap to operate the elbow lock.

Prosthetic elbow units are utilized for TH level amputations. All TH prosthetic elbow units (excluding external locking hinges) allow two degrees of freedom: flexion/extension and humeral rotation, with several control options.

1. Flexion/extension—controlled using one of the following methods:
   a. Passive, manual manipulation;
   b. Active control through a harness (i.e., body powered); or
   c. Externally powered control via myoelectric or alternate input.
2. Humeral rotation—controlled by either:
   a. Passive friction; or
   b. Externally powered humeral rotation via myoelectric or alternate input.

Elbow units can be broken down into three categories: body powered, hybrid, and externally powered.

Body powered designs require adequate strength and ROM in the residual limb to achieve the force and cable excursion necessary to operate the prosthesis. The dual control harness required to operate the body powered TH prosthesis functions as described earlier in the discussion of outside locking joints. If needed, additional components, such as a spring assist unit, may be utilized to reduce the force needed to flex the elbow.

If the amputee has sufficient strength but lacks the control cable excursion necessary to fully flex the elbow and/or operate the TD, an excursion amplifier may be added to the harness. Excursion amplifiers are small pulleys that double the amount of control cable excursion an amputee can gain from their normal ROM. However, this comes at the cost of the increased force required to operate the control cable. Typically, the shorter the limb, the less excursion is available. When the force and/or excursion available is not adequate to fully operate a body powered prosthesis efficiently, then either a hybrid or externally powered design may be indicated.

Hybrid systems typically feature elbow units that use body power to control flexion/extension, with an electric elbow lock. The TD and wrist are controlled via external power (Figure 10.7A). This system provides a greater functional envelope than the body powered design but costs more, is heavier, and is not as durable. When compared with the externally powered design, it is less expensive, lighter, and provides faster elbow response, however sufficient ROM and strength are required to flex the elbow.

Externally powered elbow designs allow the option for sequential control of the powered motion of each joint or simultaneous powered control of the elbow and either the wrist or hand (Figure 10.5C).

Sequential control utilizes the same electric input signal to control the powered functions of the elbow, wrist, and hand. A switching mechanism is employed to allow the user to cycle through the modes of control. For example, the same two electrode signals may be used, independently of each other, to control flexion/extension when the device is in elbow mode: pronation/supination when in wrist mode, and open/close when in hand mode. The user can sequentially switch modes by using muscle co-contraction or an external switch.

Alternatively, prostheses may be designed for simultaneous control of the elbow and either the wrist or hand. In this application, the elbow is typically controlled with either a linear transducer or strain gauge attached to the harness and activated with the same motions used to control body powered elbows. The difference is that there is very little force or excursion necessary to activate the motor for elbow flexion. The elbow automatically locks once motion is stopped for a given period of time, which is adjustable in the software. The elbow unlocks automatically when tension is applied to the control input a second time. The wrist rotator and TD are typically controlled with dual site EMG inputs contained in the interface and placed over the biceps and triceps, respectively. The same sequential control strategy mentioned above is utilized to allow the user to switch between wrist and hand mode.

Shoulder Disarticulation (SD)/ Interscapulothoracic (ST)

Shoulder level amputations include shoulder disarticulation, glenohumeral neck level transhumeral amputations, and interscapularthoracic amputations. These amputations are functionally devastating as the patient now effectively lacks the joints of the fingers, hand, wrist, elbow, and shoulder. Even as the number of prosthetic joints that require control increase, the number of control input options decrease.

Available prosthetic options at this amputation level include the choice of no prosthesis, passive prostheses, body powered prostheses, externally powered prostheses, and hybrid prosthesis combining passive, body powered, and externally powered components.

Given the limited function provided by prosthetic management at this amputation level, many patients choose not to wear a prosthesis. Even those who find value in a prosthesis, often do so situationally, when engaging in bimanual tasks. Daily wearing and use of a shoulder disarticulation prosthesis is uncommon, but this should not be viewed as a failure of prosthetic rehabilitation. If the prostheses enable bimanual tasks when these are required, then a level of success has been realized.

Among those who choose not to wear a full prosthesis, some individuals may choose to wear a shoulder cap. Essentially a socket and suspension harness, such caps can improve shoulder symmetry and keep clothing positioned more symmetrically on the body. Caps also provide patients with a sense of physical protection of the exposed lateral trunk, particularly if the left limb is absent, acting as an added barrier between the external environment and organs protected under the rib cage, including the heart and lungs. In some cases, patients may request a weighted shoulder cap to offset the lost mass of the upper limb.

Passive prostheses warrant consideration at this level due to the heavy nature of actively controlled prosthetic options. Comparatively lightweight shoulder, elbow, wrist, and hand components can be passively positioned by the sound side hand to allow such passive devices to enable certain bimanual activities as a stabilizing agent.

Full body powered prostheses are challenged at this amputation level by the relative lack of excursion potential but can be designed (Figure 10.6C). In the absence of an affected side elbow or shoulder joint, the only sources of cable excursion are sound side scapular abduction and chest expansion. As such, body powered components, when used, are often combined with passive and externally powered components.

Externally powered components represent an ideal solution at this amputation level as they do not require long distances of cable excursion to position the joints of the prosthesis, relying instead on myoelectric inputs and linear transducers. However, the benefits of these components are offset by the drawback of their corresponding weight. Full externally powered systems can be extremely heavy to the end user, requiring a large socket with a correspondingly large surface area to distribute the weight of the device (Figures 10.5C and 10.16).

Given the inherent limitations associated with passive, body powered, and externally powered prosthetic systems, hybrid combinations at this level are extremely common (Figure 10.7A). In most cases, the strong, functional grip of an externally powered TD is combined with a lightweight passive or body powered elbow unit.

Upper Limb Prostheses Outcomes

Given the disparity between the function of the intact upper limb and any prosthetic substitute, it is reasonable to observe that the definition of a successful prosthetic outcome differs from that associated with lower limb prosthetic rehabilitation. An international group of subject matter experts, including both upper limb prosthesis users and clinicians experienced in the provision and training of upper limb prostheses rejected several idealistic definitions of functional success in rehabilitation following upper limb amputation. These included such qualifying statements as: "the use of a prosthesis for pre-amputation job or activities," "a person's ability to perform activities to the same standards as they did before the limb loss," and "the ability to perform activities within the same time parameters as they did before." Rather, the consensus definitions of successful upper limb prosthetic rehabilitation referenced instances when a person wears their prosthesis for specific activities, demonstrates the ability to perform their own personal care/ADLs without help from other people, experiences satisfaction with their functional abilities, and is performing to the best of their ability [16].

Understanding this consensus definition for a successful outcome in upper limb prosthetic rehabilitation is important for all allied health professionals who work with this patient population to help establish and reinforce appropriate, reasonable expectations throughout the process of rehabilitation and prevent the frustrating pursuit of unattainable goals.

The conception and pursuit of unrealistic prosthetic expectations may contribute in part to the abandonment of upper limb prostheses. Reported rates of prosthetic abandonment within this population are extremely variable, with systematic review suggesting average abandonment rates of approximately 25% among adults with acquired limb absence [17] with some reports as high as 44% [18].

DEVELOPING ADVANCEMENTS IN UPPER LIMB PROSTHETICS

In addition to the concepts and principles described above, there are a number of developing advancements in upper limb prosthetics that will ultimately have a profound impact on the functional benefit and day to day usage rates of upper limb prostheses. These include improvements in control, sensory input, and suspension.

Control Strategies

The current standard in myoelectric control is dual site direct control in which two, generally antagonistic muscles provide direct control of opposing prosthetic movements such as opening and closing or flexion and extension of the elbow. Even at relatively distal amputation levels, this control approach is non-native with wrist flexors and extensors controlling prosthetic prehension. At more proximal amputations, this disparity between the controlling muscle groups and resultant prosthetic motions becomes increasingly exaggerated, with the muscles of the upper arm, shoulder girdle, and torso often being used to control movement of the prosthetic terminal devices and wrist.

In addition, at increasingly proximal amputation levels, the remaining muscle groups may be required to control movement at multiple joint segments. For example, at the shoulder disarticulation level, muscles at the chest wall and upper back might be used to control movement of the prosthetic elbow, wrist, and TD by sequentially switching control from joint segment to joint segment.

One solution to this limitation has been demonstrated with the use of Targeted Muscle Reinnervation (TMR). In this approach, proximal muscle groups are surgically divided into two or more muscle bellies separated by a border of adipose tissue. This done, the residual nerve bundles are separated out into peripheral nerves that are then individually transferred to reinnervate into targeted muscle bellies. The end result is an increase in available independent myoelectric signals that often bear a more native relationship between the controlling nerve and the resultant prosthetic movement [19].

An additional advancement is seen in the development of myoelectric control through pattern recognition. The current standard in myoelectric control is one of direct control, in which electrodes are placed immediately over the desired muscle bellies and should only receive input from a single muscle belly. In pattern recognition, an array of multiple electrodes is positioned somewhat arbitrarily around the residual limb. As the patient generates the muscle activities associated with available prosthetic movements, the processor is programmed to record and later recognize these patterns, allowing the prosthesis to perform the desired motions [19]. This control strategy increases the number of discrete myoelectric input signals available from the residual limb.

Still further accuracy and discretion in myoelectric control has been described through the combination of pattern recognition of myoelectric signals generated through muscle sites augmented through TMR [20].

Yet another developing control strategy option is that of "end-point control." This strategy allows the user to actuate multiple powered joints, in simultaneous coordinated movement, to bring the TD to a desired point in space. Rather than plan the motion of each powered joint to get the TD into a desired position, the control commands may be simplified as "hand up/down," hand left/right," "hand forward/back," etc. Endpoint control reduces the number of required control inputs in the system and can enable coordinated movement of the shoulder, elbow, wrist, and hand. This control strategy provides a new reference point for prosthetic control and has the potential to result in more anthropomorphic movements in prostheses for higher level limb absence [21].

Sensory Restoration

A considerable limitation in current upper limb prosthetic rehabilitation is the lack of sensory input from the prosthesis. While body powered devices provide a modest amount of sensory input through the control harness regarding prehensile force, myoelectric prostheses fail to provide any sensory feedback. The result is a disassociation between the user and their prosthesis, with the latter viewed as merely a tool. The restoration of sensory input from the prosthesis to the user's nervous system might serve to improve user's acceptance and performance with their device.

The greatest potential for such sensory restoration has been described through the use of implanted cuff electrodes wrapped around peripheral nerves [22]. Variations on this technique have been described in recent literature, with the longest tenured implanted electrodes reported at 40 months [22]. The integration of force and bend sensors in the prosthetic hand permit the generation of sensations related to both prehensile force and hand span. These signals are then transmitted through electrode wires that pass percutaneously to the internal cuff electrodes where they are experienced as sensory inputs by the targeted peripheral nerves. Preliminary results suggest that this sensory restoration leads to improved performance and confidence with upper limb prostheses [22].

Osseointegration

An additional limitation to modern upper limb prosthesis is the inadequate suspension experienced by many users. Particularly at more proximal amputation levels, the weight of the prosthesis creates a distractive force that would pull it away from both the residual limb and the user's body. Despite creative attempts to counter these distractive forces with harnessing, anatomic suspension, and atmospheric suction, the lack of a direct connection to the upper limb prosthesis augments the perceived weight of the device and further dissociates the user from the prosthesis.

The notion of a direct connection between the residual limb and the prosthesis has been explored through osseointegration, in which the prosthesis is attached directly to remaining bone or bones of the residual limb. While osseointegration has received much broader application in lower limb prosthetic applications, its use in association with upper limb deficiency has been explored.

For example, Jönsson et al. reported upon the introduction of osseointegration in the management of a thumb restoration, transradial limb loss and transhumeral limb loss in 1990, 1992, and 1994, respectively [23]. As of their 2011 report, the authors reported on 48 upper extremity osseointegration prosthetic fittings including cosmetic restorations, body powered and myoelectric prostheses on individuals with partial hand, thumb, transradial and transhumeral level limb deficiencies [23].

Human–Machine Gateway

Several of these advancements have been combined to produce what authors have described as the osseointegrated human–machine gateway (OHMG) [24]. In this transhumeral application the osseointegrated abutment that connects the residual humerus with prosthesis houses internal connectors through which bidirectional impulses of both motor and sensory internal neuromuscular interfaces are exchanged between the residual limb and the prosthesis. Pattern recognition algorithms can differentiate between control signals for opening and closing of the hand, pronation and supination of the wrist, flexion and extension of the wrist, and flexion and extension of the elbow [24]. This advanced prosthetic application simultaneously addresses the current limitations of control, sensory restoration, and suspension in a single, radical solution.

SUMMARY

Prosthetic rehabilitation following upper limb amputation is an extremely challenging endeavor for both the affected individual and their clinical support team. This is compounded by the relative scarcity of upper limb amputations and the resultant lack of experienced rehabilitation professionals. Optimal outcomes are currently limited by available technologies, but also require access to an experienced prosthetist to design, fabricate, and maintain the prostheses, and an engaged therapist to train the user to integrate the devices into their daily activities and habits.

REFERENCES

[1] Ziegler-Graham K, MacKenzie EJ, et al. Estimating the prevalence of limb loss in the United States: 2005 to 2050. *Arch Phys Med Rehabil.* 2008;89:422–429.

[2] Davidson JH, Khor KE, Jones LE. A cross-sectional study of post-amputation pain in upper and lower limb amputees, experience of a tertiary referral amputee clinic. *Disabil Rehabil.* 2010;32(22):1855–62.

[3] Hanley ME, Ehde DM, Jensen M, et al. Chronic pain associated with upper-limb loss. *Am J Phys Med Rehabil.* 2009;9(88): 742–754.

[4]   Desmond DM, MacLachlan M. Prevalence and characteristics of phantom limb pain and residual limb pain in the long term after upper limb amputation. *J Rehabil Res.* 2010;33:279–282.

[5]   Postema SG, Bongers RM, Brouwers MA, et al. Musculoskeletal complaints in transverse upper limb reduction deficiency and amputation in the Netherlands: prevalence, predictors, and impact on health. *Arch Phys Med Rehabil.* 2016;97(7): 1137–1145.

[6]   Jones LE, Davidson JH. Save that arm: a study of problems in the remaining arm of unilateral upper limb amputees. *Prosthet Orthot Int.* 1999;23:55–58.

[7]   Burger H, Vidmar G. A survey of overuse problems in patients with acquired or congenital upper limb deficiency. *Prosthet Orthot Int.* 2016 Aug;40(4):497–502.

[8]   Darnall BD, Ephraim P, Wegener ST, et al. Depressive symptoms and mental health service utilization among persons with limb loss: results of a national survey. *Arch Phys Med Rehabil.* 2005;86:650–658.

[9]   Ostlie K, Franklin RJ, Skjeldal OH, et al. Musculoskeletal pain and overuse syndromes in adult acquired major upper-limb amputees. *Arch Phys Med Rehabil.* 2011;92:1967–1973.

[10] Datta D, Selvarajah K, Davey N. Functional outcome of patients with proximal upper limb deficiency—acquired and congenital. *Clin Rehabil.* 2004;18(2):172–177.

[11] Desmond DM. Coping, affective distress, and psychosocial adjustment among people with traumatic upper limb amputations. *J Psychosomat Res.* 2007;62:15–21.

[12] Ostlie K, Magnus P, Skjeldal OH, et al. Mental health and satisfaction with life among upper limb amputees: a Norwegian population-based survey comparing adult acquired major upper limb amputees with a control group. *Disabil Rehabil.* 2011;33:1594–1607.

[13] Johansen H, Ostlie K, Andersen LO, Rand-Hendriksen S. Health related quality of life in adults with congenital unilateral upper limb deficiency in Norway. A cross-sectional study. *PLOS One.* 2018;13(1):e0190567.

[14] *VA/DoD Clinical Practice Guideline for the Management of Upper Extremity Amputation Rehabilitation.* Accessed October 26, 2016. http://www.healthquality.va.gov/guidelines/Rehab/UEAR/VADoDCPGManagementofUE.

[15] Resnik L, Etter K, Klinger SL, Kambe C. Using virtual reality environment to facilitate training with advanced upper-limb prosthesis. *J Rehabil Res Dev.* 2011;48(6): 707–718.

[16] Nimhurchadha S, Gallagher P, MacLachlan M, Wegener, ST. Identifying successful outcomes and important factors to consider in upper limb amputation rehabilitation: an international web-based Delphi survey. *Disabil Rehabil.* 2013;35(20):1726–1733.

[17] Biddis EA, Chau TT. Upper limb prosthesis use and abandonment: a survey of the last 25 years. *Prosthet Orthot Int.* 2007 Sep;31(3):236–257.

[18] Salminger S, Stino H, Pichler LH, et al. Current rates of prosthetic usage in upper-limb amputees—have innovations had an impact on device acceptance? *Disabil Rehabil.* 2020;44(14):3708–3713.

[19] Lipshutz RD. Targeted muscle reinnervation: prosthetic management. In: Krabich JI, Pinzur MS, Potter BK, Stevens PM, eds. *Atlas of Amputations and Limb Deficiencies: Surgical, Prosthetic, and Rehabilitation Principles,* 2016. 4th edition, pp. 339–350. American Academy of Orthopedic Surgeons, Rosemont, IL.

[20] Cheesborough JE, Smith LH, Kuiken TA, Dumanian GA. Targeted muscle reinnervation and advanced prosthetic arms. *Semin Plast Surg.* 2015;29(1):62–72.

[21] Phillips S, Resnik L, Latlief G, Fantini C. Endpoint control for a powered shoulder prosthesis. *J Prosthet Orthot.* 2013;25(4).

[22] Schiefer M, Tan D, Sidek SM, Tyler JD. Sensory feedback by peripheral nerve stimulation improves task performance in individuals with upper limb loss using a myoelectric prosthesis. *J Neural Eng.* 2016;13(1):016001

[23] Jönsson S, Caine-Winterberger K, Brånemark R. Osseointegration amputation prostheses on the upper limbs: methods, prosthetics and rehabilitation. *Prosthet Orthot Int.* 2011 Jun;35(2):190–200.

[24] Ortiz-Catalan M, Hakansson B, Branemark R. An osseointegrated human–machine gateway for long-term sensory feedback and motor control of artificial limbs. *Sci Trans Med.* 2014 Oct 8;6(257):257re6.

CHAPTER 11

Psychosocial Aspects of Amputation

Lynne B. Hansen and Keiba L. Shaw

OBJECTIVES

Upon completion of this chapter, as it relates to patients with amputation, the reader will be able to:
1. Recall terminology related to psychosocial aspects of amputation.
2. Discuss types of pain and coping strategies associated with amputation.
3. Discuss body image, social support, quality of life (QOL), changing identity, sexual role.

INTRODUCTION

The loss of (a) limb(s) creates significant psychological and sociological challenges for the person experiencing the loss, and, to some degree, the social network supporting that individual. Regardless of the etiology, amputation generates dramatic changes in all aspects of functioning and daily life—whether because of physical limitations in body structures, reduced activity levels, environmental factors, or personal and social factors [1]. Individuals with limb loss experience increased frequency and severity of stressful situations directly associated with their health condition. In addition to the impact of the trauma or underlying condition that led to amputation, amputees face additional threats: to independence and autonomy, to body integrity, to vocational and familial roles, to future goals and plans, and to economic stability. In this chapter we will explore these adversities, their impacts, and ways healthcare professionals can facilitate adaptive coping.

In order to facilitate understanding it seems prudent to begin with common language. *Body image* refers to the internal mental representation of one's own physical body, which is influenced by not only the individual's intrinsic perceptions including age, gender, and physical condition but also by extrinsic influences including the social and environmental factors within which they interact [2–4]. *Identity* is the "complex, interwoven mix" of characteristics that a person believes he/she possesses, or that are attributed to him/her by others—such as one's personal attributes personality traits; abilities; familial, societal, or employment roles; and values and ideals [5].

DOI: 10.4324/9781003526025-12

The theoretical concepts of psychosocial adaptation derive from the three basic assumptions of developmental psychology:

1. Growth occurs in every period of life, in the physical, cognitive, and emotional/social domains;
2. Both continuity and change characterize an individual's life; and
3. Behavioral analysis must consider the whole person (including personal relationships and setting).

Although the circumstances surrounding limb loss may vary, it is almost always experienced as a point of crisis: if the loss was unplanned, it likely will be experienced as traumatic; if the removal was planned (for example, because of vascular insufficiency), the actual decision to amputate is typically the last resort, and is preceded by significant efforts to salvage the limb. The situation forces the individual into a state of change, which requires the use of coping mechanisms—physiological, cognitive, behavioral, and social—to manage the dissonance and regain equilibrium. Because amputation is a permanent loss, these consequences are long-lasting and may become pathological in some cases. *Adaptation* is the ability to change in order to accommodate a variety of circumstances in an intelligent and meaningful way. When we encounter limitations in functioning, we make changes in ourselves and in our environment to address them.

Traumatic Amputation Versus Non-Traumatic/Elective Amputation

A traumatic amputation is the result of an accident or injury that results in the loss of a body part. It has been found that limbs lost as a result of traumatic injury or tumor, and those who sustain a traumatic amputation to the upper extremities, are the most vulnerable to emotional distress—more so than those whose amputations were a result of long-standing conditions [6]. Persons who have sustained traumatic amputations may experience anxiety and/or depression, sleep deprivation, silent rumination about the amputation, and overt anger and irritability [7]. Individuals who have experienced traumatic amputation should be screened for post-traumatic stress disorder/syndrome (PTSD) and depression after surgery [8].

Those individuals who have time to prepare for the loss of a limb tend to be better adjusted than those who have undergone traumatic amputation. Knowing that an amputation is necessary and being able to schedule surgery is helpful in allowing the individual to garner more detail about pre-operative and post-operative procedures. This preparation allows for an attitude of realistic acceptance and cooperation with the treatment team. However, like those who have sustained traumatic amputations, individuals who have undergone elective surgery may experience generalized anxiety, and/or depression, and may be actively grieving the loss of the limb [8].

PAIN WITH AMPUTATION

Limb loss can result in intense physical effects, including pain (see Table 11.1). A national survey found that approximately 95% of amputees surveyed said they experienced one or more types of amputation-related pain. Phantom pain was reported most often—at 79.9% of respondents, 67.7% reported stump pain, and 62.3% reported back pain. A large proportion of persons with phantom pain and stump pain reported experiencing severe pain, ranging from 7 to 10 on a Likert pain scale from 0 to 10 [9]. More recent studies continue to corroborate the finding that pain from a variety of sources is highly prevalent within the population of patients with amputation [10, 11, 12].

Phantom Limb Pain

Phantom sensations are the non-painful sensations experienced in the body part that no longer exists. They are commonly classified as neuropathic, and are assumed to be related to damage of central or peripheral neurons. Phantom limb pain (PLP), on the other hand, is thought to be triggered and exacerbated by psychological factors, with stress being implicated as having a large impact on the onset and exacerbation of PLP [13]. Cognitive factors also play a part in the modulation of PLP; patients who lack coping strategies and fear the worst when confronted with episodes of pain are more affected by the pain and report more interference than patients who cope well with their problem. Psychological variables before the amputation are also predictive of PLP. Patients who received less support before the amputation reported more PLP [14]. PLP can have overarching impact on the patient's ability to recuperate or motivation to participate in rehabilitation [7, 15]. It is not just the existence of PLP that challenges persons with amputation, but its acuteness as well: more than one-third of amputees surveyed reported PLP of severe intensity [4].

Stump pain

Stump pain (SP), also known as "residual limb pain," is localized to the remaining body part after amputation. SP is thought to be less common than PLP. The reported frequency of SP is variable, with some studies reporting prevalence at 6 months as 22%, and at 2 years as 21%, and some studies showing estimates of 10–25% [7, 15–16]. Other studies report incidence as high as 74% and SP that can persist for years, similar to PLP [17].

TABLE 11.1
Physical effects of amputation
PHYSICAL IMPLICATIONS OF THE LIMB LOSS AND PROSTHESIS USE
Prosthesis fit and use—improper fit may cause pain in the stump; sustained use of even a well-fitting prosthesis may result in pain of the lower back and/or contralateral joint
Stump effects—increased activity or ambient temperature may cause sweating or swelling that impact fit; calluses, blisters, pimples may form; scar tissue is an important consideration; stump pain may reduce willingness to use prosthesis and thereby limit mobility
Phantom limb pain—varies in frequency and duration; may become more pronounced when the person is tired, worried, or succumbing to cold/flu symptoms
Comorbidities—including conditions either underlying the amputation or arising from it, or that result in a need for stump revision
Energy consumption—weight of the prosthesis and increased energy needed for its effective use
Potential future loss—concern over potential detrimental changes to the contralateral limb because of aging or injury; fear of losing the knee joint (for those with below-knee amputation) since above-knee prostheses are associated with decreased functional efficiency and greater difficulty with ambulation
Practical Considerations
Physical surface challenges to gait and balance—wet surfaces (floor, sidewalk, shower, pool deck) or slippery surfaces (any surface with snow/ice, leaves)
Fear of falling and its consequences in lower extremity amputation—loss of confidence, increased disability with reliance on crutches, immobility
Appearance-related concerns—communal changing rooms in stores; and, with lower extremity amputation: social discomfort associated with wearing dress/skirt/shorts; and finding shoes that fit, are appropriate for the occasion (e.g., dress shoes vs. sneakers), yet do not alter gait
Additional time and planning required—challenges associated with time-bound tasks (such as being unable to run for a bus or train); sorting through solutions in "surprise" situations where forethought was not possible

SP is classically described as a sharp, burning, electrical-like, or "hypersensitivity of the skin" type of pain, which can be confined to a superficial incision, felt deep in the stump, or encompassing the entire stump [16–18]. SP can be further subdivided into postsurgical nociceptive, neurogenic, prosthogenic, arthrogenic, ischemic, sympathetically maintained, pain referred from the spine or joints, or pain secondary to abnormal stump tissue such as adhesive scar tissue or heterotopic ossification [17, 19]. While SP and PLP often occur together, SP is more bothersome immediately after amputation, whereas PLP is most dominant in the year immediately following the amputation event [16, 20].

CARE AND COPING WITH AN AMPUTATION

The type of care a person receives before and after an amputation can profoundly impact how well they compensate or cope with their new life circumstance. As previously mentioned, patients who lack coping strategies and fear the worst when confronted with episodes of pain are more affected by the pain and report more interference than patients who cope well with their problem. To explain this further, we will focus on the biopsychosocial model of stress presented by Lazarus and Folkman. These researchers describe the interaction among people and the environment, postulating that physical and psychological realms are continually engaged with each other and that all stress is a product of an inherent feedback mechanism that begins with a person's cognitive view of the world. Specifically, an individual performs a primary appraisal to analyze and evaluate whether a particular event is a threat. A complex secondary appraisal then follows, with the person analyzing his/her own ability to cope with the event. In this way, the person evaluates whether he/she has the resources—physical, psychological, and/or social—to effectively manage the event (in this case, amputation) [21, 22].

Coping Strategies

The methods of coping used by amputated persons may not be substantially different from the coping strategies used by those who are not disabled, or who suffer from other forms of disability or illness. The coping strategies individuals adopt to manage experiences associated with illness or injury play a critical mediating role in psychosocial adjustment. One study examining the coping strategies of persons with amputations identified three coping themes that revolve around the emotional reactions towards the amputation, the resulting changes to the participants' lives, and the support that enabled amputees to cope with the situation. These themes were:

- *Initial Emotional Reaction*, including subthemes of impact on self and feelings of significant others;
- *Different Life*, including subthemes of changes in lifestyle, prosthesis and discomfort, and search for meaning; and
- *Social Connections and Support*, including subthemes of family, friends, and professionals as sources of information and care [23].

Coping strategies of those who have an amputation can generally be regarded as active vs. passive, and emotion-focused and avoidant vs. problem/task-oriented and approach styles; it is suggested that emotion-focused and avoidant strategies are less adaptive [21]. Active/task-oriented strategies such as problem-solving and perceiving control over the disability have been shown to be conducive to positive psychosocial adjustment, whereas emotion-focused and passive strategies such as cognitive disengagement, catastrophizing and wishful thinking have been associated with poor psychosocial outcome [24]. Desmond and MacLachlan [25] found problem-solving to be negatively associated with anxiety symptoms, and social support-seeking was positively associated with social adaptation. Avoidance was found to be positively associated with symptoms of depression, anxiety, and intrusion, and was negatively associated with general adjustment, social adaptation, and adjustment to limitation. Of the three coping strategies, avoidance was most consistently associated with poor psychosocial adaptation to amputation. The cause of amputation has been shown to affect the degree of usage of avoidance strategies. Those with non-traumatic amputations were significantly less likely to use avoidance than those patients whose amputation was the result of traumatic injury [7]. Among individuals with amputations, avoidant and emotion-focused coping strategies (such as cognitive disengagement, which includes such strategies as denial and mental substitution) have been shown to be associated with higher levels of psychosocial and physical dysfunction [25].

Coping strategies and general coping mechanisms used by individuals appear to fluctuate across time as psychological demands change, and fall into one of five themes:

1. *Positive coping*—has beneficial health effects, such as less anxiety, anger, and depressive symptomatology. This approach both strengthens and is strengthened by a sense of control (feedback mechanism), which is central to the degree of that person's experience of helplessness, which has been demonstrated to complicate recovery. It includes the ability to cope actively with their situation, the ability to use positive reinterpretation of their situation, planning, and acceptance of their reality.

2. *Avoidance coping*—extensive use of avoidance leads to higher levels of anxiety and depression than the use of positive coping strategies [7]. Avoidance coping includes the suppression of competing activities in which the individual can no longer successfully engage. Avoidance coping can involve passive strategies such as wishful thinking, where the person chooses not to confront the problem of amputation, instead retreating into a world devoid of threatening situations.

3. *Support*—comes in the form of instrumental support where individuals seek out people who can aid them in their instrumental activities of daily living (IADLs) and emotional support, where the person who has lost a limb can find a sympathetic/empathetic ear [7]. (See also Table 11.3.)

4. *Maladaptive coping*—these strategies have been associated with worsening of a patient's physical and psychological well-being. The use of these strategies includes social withdrawal, denial, behavioral and mental disengagement, the use of alcohol or other drugs, self-criticism and blaming oneself for the amputation.

5. *Spirituality/religion*—hope, optimism, or spirituality are characteristic of this coping strategy [7, 26]. It has been suggested that spiritual beliefs may impact the experience of amputation because some religions and cultures consider it to be a mark of punishment and, in others, because it helps the amputee to find meaning and cope more effectively with the disability-related loss [27]. Limited research is available that examines these issues, and the language used in such studies must be carefully parsed. In a study examining the impact of well-being and optimism on those who have an amputation, it was demonstrated that religious affiliation had no significant impact on levels of depression in amputated patients [28]. In another study, religion—defined as a meaningful relationship with God—was not a predictor of global, physical, or social quality of life (QOL) [29]. It was found, however, that existential spirituality, defined as the belief that one's life is meaningful or has purpose, is related to global and social QOL in individuals with limb amputations.

PERSONAL AND SOCIAL IMPLICATIONS OF LIMB LOSS AND USE OF PROSTHETIC DEVICE

Body Image

A person's body image is disrupted by change in the body's appearance or by a functional change of a body part. The altered image in individuals who have a chronic condition or a sudden loss that adjusts appearance is salient to the person with a loss of limb [30]. The meaning constructed by an individual about the amputation and use of a prosthesis impacts self-concept and interactions with others. Amputation itself is an "emotionally charged experience" in which the patient feels a sense of insecurity and apprehension—both before and after the surgery, in the case of elective amputation; and in the case of traumatic amputation, this may be accompanied by an added sense of devastation over what is perceived to be a mutilation of the body. In neither case is the resolution as simple as getting a prosthesis. "Body image disturbance is the result of social values emphasizing vitality and physical appearance and fitness. Therefore amputation may be seen as a sign of failure" [27]. The discrepancy between body ideal and body reality can create a negative body image and similar negative effects on confidence and motivation [30]. Holzer et al. found that patients with lower limb amputation have lower levels of body image perception and QOL compared with a control group [3]. A significant correlation between body image and life satisfaction was found by Breakey [31], showing that the more negative the person with an amputation feels about his or her body image, the less satisfied he or she is with his/her life.

Feelings of depression, anxiety, anger, guilt, grief, and self- or other-blame are common responses to the enormous stress imposed by the loss of a limb [32–37]. Depression and anxiety have been found to be higher in upper limb amputees than in those with lower extremity limb loss, in dominant hand amputation than non-dominant hand loss, and women more so than men [38].

The presence of chronic disease, which is linked with higher levels of depression, compounds the depressive impact of amputation [39]. A study of diabetes-related amputation that controlled for other medical comorbidities demonstrated that amputation predicted greater body image disturbance, but found that "overall lower health … may better account for greater depression and poorer physical quality of life, rather than the amputation itself" [40].

The amount of time required to reach a point of acceptance of altered body image varies with personal characteristics and social support, and, indeed, some never fully resolve the dissonance between pre- and post-amputation body image. As a result, some clients may be at risk for development of clinical mental disorders: PTSD occurs in more than half of traumatic amputees but is "often overlooked because avoidance is a symptom of the disorder" [34]. Substance abuse is common, particularly among traumatic amputees and Veterans with amputation [24, 34].

Social Support

The loss of a limb challenges not only the individual's self-perception but also the way they believe others view them. It has been shown that persons, post-limb loss, who have social support and integration are more likely to have better functional outcomes and quality of life than those who do not [41]. Those closest to the patient have greater influence on responses to amputation: significant others who are fearful of what the future holds, express emotional distress, or who are unsure how to react can transmit these fears to their loved ones who have undergone amputation, who may then adopt them [23]. Typically, love and respect are most frequent expressions felt by the person undergoing amputation, especially from parents (for those who are single) and spouses (for those who are married) [41], although they also report that frustration arises if family become overprotective [42, 43].

As important as family is, the support of close and intimate friends also provides opportunities for relaxation, sharing memories, and unconditional acceptance of their amputation. Persons with amputation have stated that friends' advice, empathy, and understanding helps improve morale and allows for a more positive life outlook [43].

Stigma and Social Discomfort

Numerous negative responses of others to the person with amputation have been documented. Amputees report a "sense of being a leper" [33] resulting from offensive responses by others—such as physically recoiling from the amputee, patronizing treatment, asking intrusive questions about the injury itself or about one's capabilities afterward, losing close friends after the amputation, and derogatory comments or jokes [32, 33]. Even just one negative social interaction can have serious emotional and behavioral consequences [44]. Aside from directly stigmatizing social interactions, the well-intentioned, unconscious labeling of amputees in terms of the disability alone can result in development of a sense that one is viewed as being inferior and incompetent [43], resulting in social withdrawal. Social stigma is associated with higher rates of depression [39].

In addition to its use in restoring physical function, in many cases a prosthesis provides the ability to normalize participation in social rituals. For example, the prosthesis may allow the individual:

- to conceal or minimize bodily difference in social customs, such as shaking hands, wearing a wedding ring, or dancing;
- to avoid infantilizing behaviors, like being able to eat with a knife and fork in public;
- to minimize the extent to which the condition impacts day-to-day life; and
- to preserve the impression of being "able-bodied"—or at least avoid the impression of disability or helplessness [33, 42].

A person with amputation may exert considerable effort toward concealment of the lost limb in order to avoid stigma and retain choice about when and to whom the amputation will be revealed [30]. In a sense, the prosthesis allows them to demonstrate body competence in social functions while, at the same time, requiring "impression management" strategies, such as strategic use of clothing and daily routines. The amputee may choose a cosmetic prosthesis; the mechanical parts of the artificial limb are covered by a skin-colored cover, which may feature detailed attributes of a natural limb. For some, realism in a passive limb with little function is preferable to a limb with greater function that is less visually attractive [45]. The desire to appear "normal" may lead an amputee to continue to engage in activities of concealment even at the cost of pain and potential physical injury. Aside from its function in protecting the right to reveal one's condition on one's own terms, the use of a prosthesis may stem from a sense of obligation to avoid the discomfort of others [33]. However, not all amputees value cosmesis: those who have markedly different gait or whose prosthesis is difficult to hide may decide the effort required to conceal is not worth the bother; and others actually dislike cosmetic prostheses on principle, considering their use to indicate a failure to accept limb loss, or contributing to a culture that calls for conformity [45].

On the other hand, social factors mediate the challenges of adaptation to amputation. Upward social comparison can serve as a motivating factor for rehabilitation efforts, and downward social comparison can enhance self-esteem by causing the individual to reconsider the severity of their own situation [43].

Health literature shows an association of social support with reduced disability- and illness-related morbidity and mortality [35, 46]. Social integration, defined by Williams et al. as "the extent to which an individual participates in a broad range of social relationships," tends to be lower among the population of persons with amputation than in the population with no disability or injury, despite the relative stability of social support after limb loss. Quality of relationships appears to be more important than quantity [35]. Social support is associated with less pain and depression in a study by Hanley et al. [47], and support from family and friends provides a beneficial effect on adjustment to amputation [27, 39].

Disability Identity

For those who experience limb loss, identity is changed significantly and permanently. Society imposes specific expectations of persons with disability (PWD); whether or not to accept and internalize disability as a facet of one's identity is a primary consideration in coping and adaptation.

> While the idea of adapting to a disability tends to
> have a negative connotation ... [it] can be seen as
> a strength, as the ability to consider new situations

and manipulate our world such that we can prosper within it in our changed circumstances. With adaptation to disability can come awareness of a whole other set of strengths and abilities: We can discover, and create, whole new facets of ourselves. [5]

Those who accept disability identity (DI) may develop a positive sense of ability and belonging—empowerment—as part of the community of persons with amputation. Alternatively, they may normalize DI, viewing themselves and expecting others to view them as "just like everybody else." Some individuals reject DI [45]. If their needs for personal assistance, services, transportation, and technological aids can be met through personal or social resources, the disabling condition can more easily be deemphasized or ignored. In this case, the person may adopt a transactional perspective in which they find ways to help others as those others help them, in order to eliminate disability from the equation. If such resources are not readily available to the individual, he/she may depend on public disability programs for support. Ironically, in order to access those supports and resources that would help keep a non-disabled identity, the person must allow some other person to label them "disabled" to qualify for those services.

Prosthetic devices play an integral role in acceptance or rejection of DI; indeed, the very object viewed by one individual as an extension of self that enables physical functions and social roles may be viewed by another as a separate article, a tangible representation of disability itself and the functions and social poise that have been lost [25, 32]. The success of a prosthesis may be measured not just in terms of the physical functioning it permits or restores, but by how much it allows the user to escape the label of disability [33]. In a meta-analysis conducted by Murray and Forshaw, amputees often expressed shock and disappointment upon seeing the prosthesis for the first time because it reminded them of the permanency of their loss [42]. As described in Table 11.1, discomfort with the prosthesis may involve such physical problems as excessive sweating, skin issues, pain, and bone spurs, which can impede functional mobility and prevent proper fit. In spite of these challenges, once the adjustment period is concluded, prosthetic use is frequently welcomed as a way to regain lost independence, conceal limb loss, and manage the way they are perceived by others. Some individuals may eventually choose to flaunt the amputation site or non-cosmetic prosthesis, as a form of defiant repudiation of the societal expectation of conformity mentioned above [33, 42].

Quality of Life

Physical impairments can be accurately assessed, but they are not the only factor that predicts a patient's need for care: environmental factors, the availability of social support, and the patient's determination all affect how far an impairment will be translated into disability or handicap. Quality of Life (QOL), referring to the subjective impact of a health condition and its treatment on daily life, includes multiple domains, such as physical, social, and role functions, psychological well-being, and other domains of special relevance to the disease, if present, being investigated. It varies among different health conditions, and over time for a given patient. Various studies have yielded conflicting results on the association of amputation and QOL when compared with normative reference data [48] but higher QOL is consistently related to amputation that is more distal (below-knee amputation, or BKA; through-knee amputation, or TKA) rather than proximal (above-knee amputation, or AKA) [48, 49]. Self-reported QOL measures show physical health outcomes for traumatic amputees that are significantly lower than norms [34]. However, Unwin, Kacperek, and Clarke point out the prevalence of studies considering negative adjustment versus the relative paucity of those measuring positive adjustment; their study of predictors of positive adjustment found that social support and hope contribute significantly to positive mood and general adjustment in persons with lower limb amputation, while gender, level and cause of amputation, and age do not [50]. Likewise, body image was found not to change with level of amputation in a study by Akarsu et al. [51]. Loss of independence is a concern for individuals who undergo amputation, especially if they previously engaged in an active lifestyle incorporating sports or other physical activities. The ability to maintain some level of independence and mobility has been identified as a strong predictor of QOL among individuals with lower limb amputations [52].

QOL changes across the arc of the lifespan, as well as within the duration of a particular health challenge. Common theories of adjustment hold that a loss experience is most severe immediately after occurrence and gradually diminishes as one develops better coping skills [53]. Persons with an amputation who at first want to hide their prosthesis may change their views as they gain skill and confidence in its use over time [33, 42, 45, 54–55]. Within a given amputee's experience, there will be periods of temporary change that require further adaptation, which may be cyclical in nature—for example, the episodic development of infected heat bumps or blisters on the stump that impact ability to use the prosthesis in order to allow the sore to heal [56]. In situations where a chronic disease causes the amputation, surgery may eliminate the immediate threat but does not cure the ongoing disease process, which may cause intermittent, gradual, or sudden decline in QOL that creates a corresponding need to adapt.

Developmental Stage

The vectors of illness and disability impact the path of a person's life in complex ways [57]. The age/lifespan position of a person experiencing a disability may impact willingness to incorporate that disability into pre-existing identity, with onset at younger ages being associated with a tendency to normalize DI, and onset in the later years with rejection of DI [5].

Mackelprang and Salsgiver developed a theory that combines the integration of disability into identity over the lifespan (see Table 11.2). Amputation at a younger age may represent a change of course in life, removing or altering some of the opportunities available to that individual. If this occurs before the person has begun to make decisions and undertake training for a desired career, the amputee may simply view his/her circumstances as "the way things are." Nonetheless, there are distinct challenges for that child and his/her social circle (e.g., parents, siblings, friends, teachers) [25]. Those who fall somewhere in the middle stages of life, who have already experienced some significant transitions without disability but who will undergo future transitions *with* disability, typically experience greater turbulence in shifting roles and life adjustments [5]. For example, a young adult who adopted societal standards of beauty prior to experiencing amputation may experience considerable difficulty with accommodating his/her "non-standard" appearance into a healthy sexual identity.

"Successful aging" is typically defined in terms of absence of disease and/or disability—so for the population with amputation, it becomes necessary to reframe the idea, perhaps emphasizing psychosocial factors rather than absence of disability [57]. Of special consideration is the question, which came first—age or disability? A person experiencing "disability with age" develops a disability later in life, whether by sudden-onset (e.g., traumatic amputation) or a gradual decline in functioning due to multiple health conditions associated with aging. A person in the latter stages of life, while viewing amputation as undesirable, may nonetheless view limb loss as part of the inevitable losses that occur with aging. In the case of an elderly person whose chronic disease has caused significant disability, amputation may be accepted gratefully for its provision of improved mobility and relief of significant pain [25]. A person "aging with disability" has one or more disabilities of long duration and experiences changes in health as they get older (e.g., a person with fibromyalgia whose poorly managed diabetes leads to amputation). The person aging with disability may experience problems due to long-term overuse of mobility-related body parts, secondary complications of underlying conditions, and increases in the rate of aging for organ systems [25, 58].

TABLE 11.2	

Mackelprang and Salsgiver's Disability/Life Stage Development Concept [5] (by age at onset of disability)

Birth to 3 years: Children who are disabled from birth or who acquire a disability during their early years learn to view the world from a disability perspective: they become disabled before the development of cognitive skills that would make them aware of the difference. Parents may grieve the loss of the "perfect" baby they dreamed of, and may be overwhelmed by the child's needs and the effort required to meet those needs over the course of a lifetime. They may tend to overprotect and shelter—which helps the child develop a strong sense of trust and security in the environment but may not encourage children to learn developmental tasks appropriate to their level.

3 to 6 years: Children in this stage need to experience some sense of control over their environment and themselves—which may be made more difficult by physical dependence on parents or other caregivers. These children should be offered choices and encouraged appropriately to "take charge" of themselves so that they can gain a sense of separateness from their parents/ caregivers. It is important for these kids to be with other children—both children with the same disability and with others. The reactions of others may give children their first experience in "being different," and support and coping strategies can assist them to mitigate the effects of feeling differently.

6 to 12 years: By this age, children have internalized the view of physical beauty and body image that is prevalent in the culture around them. Children who acquire a disability during these years can have a difficult time: their bodies have changed, and they may have to modify their habits and activities to incorporate the new form. Both parents and children can experience grief for the nondisabled child they loved. These children may have not had the experiences of rejection and discrimination, and if they have developed a healthy sense of self-esteem and respect, they will be able to keep it.

12 to 18 years: The primary tasks of this stage involve developing and affirming a personal identity, increasing independence from parents, and developing a sexual identity. Frustration and ambivalence can arise from the conflict between separating from parents and dependence on parents for physical assistance, mobility, or other ADLs. Shifting roles and identity to include disability is a challenging task for a teenager, and one who believes he/she does not match the required standard of physical beauty may need assistance from others to develop a positive sexual identity. Sometimes friendships are lost, activities and interests must be refocused, and exposure to others with the same disability becomes extremely important in order to allow normalization of the condition. Teens can be helped to understand that disability is a construct of the environment, and not a personal failure in themselves.

Young adulthood: People who become disabled during the young adult years face major life adjustments because they had developed a self-image and identity prior to becoming disabled. The primary task of this stage is reaching maturity and independence. For a person with chronic illness or disability (CID), this means assuming responsibility for hiring personal attendants, organizing and managing schedules, and arranging a comfortable environment apart from parents. Awareness of community resources and support is key: existence and accessibility of jobs, educational resources, and transportation and services becomes very important. Newly developed relationships are particularly fragile and often do not survive the onset of the disability, creating a sense of loss and change even beyond the disability itself.

Middle adulthood: Middle adults who acquire a disability have a strong identity and have developed close relationships outside of the disability culture. They tend to keep their nondisabled sense of identity and do not make the shift to disability identity. In their own eyes, they are the same people they always were, just with an additional problem that does not change their basic identity, interests, or avocations. Middle adults who acquire CID frequently try to use the experience of disability as an opportunity for personal growth and a developing insight about the nature of the world.

Older adulthood: Aging greatly increases the likelihood of acquiring a disability. Most people who become disabled in older adulthood do not identify with the disability culture or with others who share the same disability. As a result, and because of the social isolation that often accompanies both disability and old age, offering social supports and resources to people who become disabled in older adulthood can be particularly helpful. People in this category tend to be more knowledgeable about needed resources and are better able to navigate the system. However, having a long-term disability may create problems that newly disabled older adults do not experience, because they are a side effect/after-effect of the disability itself. For the elderly, maintaining maximal independence is very important, as is maintaining social relationships and meaningful activities.

ROLE CHANGES

In addition to the person actually experiencing amputation, those in his/her social network have to adapt to new circumstances as well. Because all the members of a family or social system are interlocked, an individual loss destabilizes the system to some degree. Moos and Holahan identify five social coping tasks for the family experiencing a healthcare crisis like amputation:

1. Maintaining a sense of normalcy;
2. Adjusting to altered social relationships;
3. Dealing with role change;
4. Managing social stigma; and
5. Maintaining a sense of control [59].

Like the individual lifespan continuum described by Mackelprang and Salsgiver, Rolland describes the family life cycle in terms of structure-building/maintaining periods and transition periods, changing and growing over time. In either type of period, the family may experience a centripetal (pulling together) or centrifugal (pulling apart) effect [60]. Rolland proposes four rules for understanding the impact of injury or CID on a family system:

1. CID *generally* exerts a centripetal force on families. (Example: the family will typically pull together to deal with the diagnosis and treatment of cancer in one of its members.)

2. If CID occurs during centrifugal periods, it can detract from family tasks. (Example: in a couple going through divorce, the family may divert time and energy to dealing with an amputation-related crisis that would otherwise be devoted to arranging separate living quarters for parents and any resulting childcare and/or transportation changes.)

3. If CID occurs during a centripetal period, it may prolong the period. (Example: in a recently married couple, accommodation of the healthcare needs of an unexpected amputation may delay or complicate the usual family tasks of establishing which spouse takes on various household chores, the kinds of routine activities that will be carried out on weekends, etc.)

4. Normative family needs are generally subordinated to the needs of the CID of the patient. (Example: in a family with a college-bound freshman, the typical activities associated with college enrollment may be put on hold while the family attends the needs of the person with amputation.)

While basic roles (e.g., spouse, parent) may not change, the amputation may require a change in the expectations attached to those roles. For example, the parental task of taking a small child (along with diaper bag and other assorted gear) to a childcare center may require modification, suspension, or reassignment due to the functional limitations associated with the amputation of a limb. Depending on the circumstances, such modifications may be temporary or permanent and the process of deciding on how to reallocate those tasks may be contentious, as each person arrives at the point of decision from slightly different circumstances and possesses different coping skills.

Adaptation in the Sexual Role

The partners of people with amputations provide emotional and practical support in numerous ways, ranging from reassurance of acceptance to help with chores, from leisure activities to physical affection [35]. Their role in helping the person with amputation adjust to limb loss and prosthesis is well-established; the sense of being needed by a partner is accompanied by a desire to have the relationship continue in the same manner as before the amputation [42]. One characteristic of the spousal or partner role that carries particular importance is that of lover. Though rarely addressed as such, sexual activity is an activity of daily living, and is a significant factor in QOL across the lifespan [61, 62]. In the general population, sexual dysfunction is common, occurring in 40–45% of women and 20–30% of men [63]. The presence of a disability frequently increases the probability and magnitude of such difficulties, which tend to go unaddressed in routine healthcare [64]. Sexual difficulties are high on the list of problems in marriages where one partner has a chronic disease or disability [65].

In addition to the challenges that may lead to sexual dysfunction for the general population (e.g., hormonal changes, lack of emotional closeness with partner), persons with amputation may experience challenges specific to their condition, which range from mechanical problems with positioning to psychosocial concerns (grief related to the loss, body image changes that decrease confidence in desirability, changes in familial and work roles). A systematic literature review by Geertzen et al. found that the impact on sexual function differs for various amputee subgroups: persons who are single experience greater impact than those who are in stable relationships, older persons greater than younger, male more than female, and transfemoral amputees greater than transtibial amputees [62].

With regard to mobility and positioning, the level and type of amputation may hinder the individual from reaching the desired position during intercourse, maintaining stability once the position is reached, or transitioning from one position to another [62]. For example:

- A transhumeral or transfemoral amputation may impede one's ability to engage in intercourse using the missionary position.

- Amputation of a hand or arm may impact the ability to stimulate oneself or one's partner through caressing or masturbation.

- Sex in the shower, bath, or pool may require much more attention and effort than before amputation.

More forethought may be required for sex in general, even if only to consider what to do with the prosthesis while engaging in sexual activity [66]. Amputees may experience cramps, stump pain, prosthesis-associated discomfort, and/or phantom pain, any of which can have a dampening effect on libido and may reduce or prevent sexual activity [62]. Chronic illness itself—or the medication to treat it—may have unwanted sexual side effects (e.g., decreased libido, erectile dysfunction, vaginal dryness, bad breath from chemotherapy). A consistent theme in discussions of sexuality is the emphasis by the amputee on the way the partner reacts to the amputation [66].

Adaptation in the Vocational Role

The role of occupation is highly valued in society, affecting identity, social status, and QOL [42]. Limb loss interrupts this role, at least temporarily and sometimes permanently. The use of differing definitions of successful return-to-work (RTW) complicates comparison of research studies; nonetheless, numerous studies do show that persons with limb loss experience significant effects in employment and only about 20% return to their pre-amputation job [34, 67–72]. In one study, over half stopped working in the first 2 years after amputation, with three-quarters of those indicating the reason was amputation-related, and more than one-quarter had problems finding employment due to amputation [67]. An examination of multiple studies and a systematic review found the average time before RTW following traumatic amputation is approximately 1 year [34], but the impact for some is considerably longer-lasting: even 7 years post-amputation, just over half of traumatic amputation participants in one study had returned to work—and those who did experienced performance limitations 20–25% of the time [68]. The impact seems to be less severe for those with congenital limb absence than for acquired amputation, perhaps because of the extended time for selection of and preparation for an occupation that matches one's functional abilities in the former, as opposed to the relatively shortened (and in the case of trauma, non-existent) opportunity experienced by those who undergo amputation after entry into a vocation [72]. Those with higher levels of education tend to have greater likelihood of employment after amputation, which could be reflective of higher expectations of rehabilitation or higher adaptability [68].

Most amputees who do RTW are employed only part-time or take on roles that are less physically demanding than pre-injury jobs, which often requires retraining [34, 67]. Physical challenges in completing job tasks differ by type of amputation, and range from decreased walking speed, endurance, and balance (lower limb amputation), to decreased weight/torque support capacity and fine motor limitations (upper limb amputation) [70]. Persons with amputation report other specific work challenges, including salary reduction after amputation, difficulty getting the job accommodations or workplace modifications they need, and discrimination (e.g., fewer promotion opportunities) [67, 68, 70]. In the United States, employment discrimination is identified more frequently by persons with amputation who are male, who fit in the outermost segments of typical employment age (i.e., under 20 or over 65 years of age), who are employed by small companies (<200 employees), and who work in manufacturing, construction, or transportation industries. The type of discrimination experienced tends to be related to hiring, promotion, and job training [70].

In addition to its implications for financial security and social connections, completing productive work is an important part of identity, perceived QOL, and adjustment for persons with amputation [1, 39, 72]. Though noting the difficulty in parsing cause versus effect, Sinha, van den Heuvel, and Arokiasamy report an association in amputees between unemployment, lower social adjustment, and functional and social restrictions [1].

PSYCHOSOCIAL INTERVENTIONS WITH AMPUTATION

The complex medical care required for amputation can leave the patient feeling powerless and overwhelmed [56]. During inpatient care, the treatment of patients with amputation typically centers on regaining physical function and mobility through the use of prosthetic devices. The early involvement of rehabilitation professionals is useful for advice giving on prosthetic options, maintaining and improving muscle strength, range of motion, mobility and ability to maintain activities of daily living [7, 42, 73].

While improvement of functional outcomes following amputation is necessary, that alone is not sufficient. In order to improve QOL, rehabilitation must address the holistic needs of the individual, taking into account the psychosocial aspects of amputation and renegotiation of identity [55, 56, 74]. For planned amputations, the interprofessional rehabilitation team should engage in psychoeducational interventions, such as education, support, and counseling, before and immediately after the amputation to help the patient understand and manage stress and emotions about the surgical and recovery processes to come [25, 32, 55].

Patient Education

In the course of recommending and preparing for amputation, clinicians discuss with clients the surgical procedure, along with the preparations and events that surround it. In addition to questions about the actual surgical procedure, patients with amputation must be educated on the physical management of the amputation site and stump, potential complications, and what activities compose rehabilitation [32]. Patients who intend to use a prosthesis have additional pragmatic questions: What will the prosthesis look like? What functions will it restore? What care and maintenance are required?

Learning how to accomplish routine tasks after limb loss, and how to use the prosthesis (if elected) gives the individual a renewed sense of control and body competence. As the person transitions from the hospital to the home environment, the reality of the challenges inherent in each new location, task, and social interaction sets in and the person must continue figuring out how to manage. Success and satisfaction with the use of a prosthesis is associated with absence of emotional problems and better social integration [33]. In circumstances where the amputee has low social support and complex health issues that present multiple difficulties beyond the amputation itself, it may be appropriate to consider extending the transition period from hospital to home [39].

Counseling

There is widespread acceptance that counseling is needed immediately before and after amputation. As they try to anticipate the unknown, patients have vague and uninformed expectations about the recovery process. They may not be able to anticipate which questions to ask and may rely on clinicians to tell them what they need to know. Coping is enhanced by knowing what to expect rather than fearing the unknown [32], and it is important to address expectations such that the client is informed and engaged in the process of rehabilitation [55].

In addition to exploration and development of realistic rehabilitation expectations, a counselor can facilitate positive social comparisons before and after amputation, helping the client frame their limb loss in the context of both "worst possible loss" and the inevitability of loss over the span of a lifetime, without diminishing its significance in that individual's experience: as an amputee in Gallagher and MacLachlan's qualitative study stated, "everybody has their area of weakness. You get it somewhere along the line … Nobody ever escapes completely. There is always something" [32].

Counseling should include guidance in the development of coping skills, and instruction and rehearsal on pragmatic social skills of immediate concern to the person with amputation (e.g, managing social interactions, responding to questions) [25, 42, 55]. This therapy can pave the way for the client to direct at least some energy to recovery and adjustment that otherwise would be spent on managing worry and stress [32].

Some research indicates that periodic follow-up after discharge is beneficial for continued adjustment, given the long-term nature of the physical, social, and psychological after-effects of limb loss [32, 39, 75]. This may be particularly helpful for those amputees whose reduced participation in social activities leads to deterioration of relationships based on formerly shared roles [35]. The permanence of limb loss means that as time elapses, the issues associated with amputation will evolve, and the need for counseling may recur [32].

Family and Social Support

Given the impact on the individual and family, as well as the importance and potential impact of family and social support described above, those in the immediate social circle should be included in rehabilitation planning as completely as possible [32, 42]. Members of the client's network can offer several types of social support, depending on the nature of the relationship, the personal characteristics of the family member or friend, and resources available (Table 11.3) [35].

Particularly in the early days of recovery, amputees report feeling isolated. In part, this may be true simply because of their hospitalization and resulting absence from the usual settings (e.g., workplace, leisure activities). In addition to this, however, immediate family and friends who surround the person in the hospital may experience feelings of helplessness and uncertainty about the type of comments that would be perceived as helpful by the amputee—and their self-edited remarks result in conversations that seem less genuine and emotionally connected [35]. Family and friends may need guidance to focus on future function instead of loss, especially if there was disagreement in the social circle over the person's decision to amputate [33]. Their participation in patient education and counseling can facilitate the provision of appropriate support, reassurance, and encouragement, while enabling them to recognize the importance of balancing the amputee's early need for assistance with the development of independence in order to regain a sense of body competence [32, 39, 47].

TABLE 11.3
Dimensions of perceived social support [35]

TYPE OF SUPPORT	SAMPLE ACTIVITIES
Emotional support	Sympathetic listening, reassurances of caring, and acceptance
Instrumental support	Practical help with transportation, chores, childcare, or finances
Informational support	Advice and guidance
Companionship support and company	Social and leisure activities
Affection	Comforting and physical affection

Contact with an Established Amputee

Persons who have been through amputation and have experienced success in life after amputation provide an incredibly valuable perspective for the person considering or recently experiencing amputation. They can serve as positive models and motivators [32, 44, 56]. Peer group support from others having similar experiences of limb loss has been shown to contribute to improved morale [43]. In at least one study, talking to person with amputation was considered by the patients to be more beneficial than talking to doctors, who were often unable to answer the questions that they wanted to ask [32].

Early Contact with the Prosthetist

As mentioned previously, questions abound regarding the prosthetic device under consideration. The desired outcome of prosthesis use is that the client will be fitted with a comfortable, durable appliance that will enhance mobility and ability of the user. Because there are so many physical variables in the body and health of the person using the device, as well as in the design and function of the prosthesis, the development of a trusting, candid partnership between patient and prosthetist is critical. Hence, involvement of the prosthetist early in the process is beneficial for helping the patient develop a frame of reference for the role of the prosthetist and for assisting in the formation of realistic expectations of the device and rehabilitation process [32, 55]. Some challenges that a prosthetist is especially suited to discuss include:

- physical and practical considerations related to prosthesis use, fit and comfort (see Table 11.1);
- importance of reliability and immobility/dependence on others if function of the prosthetic device is interrupted;
- noise made by the prosthesis and awkward social interactions that may result;
- activities facilitated by the type of prosthesis selected (e.g., type/height of shoe and heel, swimming); and
- expense associated with various options [32].

Vocational Rehabilitation

Rehabilitation aims to maximize the client's independent function, personally and in social roles. MacKenzie et al. cite RTW as one of the most important outcomes of treatment to evaluate, since most persons who experience amputation are in the workforce beforehand [68]. The field of vocational rehabilitation is founded on the notion that everyone is employable if provided the appropriate supports. These may include compensatory strategies, job coaching, assistive technology, medical management, and job restructuring. For example, the provision of parking close to the worksite allows conservation of energy for the person with lower limb amputation, as would moving the workstation closer to restrooms and break rooms. Establishing a schedule of breaks and task switches (such as periodically alternating between gross motor tasks and fine motor tasks) may make a particular set of work responsibilities more manageable for a person with upper extremity amputation. For those whose work relies significantly on appearance and personal contact, a cosmetic prosthesis for work may be helpful [71, 72]. Table 11.4 identifies job aids and assistive devices for persons with different types of amputation. Predictors of RTW success vary, depending on the nature of the study question (see Table 11.5), but persons with amputation highly value the ability to regain work identity, making vocational rehabilitation a critical part of the reintegration process [1, 45, 68, 76].

TABLE 11.4

Workplace assistive devices [70, 76]

UPPER EXTREMITY AMPUTATION	LOWER EXTREMITY AMPUTATION
Orthotic writing aids—grip aid, writing cuff	Ambulation aids—rolling seat, wheelchair, cane, powered scooter
Alternative computer input devices—trackball mouse, one-handed keyboard, speech-to-text software	Standing supports—task stool, anti-fatigue mat, sit/stand stool
Tool grips—grasping cuff or orthosis, tool wrap and glove, vise, foot control, pistol grip attachment, digital distance measuring device	Climbing assistance—stair lift, climbing wheelchair, rolling safety ladder with handrails, work platform, hydraulic personnel lift
Lifting and carrying devices—tailgate lift, hoist, compact lifting device, lightweight cart, shoulder bag, scooter with carrying basket	Lifting and carrying devices—material handling lift, hoist, powered cart/scooter, hydraulic lift cart, lightweight cart with large wheels
Driving aids—steering knob, power-assisted steering, grip glove, steering wheel cover, remote engine starter	Driving aids—hand controls, automatic clutch, left-foot gas pedal, automatic transmission
Telecommunications aids—speaker phone, phone with programmable number storage, phone holder, telephone headset	

TABLE 11.5

Factors associated with re-employment/return-to-work [34,67–70]

INCREASED LIKELIHOOD

Younger age	Lower level of amputation
Higher level of education	Prompt fitting with prosthesis
Non-smoker	Comfort of prosthesis fit
Extroversion	Early (3 month) assessments of pain and physical functioning
Average to high self-efficacy	Psychological acceptance of limb loss
Substantial pre-injury job tenure	Psychological acceptance and use of prosthesis
High job involvement	Participation in work-hardening program
Extensive social network	Positive workplace accommodation beyond prosthetics
Participation in vocational counseling	

REDUCED LIKELIHOOD

Advancing age	Intense/persistent stump pain
Co-morbidities	Intense/persistent phantom limb pain
Multiple amputations	Involvement in litigation for compensation
Higher level of amputation	Prolonged depression or psychological distress related to body image

Discussion of Sexual Function

There is considerable evidence that persons with disability want sexual information from healthcare professionals [61, 77–80]. Assessment of sexual functioning should be integral to the rehabilitation process—not just as a question asked once but rather as a discussion that recurs systematically over time and transitions; where possible, partners should be included in these conversations [62, 65]. By discussing sex as a common topic, professionals diminish the sense of taboo that inhibits amputees and their partners from asking uncomfortable questions. Normalizing the discussion of sex by introducing it early in the rehabilitation process gives permission for the client to bring up sexual problems or concerns throughout the journey of reintegration, as trust and familiarity with clinicians grow. A subsequent verbal check-in on sexual functioning immediately before or after the patient goes home may be appropriate, as that environment may be the first in which sexual partners feel comfortable engaging in sexual activity [66].

Healthcare providers' self-perceived lack of knowledge about sexuality, and anxiety when discussing sexual concerns is widespread. Healthcare providers receive relatively little training on sexuality education and discussion of sexual problems, despite the significance of the sexual role in one's identity. This may lead to insecurity about one's knowledge base, and embarrassment may lead to avoidance of the subject [77, 80–82]. Many healthcare providers

believe these discussions are someone else's responsibility [83], and in interprofessional teams, each member may believe that a different team member has greater knowledge and should address this topic. Although a majority of providers agree that they bear responsibility for addressing sexuality, two-thirds reported they had not done so with their recent lower extremity amputation patients [65]. Other challenges that may inhibit the healthcare provider's ability or willingness to engage in discussion of sexuality include inadequate privacy for sensitive discussions and limited time; for example, with the current focus on reducing length of hospital stays. The net outcome is that both provider and patient avoid the discussion of sexual health in spite of its widespread importance, resulting in inadequate sexual healthcare [64, 65]. This is underscored by the report in Verschuren et al. that "almost all participants did remember the first time they had sex again after the [lower limb amputation], even when the amputation had taken place years ago" [65].

Several frameworks have been developed to assist healthcare professionals with screening for sexual problems (see Table 11.6). While formal training may help boost clinicians' confidence, any provider can initiate the dialogue and carry out a meaningful discussion about sexuality, if he/she possesses the following.

1. Willingness and ability to talk about sexual topics in an open and comfortable fashion.

2. Awareness of the variety of human sexual practices and concerns.

3. Ability to separate one's personal beliefs and values from those of clients.

4. Skill at taking an appropriately detailed sexual problem history.

5. Ability to convey accurate information, make specific suggestions, and refer when appropriate [84].

The last point in this list is key: there may occasionally be questions or situations in which the clinician truly does not have the knowledge or skill to help. In these cases, it may be necessary to refer to a specialist in sexual health—but these situations are relatively rare [85].

The use of "bridge" statements or questions lets any member of the team to broach sexual topics into the interview in a way that minimizes awkwardness. This can be as direct as saying, "It is common for people in your situation to have concerns about sexual functioning after amputation. What concerns do you have?" Or the provider can open the conversation more obliquely by saying, "How has your injury/surgery changed the types of things you and your partner do together?" Reporting to the patient the findings of basic lab screenings and medication reviews opens the door for the provider to bring up any associated sexual implications (e.g., hormonal or metabolic imbalances, side effects or cross-reactions). Throughout these interactions, the clinician should encourage the client to be open and honest, and take care to ensure that he/she feels like an equal. Generally speaking, open-ended questions are more useful than yes/no questions. Each question should be followed by a period of silence to allow the client time to reflect on the answer and mentally phrase it in language with which he/she is comfortable. Questions should be asked one at a time, beginning with the least sensitive (e.g., medication questions before position questions). Once the conversation is underway, the clinician should be direct; should use language that is appropriate, avoiding both jargon and euphemisms; and should not make judgments or impose his/her own values on the patient [85].

By considering sexuality to be an ADL, rehabilitation clinicians can incorporate the subject into routine conversations with clients and ensure it is not disregarded. The omission of sexual assessment in the rehabilitation process "may reinforce larger societal messages that devalue or marginalize individuals with amputations" [61].

TABLE 11.6			
Models to screen for sexual problems			
EX-PLISSIT MODEL [90]		**ALLOW MODEL [91]**	
Ex(tended)	Permission-giving is the core of each stage, so that at any point the patient may ask questions or concerns; not all questions have to be answered in a single session. The purpose of continued permission-giving is to normalize sexuality.	*Ask*	Ask the client about sexual activity and function.
Permission	Ask the patient for permission to discuss sexual issues and give them permission to discuss sexual concerns at any time. If appropriate, seek permission to discuss with the client's partner.	*Legitimize*	Legitimize the client's concerns by acknowledging them as relevant within their rehabilitation program.
Limited Information	Offer a way to begin the discussion of sexuality. Clinicians can provide facts that are relevant but limited in scope, such as possible complications and contraindications. It may be beneficial to include the partner (with permission) in order to ease fears about hurting client and dispel myths about sex/disability.	*Limitations*	Address the healthcare provider's limitations presented by lack of knowledge and/or discomfort in the discussion.
Specific Suggestions	Set therapeutic goals and make specific behavioral suggestions for adapting sexual activity.	*Open*	Open discussions about sexual issues for additional assessment and the provision of referrals to a specialist.
Intensive Therapy (Usually reserved for sex therapists, urologists, gynecologists.)	This level of counseling may be needed at any point, and it should ***not*** be assumed that this counseling is needed only if previous levels of assistance have been insufficient. However, this level of therapy is required by relatively few clients.	*Work*	Healthcare provider(s) and client work collectively to develop or while implementing a treatment plan.

SUMMARY

Limb loss presents a significant crisis and requires adjustment in numerous arenas of human experience. This chapter has looked beyond the physical effects described in other chapters, examining the challenges and implications of amputation and prosthesis use on identity and QOL, which are substantial. In addition, the chapter has provided recommendations for intervention by the members of the interprofessional team that can contribute to an individual's coping and adjustment to these long-lasting difficulties [32].

Body Dysmorphic Disorder and Body Integrity Identity Disorder [86-89]

Body dysmorphic disorder (BDD) is a mental disorder in which a person believes that a specific part of the body is diseased or extremely ugly, causing intense embarrassment and shame, although others do not find anything noticeable about the body part. It is a chronic and unremitting condition with onset typically during adolescence, and is characterized by compulsive and time-consuming behaviors related to the body part in question—such as constant mirror checking, comparing with others, camouflaging, touching or skin-picking, and seeking reassurance from others—for the purpose of reducing anxiety or distress, without deriving pleasure from those behaviors. The individual may seek non-psychiatric care to improve appearance (e.g, plastic surgery). BDD is included in the *DSM-5* in the diagnostic category of Obsessive Compulsive Related Disorders.

Body integrity identity disorder (BIID) is a chronic psychiatric condition in which a person's subjective experience of the body does not match the structure of the physical body: despite the absence of a disabling condition, the person believes his/her true identity is that of a person with disability. As a result, the individual experiences severe distress and disruption of everyday life, leading to persistent preoccupation with the desire to correct the perceived mismatch through spinal cord injury or amputation of the limb that "doesn't belong." For those whose focus is elimination of a limb, the individual may spend significant periods of time pretending to have an amputation by binding or camouflaging the limb in order to experience the pleasurable or calming effects of being disabled. The person may go so far as to cut off the offending body part themselves or may seek to force amputation by intentionally damaging it (e.g., shooting, freezing), either catastrophically or by repeated intentional injury over time. Awareness of the stigma surrounding these behaviors makes it uncommon for these individuals to seek help from medical or psychiatric professionals. The condition is relatively rare, with onset in childhood (before adolescence). Both psychiatric and neurobiological causes have been theorized. Although BIID is not included as a specific diagnosis in the *DSM-5*, research finds growing evidence of this condition and associated behaviors.

REFERENCES

[1] Sinha R, van den Heuvel WJ, Arokiasamy P. Adjustments to amputation and an artificial limb in lower limb amputees. *Prosthet Orthot Int.* 2014;38(2):115.

[2] Horgan O, MacLachlan M. Psychosocial adjustment to lower-limb amputation: a review. *Disabil Rehabil.* 2004;26: 14-15, 837-850.

[3] Holzer LA, Sevelda F, Fraberger G, et al. Body image and self-esteem in lower limb amputees. *PLOS One.* 2014;9(3):e92943.

[4] Taleperos G, McCabe MP. Body image and physical disability personal perspectives. *Soc Sci Med.* 2002;54:971–980.

[5] Rothman JC. *Social Work Practice Across Disability*, 2003. Pearson Education, Boston, MA.

[6] Price EM, Fisher K. Further study of the emotional needs of amputees. *J Prosthet Orthot.* 2007;19(4):106–110.

[7] Andersson M, Deighan F. Coping strategies in conjunction with amputation: a literature study, 2006. Independent thesis, Karlstad University, Sweden.

[8] Dadkhah B, Valizdeh S, Mohammadi E, Hassankhani H. Psychosocial adjustment to lower-limb amputation: a review article. *HealthMED.* 2013;7(2):502–507.

[9] Ephraim PL, Wegener ST, MacKenzie EJ, et al. Phantom pain, residual limb pain, and back pain in amputees: results of a national survey. *Arch Phys Med Rehab.* 2005;86:1910–1919.

[10] Rich T, Phelan H, Gravely A, et al. Examining patient reported outcome measures for phantom limb pain: measurement use in a sample of veterans with amputation. *Disabil Rehabil.* 2024 May;30:1–9.

[11] Highsmith MJ, Goff LM, Lewandowski AL, et al. Low back pain in persons with lower extremity amputation: a systematic review of the literature. *Spine.* 2019;19:552–563.

[12] Sadowski PK, Battista S, Leuzzi G, et al. Low back pain in people with lower limb amputation: a cross-sectional study. *Spine* (Phila Pa 1976). 2022 Nov 15;47(22):1599–1606.

[13] Subedi B, Grossberg GT. Phantom limb pain: mechanisms and treatment approaches. *Pain Res Treat.* 2011;Article ID 864605.

[14] Flor H. Phantom-limb pain: characteristics, causes, and treatment. *Lancet Neurol.* 2002;1:182–189.

[15] Mohta M, Sethi AK, Tyagi A, Mohta A. Psychological care in trauma patients. *Injury.* 2003;34:17–25.

[16] Davis RW. Phantom sensation, phantom pain, and stump pain. *Arch Phys Med Rehab.* 1993;74:79–91.

[17] Ehde DM, Czerniecki JM, Smith DG, et al. Chronic phantom sensations, phantom pain, residual limb pain, and other regional pain after lower limb amputation. *Arch Phys Med Rehab.* 2000;81:1039–1044.

[18] Hsu E, Cohen SP. Postamputation pain: epidemiology, mechanisms, and treatment. *J Pain Res.* 2013;6:121–136.

[19] Jensen TS, Krebs B, Nielsen J, Rasmussen P. Immediate and long-term phantom limb pain in amputees: incidence, clinical characteristics, and relationship to pre-amputation pain. *Pain.* 1985;21:267–278.

[20] Schley MT, Wilms P, Toepfner S, et al. Painful and nonpainful phantom and stump sensations in acute traumatic amputees. *J Trauma.* 2008;65(4):858–864.

[21] Lazarus RS, Folkman S. *Stress, Appraisal and Coping*, 1984. Springer Publishing Company, New York.

[22] Lazarus RS. Coping theory and research: past, present, and future. *Psychosom Med.* 1993;55:234–247.

[23] Grech C, Debono RF. The lived experience of persons with an amputation. *Malta J Health Sci.* 2014;54–59.

[24] Desmond DM, MacLachlan M. Coping strategies as predictors of psychosocial adaptation in a sample of elderly veterans with acquired lower limb amputations. *Soc Sci Med.* 2006;62:208–216.

[25] Desmond D, MacLachlan M. Psychological issues in prosthetic and orthotic practice: a 25 year review of psychology in Prosthetics and Orthotics International. *Prosthet Orthot Int.* 2002;26(3);182–188.

[26] Livneh H, Antonak RF, Gerhardt J. Multidimensional investigation of the structure of coping among people with amputation. *Psychosomatics.* 2000;41(3):235–244.

[27] Stancu B, Rednic G, Grad NO, et al. Medical, social and Christian aspects in patients with major lower limb amputations. *J Study Relig Ideol.* 2016;15(43):82–101.

[28] Dunn DS. Well-being following amputation: salutary effects of positive meaning, optimism, and control. *Rehabil Psychol.* 1996;41(4):285–302.

[29] Peirano H, Franz RW. Spirituality and quality of life in limb amputees. *Int J Angiol.* 2012;21:47–52.

[30] Green T. Understanding body image in patients with chronic oedema. *Br J Community Nurs.* 2008;13(10):S15–S18.

[31] Breakey J. Body image: the lower-limb amputee. *J Prosthet Orthot.* 1997;9(2):58–66.

[32] Gallagher P, Maclachlan, M. Adjustment to an artificial limb: a qualitative perspective. *J Health Psychol.* 2001;6(1):85–100; 015314.

[33] Murray CD. The social meanings of prosthesis use. *J Health Psychol.* 2005;10(3):425–441.

[34] Perkins ZB, De'Ath HD, Sharp G, Tai NM. Factors affecting outcome after traumatic limb amputation. *Brit J Surg.* 2012;99:75–86.

[35] Williams RM, Ehde DM, Smiths DG, et al. A two-year longitudinal study of social support following amputation. *Disabil Rehabil.* 2004;26(14/15):862–874.

[36] Vranceanu A, Bachoura A, Weening A, et al. Psychological factors predict disability and pain intensity after skeletal trauma. *J Bone Joint Surg Am.* 2014;96(3):e20(1)–e20(6).

[37] Ranti BO, Adebayo OO, Saheed Y, Olukayode A. Early psychosocial impact and functional level following major lower limb amputations. *Int J Dev Res.* 2015;5(1):3098.

[38] Desteli E, İmren Y, Erdoğan M, et al. Comparison of upper limb amputees and lower limb amputees: a psychosocial perspective. *Eur J Trauma Emerg S.* 2014;40(6):735.

[39] Washington ED, Williams AE. An exploratory phenomenological study exploring the experiences of people with systemic disease who have undergone lower limb amputation and its impact on their psychological well-being. *Prosthet Orthot Int.* 2016;40(1):44.

[40] McDonald S, Sharpe L, Blaszczynski A. The psychosocial impact associated with diabetes-related amputation. *Diabet Med.* 2014;31:1424–1430.

[41] Hawkins AT, Pallangyo AJ, Herman AM, et al. The effect of social integration on outcomes after major lower extremity amputation. *J Vasc Surg.* 2016;63:154–162.

[42] Murray CD, Forshaw MJ. The experience of amputation and prosthesis use for adults: a metasynthesis. *Disabil Rehabil.* 2013;35:14:1133–1142.

[43] Hamill R, Carson S, Dorahy M. Experiences of psychosocial adjustment within 18 months of amputation: an interpretative phenomenological analysis. *Disabil Rehabil.* 2010;32(9):729–740.

[44] Oaksford K, Frude N, Cuddihy R. Positive coping and stress-related psychological growth following lower limb amputation. *Rehabil Psychol.* 2005;50:266–277.

[45] Murray CD. Being like everybody else: the personal meanings of being a prosthesis user. *Disabil Rehabil.* 2009;31(7):573–581.

[46] Khademi M, Gharib M, Rashedi V. Prevalence of depression in the amputated patients concerning demographic variables. *Iran J Public Health.* 2012;4(2):12–17.

[47] Hanley MA, Jensen MP, Ehde DM, et al. Psychosocial predictors of long-term adjustment to lower-limb amputation and phantom limb pain. *Disabil Rehabil.* 2004;26(14/15):882–893.

[48] Barnett CT, Vanicek N, Polman RC. Temporal adaptations in generic and population-specific quality of life and falls efficacy in men with recent lower-limb amputations. *J Rehabil Res Dev.* 2013;50(3):437–448.

[49] Penn-Barwell JG. Outcomes in lower limb amputation following trauma: a systematic review and meta-analysis. *Injury.* 2011;42:1474–1479.

[50] Unwin J, Kacperek L, Clarke C. A prospective study of positive adjustment to lower limb amputation. *Clin Rehabil.* 2009;23(11):1044–1050.

[51] Akarsu S, Tekin L, Safaz I, et al. Quality of life and functionality after lower limb amputations: comparison between uni- vs. bilateral amputee patients. *Prosthet Orthot Int.* 2013;37(1):9.

[52] Asano M, Rushton P, Miller WC, Deathe BA. Predictors of quality of life among individuals who have a lower limb amputation. *Prosthet Orthot Int.* 2008;32(2):231–243.

[53] Bhutani S, Bhutani J, Chhabra A, Uppal R. Living with amputation: anxiety and depression correlates. *J Clin Diagn Res.* 2016;10(9):9.

[54] Murray C. An interpretive phenomenological analysis of the embodiment of artificial limbs. *Disabil Rehabil.* 2004;26:963–973.

[55] Ostler C, Ellis-Hill C, Donovan-Hall M. Expectations of rehabilitation following lower amputation: a qualitative study. *Disabil Rehabil.* 2014;36(14):1169.

[56] Livingstone W, van de Mortel TF, Taylor B. A path of perpetual resilience: exploring the experience of a diabetes-related amputation through grounded theory. *Contemp Nurse.* 2011;1,20.

[57] Yorkston KM, McMullan KA, Molton I, Jensen MP. Pathways of change experienced by people aging with disability: a focus group study. *Disabil Rehabil.* 2010;32(20):1697–1704.

[58] Chung A. Exploratory study on challenges faced by ageing persons with physical disabilities. *Asia Pac J Soc Work.* 2011;21(1):89–96.

[59] Moos RH, Holahan CJ. Adaptive tasks and methods of coping with illness and disability. In: Martz E, Livneh H, eds. *Coping with Chronic Illness and Disability: Theoretical, Empirical, and Clinical Aspects,* 2007. Springer, New York, pp. 107–126.

[60] Rolland J. Mastering family challenges in illness and disability. In: Walsh F, ed. *Normal Family Processes: Growing Diversity and Complexity,* 2003. 3rd edition. The Guilford Press, New York.

[61] Henderson AW, Turner AP, Williams RM, et al. Sexual activity after dysvascular lower extremity amputation. *Rehabil Psychol.* 2016;61(3):260–268.

[62] Geertzen JB, Van Es CG, Dijkstra PU. Sexuality and amputation: a systematic literature review. *Disabil Rehabil.* 2009;31(7):522–527.

[63] Lewis RW, Fugl-Meyer KS, Bosch R, et al. Epidemiology/risk factors of sexual dysfunction. *J Sex Med.* 2004;1(1):35–39.

[64] Valvano AK, West LM, Wilson CK, et al. Health professions students' perceptions of sexuality in patients with disability. *Sex Disabil.* 2014;32:413–427.

[65] Verschuren JE, Zhdanova MA, Geertzen JH, et al. Let's talk about sex: lower limb amputation, sexual functioning and sexual well-being: a qualitative study of the partner's perspective. *J Clin Nurs.* 2013;22(23/24):3557–3567.

[66] Verschuren JE, Geertzen JH, Enzlin P, et al. People with lower limb amputation and their sexual functioning and sexual well-being. *Disabil Rehabil.* 2015;37(3): 87–193.

[67] Burger H, Marinček Č. Return to work after lower limb amputation. *Disabil Rehabil.* 2007;29(17):1323–1329.

[68] MacKenzie EJ, Bosse MJ, Kellam JF, et al. Early predictors of long-term work disability after major limb trauma. *J Trauma.* 2006;61:688–694.

[69] Cater JK. Traumatic amputation: psychosocial adjustment of six army women to loss of one or more limbs. *J Rehabil Res Dev.* 2012;49(10):1443–1455.

[70] West SL, McMahon BT, Monasterio E, et al. Workplace discrimination and missing limbs: The National EEOC ADA Research Project. *Work.* 2005;25:27–35.

[71] Burger H, Maver T, Marinček Č. Partial hand amputation and work. *Disabil Rehabil.* 2007;29(17):1317–1321.

[72] Postema SG, Bongers RM, Brouwers MA, et al. Upper limb absence: predictors of work participation and work productivity. *Arch Phys Med Rehab.* 2016;97:892–899.

[73] Eldar R, Jelić M. The association of rehabilitation and war. *Disabil Rehabil.* 2003;25(18):1019–1023.

[74] Schaffalitzky E, Gallagher P, Maclachlan M, Wegener ST. Developing consensus on important factors associated with lower limb prosthetic prescription and use. *Disabil Rehabil.* 2012;34(24):2085–2094.

[75] Hill A, Niven CA, Knussen C, McCreath SW. Rehabilitation outcome in long-term amputees. *Br J Ther Rehabil.* 1995;2(11):593–598.

[76] Job Accommodation Network. Job accommodations for people with amputations. *Effective Accommodation Practices Series,* 2012. Accessed December 31, 2016. http://askjan.org/media/ampu.htm.

[77] McAlonan S. Improving sexual rehabilitation services: the patient's perspective. *Am J Occup Ther.* 1996;50(10):826–834.

[78] O'Dea SM, Shuttleworth RP, Wedgwood N. Disability, doctors, and sexuality: do healthcare providers influence the sexual well-being of people living with a neuromuscular disorder? *Sex Disabil.* 2012;30:171–185.

[79] Haboubi NHJ, Lincoln N. Views of health professionals on discussing sexual issues with patients. *Disabil Rehabil.* 2003;25(6):291–296.

[80] Gianotten W, Bender J, Post M, Höing M. Training in sexology for medical and paramedical professionals: a model for the rehabilitation setting. *Sex Relation Ther.* 2006;21(3):303–317.

[81] Pynor R, Weerakoon P, Jones MK. A preliminary investigation of physiotherapy students' attitudes towards issues of sexuality in clinical practice. *Physiotherapy.* 2005;91(1):42–48.

[82] Solursh DS, Ernst JL, Lewis RW, et al. The human sexuality education of physicians in North American medical schools. *Int J Impot Res.* 2003;15, Suppl 5:S41–S45.

[83] East LJ, Orchard TR. Somebody else's job: experiences of sex education among health professionals, parents and adolescents with physical disabilities in Southwestern Ontario. *Sex Disabil.* 2014;32:335–350.

[84] Bullard DG, Caplan H, Derzko C. Sexual problems. In: Feldman MD, Christensen JF, Satterfield JM, eds. *Behavioral Medicine: A Guide for Clinical Practice,* 2014. 4th edition. McGraw-Hill Education, New York.

[85] International Encyclopedia of Rehabilitation [website]. Accessed July 1, 2017. http://cirrie.buffalo.edu/encyclopedia/en/.

[86] Blom RM, Hennekam RC, Denys D. Body Integrity Identity Disorder. *PLOS One.* 2012;7(4):e34702.

[87] First MB, Fischer CE. Body Integrity Identity Disorder: the persistent desire to acquire a physical disability. *Psychopathology.* 2012;45:3–14.

[88] Enander J, Andersson E, Mataix-Cols D, et al. Therapist guided internet based Cognitive Behavioural Therapy for Body Dysmorphic Disorder: single blind randomised controlled trial. *Brit Med J.* 2016;352:i241.

[89] Weingarden H. Anxiety and shame as risk factors for depression, suicidality, and functional impairment in Body Dysmorphic Disorder and Obsessive Compulsive Disorder. *J Nerv Ment Dis.* 2016;204(11):832–839.

[90] Taylor B, Davis S. The Extended PLISSIT Model for addressing sexual wellbeing of individuals with an acquired disability or chronic illness. *Sex Disabil.* 2007;(25):135–139.

[91] Hatzichristou D, Rosen RC, Broderick G, et al. Clinical evaluation and management strategy for sexual dysfunction in men and women. *J Sex Med.* 2004;1(1):49–57.

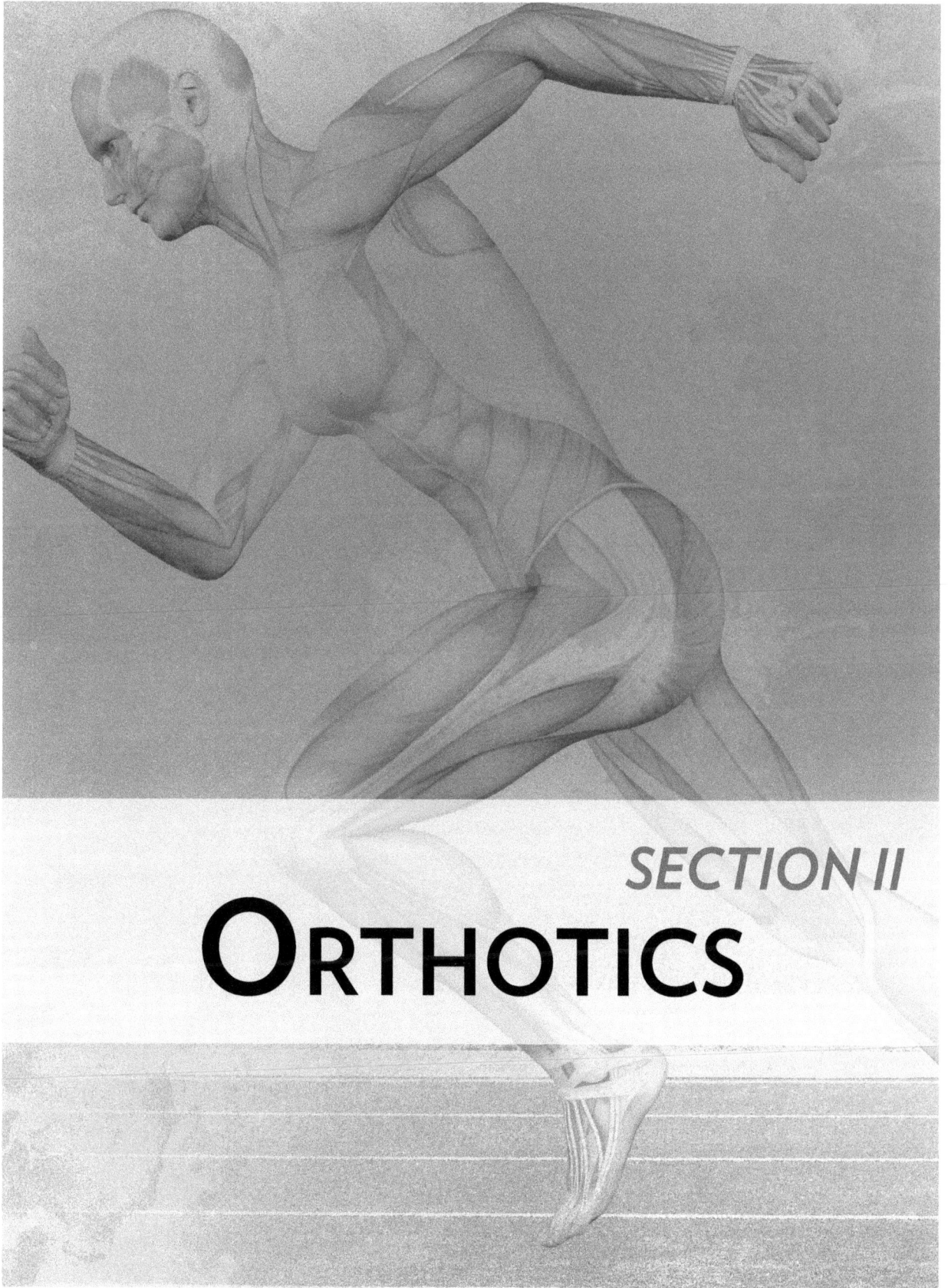

ORTHOTICS

CHAPTER 12

Overview of Pathologies for which Orthoses are Commonly Recommended

John H. Seiverd, Gail A. Latlief, and Marissa R. McCarthy

OBJECTIVES

Upon completion of this chapter, the reader will be able to:
1. Recall common pathologies for which orthoses are commonly recommended.
2. Recall the etiology associated with pathologies for which orthoses are commonly recommended.
3. Recall the epidemiology associated with pathologies for which orthoses are commonly recommended.
4. Recall common impairments and potential benefits of orthoses associated with pathologies for which orthoses are commonly recommended.

INTRODUCTION

This chapter discusses pathologic conditions that typically manifest or present with impairments and functional limitations for which an orthosis or orthotic assistive device are commonly indicated or recommended. The conditions discussed within this chapter can be organized and categorized into five main groups: (1) neurologic/neuromuscular, (2) musculoskeletal, (3) traumatic, (4) metabolic or rheumatologic, and (5) pediatric. Specific orthoses and prostheses related to these conditions, including the indications, prescription, and implications, are explained throughout this text in further detail. This chapter is in no way all-inclusive and is intended to provide merely an overview of those conditions that may necessitate the use of an orthosis.

NEUROLOGIC/ NEUROMUSCULAR DISORDERS

Stroke

Epidemiology, Etiology, and Presentation

Stroke is the most common neurologic emergency, and it is the leading cause of disability in the United States [1]. It is also known as a cerebrovascular accident (CVA) or brain attack. Risk factors include hypertension, hyperlipidemia, poorly controlled diabetes mellitus, obesity, substance abuse, and atrial fibrillation. Non-modifiable

DOI: 10.4324/9781003526025-14

risk factors include a family history of cerebrovascular disease, sickle cell disease, or hypercoagulable states. Ethnic populations, such as African-Americans and Hispanics, are more likely to have cerebrovascular disease than Caucasians. Advanced age and male sex are also other non-modifiable risk factors.

Cerebrovascular disease results from a pathologic process of the blood vessels. Cerebrovascular disease and stroke are often used interchangeably. The term stroke refers to the sudden onset of a focal neurologic deficit caused by cerebrovascular disease. Strokes are classified as either ischemic (85%) or hemorrhagic (15%). Ischemic strokes can be due to large artery atherosclerosis, cardio-embolic causes like atrial fibrillation, and small vessel disease or lacunar infarcts. Other less common causes of ischemic stroke include vessel dissection, venous thrombosis, drugs, and cryptogenic (cause is unknown) [2]. Hemorrhagic strokes are most often caused by hypertension.

There are signs and symptoms characteristic of vascular lesions in the various arterial territories of the brain. Presentation of strokes varies according to the underlying etiology [3]. Early initiation of rehabilitation after acute stroke is associated with improved functional outcome at discharge and shorter rehabilitation length of stay [4]. The primary goal of rehabilitation is to prevent complications, minimize impairments, and maximize function. Rehabilitation involves a multidisciplinary team including physical therapy, occupational therapy, speech therapy, neuropsychology, recreation therapy, nursing, social work, and other disciplines.

Rehabilitation Aim and Orthotic Considerations

Common post-stroke complications include spasticity and post-stroke shoulder pain. Spasticity, a velocity dependent resistance to stretch, occurs post stroke and often leads to contractures and deformity. Prevention measures include early mobilization, range of motion activities, proper positioning, and use of braces. Contractures can be treated using splinting, serial casting, or surgical correction. Post-stroke shoulder pain and subluxation (partial dislocation) is also a complication. Prevention is accomplished through careful monitoring, proper positioning, shoulder harness/sling or taping, trauma prevention, avoidance of uncontrolled abduction and overhead pulley use, and precautions during transfers.

Motor assessments happen at the impairment and functional level. Components include strength, active and passive range of motion, muscle tone, gross and fine motor coordination, balance, apraxia, and mobility. Motor function is addressed with strengthening, balance and gait training, orthoses (i.e. ankle foot orthoses), transcutaneous electrical nerve stimulation (TENS), robot-assisted movement therapy, constraint-induced movement

therapy, body-weight-supported treadmill training, and upper extremity interventions in order to improve function [5]. Team members including physical therapists provide assistance with ordering functionally appropriate durable medical equipment (DME) and instructions for home exercise programs. Ongoing management may include a regular exercise program, walking aids and/or wheelchair, adaptive devices for activities of daily living (ADLs), and home modifications [6].

Post-Polio

Epidemiology, Etiology, and Presentation

The polio virus is an RNA enterovirus that invades the central nervous system (CNS) in about 5% of clinical infections, causing varying degrees of paralysis in about 2% of patients [7]. Acute paralytic polio is characterized by sudden onset of paralysis with a febrile illness. Following the acute infection, recovery of strength and function occurs over a period of months to years. Post-polio syndrome (PPS) is defined as a neurologic disorder that can occur in survivors of paralytic polio after a period of functional stability of usually 15 years or more, characterized by new weakness or muscle fatigability, with or without generalized fatigue, muscle atrophy, or pain in muscles and/or joints [8]. Presentation of PPS can be insidious or acute. Acute presentation may be associated with trauma, surgery, a period of immobility, or an increase in activity. PPS is more often classified as a slowly progressive neuromuscular disease with a clinical presentation of functional declines and plateaus.

The most widely accepted hypothesis for PPS was proposed by Weichers and Hubbell [9]. They believe re-innervation of denervated muscle fibers during the recovery phase of acute polio results in giant motor units. Due to the slow loss of anterior horn cells with normal aging, motor units undergo continuous remodeling. As more motor units are lost, the ability of neighboring motor units to re-innervate the denervated muscle fibers is not sufficient to maintain the balance so weakness results.

Rehabilitation Aim and Orthotic Considerations

PPS is often associated with musculoskeletal problems. New weakness may present as a change in gait, loss of function, easy fatigability, or increased number of falls. There is a wide variability in degree of weakness between agonist and antagonist muscles within a limb and between limbs which alters body mechanics. These imbalances can result in spine and joint deformities, accelerated degeneration, and soft tissue overuse syndromes. Secondary radiculopathies and compression neuropathies can be common. Electromyography (EMG) may assist in identifying compression neuropathies, radiculopathies, other neurologic conditions, or myopathies.

Functional mobility should be observed for muscle substitutions and compensatory strategies. Clinical gait analysis with and without orthotics and assistive devices is important for identification of mechanical stress on weak muscles and to assess fall risk. Post-polio patients should decrease stress on specific muscles by activity modification or use of orthoses and assistive devices, and/or initiate a targeted exercise program. A classification for exercise prescription was developed by the National Rehabilitation Hospital (NRH) [10]. Care must be taken with any polio-affected muscle, pacing activity with rest and watching for signs of overuse. Energy conservation techniques may include use of orthotics (i.e. knee ankle foot orthoses [KAFOs] or AFOs), assistive devices, and mobility aids. Rehabilitation interventions can prevent or improve the musculoskeletal disorders to help minimize symptoms. There is no evidence that PPS can be avoided through preventive measures.

Spinal Cord Injury (SCI)

Epidemiology, Etiology, and Presentation

A spinal cord injury (SCI) refers to an insult to the spinal cord resulting in impaired motor, sensory, and/or autonomic function below the injured spinal cord level. Injury to the cervical segments through the first thoracic segments typically results in impaired function to both the arms and the legs, referred to as *tetraplegia*. Injury to the thoracic, lumbar, or sacral segments of the spinal cord causes *paraplegia*, typically resulting in impaired function in the legs. Motor vehicle accidents are the most common cause of SCI, followed by falls, acts of violence, and sports injuries.

In the United States there are 12,000 new cases each year [11]. Although traumatic SCI primarily affects young males between the ages of 15 and 35, the age at injury has been steadily increasing [12]. The incidence peaks in young adulthood and declines thereafter, though there appears to be a secondary rise in incidence among the elderly. Falls are the leading cause of SCI among persons aged >60. The most common injury category is incomplete tetraplegia followed by incomplete paraplegia, complete paraplegia, and complete tetraplegia. Of all injuries, 34% are complete, 66% are incomplete [12].

The level and completeness of SCI should be determined with a careful sensory examination for light touch and pin prick at key sensory points, and motor examination of designated key muscles bilaterally. The neurological completeness of SCI is classified according to the American Spinal Injury Association (ASIA) Impairment Scale [12, 13].

Rehabilitation Aim and Orthotic Considerations

Motor and sensory recovery depends on the extent and location of the insult. Persons with incomplete SCI recover faster and to a greater extent than do those with complete injuries. Regardless of level and completeness of injury, most recovery occurs within the first 6 months after injury [14]. The primary goals during the rehabilitation period are to educate the person and family about SCI, prevent secondary complications, improve function, and prepare the person for integration into the community. Therapy goals include increasing tolerance to the upright position, exercises for strength, balance, and endurance, improving function in ADLs, bed mobility, transfers, wheelchair training, gait training, as appropriate, and bowel/bladder management training. Spasticity may become a barrier to functional improvement and could cause contracture and skin breakdown. Interventions include splinting, stretching, and electric stimulation to help improve range of motion and strengthen weakened muscles. Functional electric stimulation (FES) is a newer concept and practice in the rehabilitation of SCI. Upper-extremity devices (i.e. NESS H200. Bioness. Valencia, CA, U.S.A.) and lower-extremity devices (i.e. NESS L300. Bioness. Valencia, CA, U.S.A.; WalkAide, ACP-Accelerated Care Plus, Reno, NV, U.S.A.) exist for the treatment of functional deficits [15]. Exoskeleton units have been developed to allow for ambulation with the use of assistive devices in those with limited leg strength [16, 17]. There is controversy regarding outcomes in body-weight-supported treadmill systems versus overground ambulation training [17]. Spinal orthoses are used for stable spine fractures, post-operative control of fractures, and post-surgical care of spinal fusion or reconstruction. Immobilization orthoses are primarily used for spinal trauma, with or without surgical intervention, as well as post-spinal reconstruction surgeries, including fusions. There are cervical orthoses (CO), thoracic and thoracolumbosacral orthoses (TLSO), the Milwaukee brace—cervicothoracolumbosacral orthoses (CTLSO), and sacral orthoses. The clinician must first diagnose the underlying condition and decide if orthotic treatment is required.

Traumatic Brain Injury (TBI)

Epidemiology, Etiology, and Presentation

The definition of traumatic brain injury (TBI) is a disruption of brain function due to an external force or blow to the head resulting in a decreased level of consciousness, memory loss before or after injury, alteration of mental status, neurologic deficits, or intracranial lesion [18, 19]. The most common cause of TBI is falls (49.1%) and motor vehicle crashes (24.5%). Other causes are less common and include unknown/other, struck by/against an object, and assaults. Penetrating injuries, such as gun-shot wounds, are a less frequent cause. Falls were the most frequent cause in young children and older adults, whereas motor vehicle collisions were the most frequent cause in those 15–24 years old [20]. Active duty service members have blast brain injury as the most common type of war-related TBI [21]. Approximately 1.7 million people have TBI annually in the United States; 1.365 million are treated and released from an emergency department, 275,000 are hospitalized, and 52,000 die [20]. The rate was highest among those 4 years old or less, followed by those 15–24, and those over 75. Males have 1.4 times as many TBIs as females among all age groups. Mortality is higher in patients over the age of 75. Firearms (34.8%), motor-vehicle (31.4%), and fall-related TBIs (16.7%) are the leading causes of TBI-related death by etiology [22].

The natural history of TBI varies with regard to amount and speed of recovery. A patient with TBI can start out in a vegetative state with no purposeful behavior. This state can progress to a minimally conscious state with intermittent purposeful behaviors. As patients continue to improve, recovery will be observed to varying degrees in motor control, memory, and behavior. Similar to stoke, TBI patients will have deficits related to certain areas of the brain that are affected.

Rehabilitation Aim and Orthotic Considerations

The rehabilitation team is encouraged to use outcome measures to assess objectively function and potential orthotic need. Measures such as the Functional Independence Measure (FIM) are useful in such cases. The FIM contains 18 items with 13 covering ADLs, mobility, bowel/bladder, and five covering communication and cognition. These tests are scored from total assistance (1) to complete independence (7). The Functional Assessment Measure is an adjunct to the FIM that adds 12 items to assess more adequately domains affected in TBI including behavioral, cognitive, communication, and community function measures [23]. Similar to stroke, TBI patients can suffer from hemiplegia, spasticity, quadriplegia, monoplegia, and are at risk for contractures and deformities. Depending on the presenting deficits, a range of orthoses and assistive devices may be indicated. These may include shoulder slings, lap boards, hand splints, wheelchairs, or lower extremity orthoses. Prudent care is necessary to help

prevent skin breakdown or complications especially in severely impaired, low mobility patients. Again, strength, active and passive range of motion, tone, gross and fine motor coordination, balance, apraxia, and mobility are assessed. Motor function is addressed with strengthening, balance and gait training, orthoses, transcutaneous electrical nerve stimulation (TENS), robot-assisted movement therapy, constraint-induced movement therapy, and body-weight-supported treadmill training, and upper extremity interventions in order to improve function when indicated.

MUSCULOSKELETAL CONDITIONS

Epidemiology, Etiology, and Cost

Musculoskeletal conditions involve joints, muscle, bone, cartilage, or connective tissues (tendons, ligaments, fascia, joint capsules, intervertebral discs, etc.). At some point, these conditions affect more than 78% of people in the United States over the age of 18 [24]. The three most commonly reported musculoskeletal conditions are back pain, injury/trauma, and arthritis. Musculoskeletal complaints account for approximately 20% of primary care provider visits, overall [24–27]. Common conditions from injuries and accidents discussed within this section include: bruises/contusions, strains, sprains, overuse, and fractures. Systemic, genetic, and metabolic musculoskeletal conditions include arthritis, osteoporosis, spinal deformity, and joint pain (arthralgias), and are discussed in additional detail in the Metabolic and Rheumatologic section that follows.

Musculoskeletal diseases cost the US over $980.1 billion dollars in 2011, which equated to 5.76% of the annual gross domestic product (GDP) [24]. In 2012, 1 in 8 people of working age reported losing work days due to a musculoskeletal condition—a total of 216 million days [24]. For those individuals over age 65, physical work appears to have a positive impact on overall health [24, 28]. However, depending on the type of work being performed it may or may not be good for someone with a musculoskeletal disorder. Although physical activity and general aerobic activity, such as walking, all have positive health benefits, some jobs may require repetitive or specific motions or activity that can become problematic. Some highly repetitive and occupational activities have been linked with an association of increased risk for musculoskeletal problems. Frequent kneeling, squatting, climbing, and heavy lifting have been associated with higher incidence of knee osteoarthritis (OA) [29]. Frequent occupational kneeling and squatting are associated with a higher risk of meniscal injury [29]. Heavy lifting and squatting are risk factors for the development of hip OA, and frequent lifting, bending, or twisting have been associated with higher incidents of low back pain (LBP) [28].

Strains, Sprains, Fractures, Joint Pain, and Overuse Syndromes

Strains and Sprains

Strains and sprains are common in most primary care and rehabilitation settings. Strain is a term used to describe an injury to a tendon or muscle. Tendons are collagenous soft tissue that can be cord-like and connect muscle to bone. They can also be thick, flat, and fibrous and connect muscle to muscle or muscle to fascia. Injuries to tendons can be acute or become chronic, as is the typical case with repetitive or overuse conditions. Evaluation and treatment, especially when overuse is suspected, should focus on identifying the cause and modifying the behaviors or activities that are contributing or causing the irritation. The phases of tendon healing involve an inflammatory phase, a proliferation phase, and a remodeling phase. Intervention should be dependent on which phase of healing the condition is presently in. In the acute phase, Rest, Ice, Compression, and Elevation (or "RICE") are commonly utilized. Chronic conditions involving tendons are known as a tendinosis, which implies a chronic degeneration.

Injury to a ligament or ligamentous tissues is known as a sprain. Sprains are classified in degrees (1st degree, 2nd degree, 3rd degree) and are most common in the ankle, knee, and fingers. Signs and symptoms typically include pain, edema, calor (localized increased body heat), ecchymosis, loss of function, and can include hypermobility or instability, dislocation, and subluxation. Prognosis is highly variable depending on the extent of tissue damage, biomechanical disruption, and the overall impact on pain levels and function. Many types of orthoses are available to treat sprains and strains, from compressive garments and sleeves, to soft and rigid braces for the joints and spine to promote alignment and stability.

Fractures

A defect in the bone continuity is known as a fracture. Fractures can be a small crack or complex, broken into many pieces (comminuted). There are four main categories: sudden impact (most common), stress/fatigue, pathologic, and open versus closed. Signs and symptoms include pain, tenderness, edema, ecchymosis, loss of function and mobility, and may include deformity. Prognosis is typically a predictable healing pattern, unless there are underlying pathologic processes present. Fractures are typically immobilized in a rigid orthosis or cast for a period ranging from 4 to 8 weeks. Those who smoke cigarettes have significantly delayed healing times and may require several more days or weeks to heal as compared with someone who does not smoke [30].

Shoulder, Arm, and Wrist

Carpal tunnel syndrome (CTS) is a peripheral nerve lesion or irritation caused by a compression of the median nerve within the carpal tunnel of the wrist. The etiology in many cases can be contributed to repetitive finger movements or grasping vibrating tools. The signs and symptoms can include numbness, tingling, burning, and lack of sweating in the median nerve distribution of the hand. In more severe or chronic cases, weakness (paresis) and atrophy of the thenar muscles is also possible. The condition is most common in individuals over the age of 30 and affects more females than males. Job or activity modification with night splinting of the wrist can be helpful. Surgery is also an option but carries many risks [31].

Rib/Costal Conditions

Rib fractures are common in sports, after a fall, and during a motor vehicle accident (MVA). After rib fracture, coughing and general mobility can cause significant discomfort. A simple abdominal binder or rib belt snugly secured around the ribs can often offer compression and support that reduces pain and discomfort. Unless they are significantly displaced, compromising the pleural space, or causing breathing issues, surgical intervention is typically not indicated.

Injury Prevention and Prophylactic Orthotic Use

With their vast education in biomechanics, physiology, tissue healing, pain science, and biopsychosocial approaches to condition management, physical therapists are positioned and prepared to play a key role in the prevention of injuries. Injury prevention strategies typically involve patient education, self-management (i.e. stretching, icing, therapeutic exercise, etc.), activity modification, environmental considerations, and can involve orthotics/bracing and assistive devices. The physical therapist's role in collaborating with referring physicians and orthotists to determine biomechanical and functional issues is vital in assessing orthotic need and facilitating a successful rehabilitative outcome.

TRAUMATIC CONDITIONS/ TRAUMA

Polytrauma

Epidemiology, Etiology, and Cost

The definition of polytrauma is injuries that affect two or more body systems or organs, with one of the injuries usually being a TBI, and at least one of the injuries being potentially life-threatening in severity. These injuries can lead to impairments in physical, cognitive, psychological, or psychosocial functioning [32]. The terminology has been around for some time. In 2005 the Veterans Health Administration described polytrauma as a prominent clinical phenomenon. With over a decade's worth of combat in the Middle East there had been a surge in polytrauma injuries. There was unprecedented exposure to blasts, changes to body armor, improved survival, and a new set of wounds with protracted and complex recovery periods [33].

Polytrauma injuries dominate resources. In the United States, trauma accounts for more than 26 million emergency department visits and more than 2 million hospital admissions every year. The economic burden of trauma has been estimated at more than $671 billion annually [34]. The processes underlying other complex injuries, including traumatic limb loss and limb salvage, vary by injury type. Patients recovering from musculoskeletal injuries, who may require multiple additional surgeries to optimize bone healing, often experience pain and impaired mobility [35].

Rehabilitation Aim and Orthotic Considerations

Limb salvage patients, those who retained their limbs despite massive trauma, often have a long rehabilitation course. Due to the nature of their injuries, they can have damage to muscles, nerves, and joints leading to debilitating pain and decreased mobility. In 2009, rehabilitation specialists within the Department of Defense observed an alarming number of wounded warriors who, following limb salvage, requested delayed amputation(s), with many patients electing to have limbs amputated due to pain. In response, the team developed the *Return to Run* Clinical Pathway. Members of this team studied prostheses designed for running and designed the Intrepid Dynamic Exoskeletal Orthosis (IDEO). The orthosis has a footplate that fits into a shoe, a brace that stabilizes the ankle, and carbon fiber rods that extend proximally along the posterior leg to a cuff positioned just below the knee. Those using the IDEO have to learn to run on the 1st metatarsal head (i.e. the ball of the foot) and the IDEO helps them "spring" forward [36]. The IDEO was one recent orthotic development associated with rehabilitation following highly visible polytrauma cases in high functioning patients. Numerous other orthoses may be useful in polytrauma cases.

Amputation

Limb amputations are typically a result of peripheral vascular disease (PVD), chronic venous insufficiency, diabetes mellitus, infection, tumor, trauma, or limb deficiency. Post-operatively, limb wrapping with a compressive elastic wrap or shrinker can help control edema and pain, while preparing the residual limb for prosthesis. Sometimes a solid or rigid shell orthosis can be fabricated to protect the healing limb during the healing phase and further prepare the limb for acceptance of a prosthetic limb. A significant portion of this text is devoted to management of the patient with amputation. This section serves as a reminder that orthoses may have a role in caring for patients who may be facing amputation.

METABOLIC AND RHEUMATOLOGIC CONDITIONS

Diabetes Mellitus and Diabetic Neuropathy

Epidemiology, Etiology, and Presentation

In 2021, more than 38 million Americans, or 11.6% of the population, had diabetes mellitus. Approximately half of those diagnosed with diabetes mellitus for longer than 25 years will develop diabetic neuropathy. The primary risk factor for diabetic neuropathy is poorly controlled diabetes mellitus from high blood sugar [37]. Peripheral neuropathy initially produces sensory disturbances of the distal limbs in a stocking glove distribution as opposed to along any specific nerve distribution. It may subsequently result in distal motor weakness and absent ankle reflexes. Neuropathy can cause decreased pain and temperature sensation but can also cause burning pain, usually in the feet [38, 39]. Loss of pedal sensation from diabetic neuropathy may result in skin wounds and ulceration. The vascular and immunologic disorders make these wounds susceptible to infection. Other complications include neuropathic arthropathies (Charcot joints) and entrapment neuropathies, such as carpal tunnel syndrome.

Diabetic polyneuropathy often advances and results in further sensory loss with progression to weakness and atrophy in a distal to proximal distribution. Proprioceptive deficits should be tested with Romberg, tandem gait, and one-leg stand tests. Vibratory sensation is often the first sensory finding in diabetic neuropathy. Deep tendon reflexes and strength at the ankle should be documented. A skin examination to detect redness, callouses, and ulcers is necessary. Inspection should assess for boney irregularities and muscle atrophy. Diabetic neuropathy increases the risk of amputation 1.7-fold, and more than 80% of amputations are related to a foot ulcer or other injury. Following a diabetes-related amputation of one limb, the risk of amputation for the corresponding limb is 50% over 5 years [38, 39].

Other causes of polyneuropathy include renal and liver disease. Vitamin deficiencies, toxins, infectious diseases, autoimmune conditions, endocrine disorders, paraneoplastic syndromes, and monoclonal gammopathies can also cause neuropathy. Inherited disorders like Charcot Marie Tooth disease and idiopathic causes account for about 20–25% of patients with a peripheral neuropathy [40, 41]. Physical examination focusing on limb inspection, strength, sensation, reflexes, balance, and gait is paramount. These patients are at increased risk for falls [42].

Rehabilitation Aim

Ultimate goals of treatment are maintenance of function, quality of life, and limb preservation. There is strong evidence that anticonvulsants are beneficial, particularly pregabalin. There is moderate evidence supporting antidepressants, capsaicin, and opioids to treat pain [43].

Common impairments include balance and gait disturbances, falls, and increased fatigue. Assessment for orthotics, gait aids, and wheelchairs is often necessary. Home evaluations help determine equipment needs such as shower chairs and grab bars in the bathroom, railings on stairs, and other adaptions. ADL deficits include impaired hand function, resulting in difficulty with fasteners, handwriting, eating, caregiving, and homemaking. Upper extremity orthosis and adaptive tools can assist persons with neuropathy to maintain their independence.

Rheumatologic Conditions and Arthritis

Epidemiology, Etiology, and Cost

Inflammatory arthritides are inflammatory diseases affecting the synovial joints and related structures. Presentation includes one, few, or many joints. The condition may be acute or chronic. Inflammatory connective tissue diseases including rheumatoid arthritis and systemic lupus erythematosus, crystal-induced inflammatory arthritis like gout, seronegative spondyloarthropathies such as ankylosing spondylitis and psoriatic arthritis, and infectious arthritis like gonorrhea, tuberculosis, and osteomyelitis may affect the joints [44]. Osteoarthritis (OA) of the knee is the most common type of arthritis diagnosed affecting approximately 13% of women and 10% of men over age 60. The prevalence increases to 40% over age 70 [45]. The average annual direct cost per person related to arthritis is $11,000 whereas the U.S. absenteeism costs are $10.3 billion, and the total costs are $136 billion [46].

Certain populations are at increased risk for joint disease. Severity varies by disease, age, and gender. In inflammatory connective tissue diseases like rheumatoid arthritis, 75% are women; peak age is 25 to 50; it is more common in those of European descent. Systemic lupus erythematosus (SLE) is three times higher in African Americans and the female:male ratio is 9:1. Psoriatic arthritis and ankylosing spondylitis are more common in younger populations [47].

Joint pain is the most common presenting complaint. Onset and duration help differentiate acute inflammatory from non-inflammatory arthritis. Constitutional symptoms such as fatigue, weight loss, and/or fever suggest systemic disease. Examination of all joints, peripheral and axial, for pain, effusion, synovitis, deformities, range of movement, and strength is necessary. Mobility, ADLs, and social skills are also important to assess. Performance-based outcome measures such as the timed up and go and the 6-minute walk test may be useful. Patient reported outcome measures such as the health assessment questionnaire (HAQ) may also be useful to assess perceived mobility, self-care, and pain, and to assist in forecasting later function and morbidity [48].

Rehabilitation Aim

The Rheumatic Disease Treatment Pyramid (revised) includes rehabilitation interventions. Individualized treatment plans are most effective when initiated early in the disease process. Early engagement of the patient and family improves compliance [49]. Early rehabilitation includes orthoses, splints, joint protection, energy conservation, strengthening, stretching, and local modalities. Rehabilitation interventions, including activity pacing, can reduce joint inflammation. During acute joint flare-ups, passive ROM, where the patient's extremities are moved without muscle activation, should be avoided. Exercises should target specific goals for specific joints. Appropriate exercise can assist in maintaining strength, ROM, bone mineralization, endurance, aerobic capacity, bone density, and can assist in minimizing atrophy associated with inactivity. Isotonic exercises (moving a constant mass through a ROM) are ideal for joints without deformity or acute inflammation. Isometric exercise (contracting a muscle without movement) limits joint stress, maintains and restores strength, and is recommended for mechanically disrupted joints. Stretching exercises are appropriate for restoring ROM in the absence of acute inflammation. Aquatic therapy can deliver pain control, decrease joint stress, and enhance relaxation. Heat can offer muscle relaxation, pain reduction, and decreased stiffness. Cold decreases pain, muscle spasm, and local tissue metabolism. Orthoses and splints afford rest, reduce joint loads, and improve joint stability. In acute and subacutely inflamed joints, splints and orthoses can facilitate maintenance of proper segmental alignment. Ring orthoses may assist in mitigating finger deformity. Joint replacement surgery is indicated in select cases of severe structural damage, refractory pain, or disability.

Osteoporosis

Epidemiology, Etiology, and Presentation

The National Osteoporosis Foundation (NOF) has estimated that more than 9.9 million Americans have osteoporosis, and an additional 43.1 million have low bone density. More than 2 million fractures are attributed to osteoporosis annually. Hip fractures account for 14% of fractures and 72% of fracture costs. The cost of care is expected to rise to $25.3 billion by 2025 [50].

The World Health Organization defines osteoporosis as a bone mineral density at the hip or lumbar spine that is at least 2.5 standard deviations below the mean T-score of a young-adult female reference population [51]. Osteoporosis results from changes in the bone remodeling process. Osteoporosis can be either primary or secondary in etiology. Postmenopausal osteoporosis occurs in women aged 50–65 years with a phase of accelerated bone loss, and age-associated or senile osteoporosis occurs in women and men older than 70 years with bone loss associated with age. Secondary osteoporosis is a result of medical conditions or treatments that alter bone remodeling [52]. Peak bone mass is achieved by age 18–25. With age, daily bone remodeling occurs. Effective remodeling depends upon a balance between bone resorption and bone deposition.

Risk factors for the development of osteoporosis include age, race (being Caucasian or Asian), body mass index, genetic factors, and pre-existing medical conditions. Social risk factors include cigarette smoking, alcohol abuse, and lack of exercise. Nutritional and hormonal risk factors include diets low in calcium or vitamin D, excess vitamin A, high salt intake, low estrogen levels in women, and low testosterone levels in men.

Rehabilitation Aim

Hip fractures are associated with an 8.4 to 36% excess mortality within 1 year, with a higher mortality in men than in women [53]. Vertebral compression fractures may result in pain, disability, and mortality. Additionally, wrist or distal radial fractures can interfere with ADLs [50]. Risk factors for falls should be reduced. Early identification and treatment of patients with osteoporosis are essential. Weight bearing exercise is recommended to prevent and treat the loss of bone mass, help postural stability, and prevent falls [54]. By facilitating proper segmental alignment, orthoses may have a preventive role. Post fracture, they may have a therapeutic role in terms of protection, ROM, and again through facilitation of proper segmental loading.

PEDIATRIC CONDITIONS

Cerebral Palsy

Epidemiology, Etiology, and Cost

Cerebral palsy (CP) is a non-progressive, congenital condition that can affect motor control or movement, muscle tone, coordination, sensation, posture, communication, behavior, and cognition. It is typically caused by malformation or damage to the developing brain either before or at birth. The prevalence of CP in the USA has been reported at 3.1 cases per 1,000 (1 in 323 8-year-old children), in 2008. Overall prevalence appears to be higher for males than females by a ratio of 1.5:1. Studies have reported approximately 58% of children with CP walk independently, 11% walk with an assistive device, and 31% have limited or no walking ability. Approximately 41% of those affected by CP also have co-occurring epilepsy [55].

Patients with CP can present with the following problems: motor weakness, spasticity or "spastic CP," discoordination, hearing difficulty, visual problems, cognitive deficits, emotional regulation, learning disability, and epilepsy. Risk factors for CP include low birth weight, premature birth, disruption of blood or oxygen flow to the developing brain, maternal infection, and birth defects within the central nervous system (CNS). The overall lifetime cost for raising a child with CP is approximately 1 million U.S. dollars. In 2003, the estimated combined lifetime cost for all people with CP who were born in the U.S.A. in the year 2000 was $11.5 billion [56].

Factors associated with CP include low birth weight, premature birth among low-birth weight infants, and history of asphyxia and/or brain damage. Assessment should include physical and cognitive function with a focus on gathering information and evidence about existing and potential problems that affect ADLs.

Rehabilitation Aim and Orthotic Considerations

CP cannot be cured but treatment can help. Physical therapy (PT) typically plays a central role in the management of CP and there is moderate evidence within the literature to suggest that PT is beneficial [57]. PT intervention should focus on normalizing movement, safe mobility, gait speed, function, and reaching the child's full potential for independence. Patients who are non-ambulatory will likely have seating and mobility needs. There are a myriad of seating systems and wheelchairs available on the market, in both manual and power versions.

For patients who are ambulatory, gait training is the most effective intervention for improving gait speed, which correlates directly with quality of life [57–59]. Evaluation and prescription of the most appropriate and safest assistive device should be a priority for the PT.

For individuals with CP, increased hip muscle imbalance and muscle tone can lead to hip problems such as dislocations, subluxations, and decreased ROM. The goal of treatment and orthotic management in those suffering with hip problems is to prevent hip pain, prevent subluxation or dislocation, improve ROM, maximize muscle function, and encourage safe and independent mobility [57–59]. There are many different types of hip orthoses in the way of braces and garments. Thus, it is imperative that the PT, physician, orthotist, and other interdisciplinary team members work closely together to optimize outcomes in a patient-centered approach. This would be considered best practice [57–59]. Orthoses may be useful to facilitate optimal posture, balance, ambulation, or other functional activities.

Muscular Dystrophy

Epidemiology, Etiology, and Cost

Muscular dystrophy (MD) is a group of inherited genetic diseases that progress over time and affect proteins within muscles that ultimately leads to weakness and muscle loss. There are more than 30 known forms of MD. Some forms appear in young children, whereas other forms first appear during adulthood. The two most common pediatric forms are Duchenne muscular dystrophy (DMD) and spinal muscular atrophy (SMA). DMD primarily affects boys with an incidence estimated at 1 in 3,600 to 1 in 6,000 live male births, while the estimated incidence of SMA is between 1 in 6,000 to 1 in 10,000 live births. DMD accounts for over 50% of all MD cases and is the most severe childhood form of MD. Boys typically begin to show symptoms between ages 3 to 5 years as weakness begins in the upper legs and pelvic muscles. As proximal muscle weakness progresses or worsens, there are predictable adaptations and compensations that occur. Those affected usually lose the ability to ambulate by the second decade of life, or earlier. Boys with DMD often need a respirator to breathe as the disease progresses and many die in their late teens and early 20s from cardiac and breathing problems or infection [60, 61].

The total estimated cost in 2013 for patients within the U.S. for all forms of MD combined was $1.07 to $1.37 billion per year [62]. In 2012, the total societal cost within a group of international patients diagnosed with DMD was estimated between $80,012 and $120,910 (international dollars) per patient, per annum, and increased with disease progression. Related household burden for patients with DMD was estimated between $58,000 and $71,900. Thus, the disease carries a high burden of cost for affected families and the healthcare system [62]. Studies suggest that interventions that slow the progression of disease, keep patients walking longer, and reduce overall care requirements could significantly reduce the overall costs of these diseases [62].

Rehabilitation Aim and Orthotic Considerations

Currently, there is no cure or ability to reverse MD. However, certain therapies and medications can help treat some of the problems associated with MD and contribute toward improving the quality of life for those affected. Early PT intervention with therapeutic exercises and activities may be beneficial as the disease progresses [60]. PTs prescribe appropriate activities, provide non-pharmacologic pain management options, and assess for appropriate assistive devices and equipment needs (i.e. crutches, walkers, wheelchairs, home modifications, etc.) to promote safety and independence with mobility and ADLs. They also educate patients and caregivers to help reduce caregiver injury and burden as the disease slowly renders the patient more dependent.

Orthotists and PTs play a vital role to help extend or prolong independent ambulation in patients with MD. Patients typically progress from independent ambulation to assisted ambulation and eventually to reliance upon a wheelchair. Prudence should be exercised when considering orthotic bracing for patients with DMD, especially while they are still ambulatory. Daytime bracing should generally be avoided, as this places excessive forces on increasingly weakening muscle groups during the stance phase of gait (namely the quadriceps muscles). Thus, inappropriate prescription of daytime AFOs in patients with functional gait can detrimentally weaken lower extremity muscles and compromise the period of time that the child is independently ambulating. Compliance with night-time AFOs can help with controlling equinovarus and heel cord deformities, or plantarflexion contractures, within the feet and ankles. Passive stretching regimens along with night-time AFO use should be prescribed to help minimize the typical progression of equinovarus formation that could negatively affect independent or assisted standing and ambulation. Once a patient becomes reliant upon a wheelchair for mobility, orthotic intervention for the foot and ankle should be considered to control progression of equinovarus foot deformities and encourage anatomic alignment of the tarsal joints [63–65].

Spina Bifida

Epidemiology, Etiology, and Cost

Spina bifida is a treatable condition of the spine. It is classified as a defect within the neural tube and occurs in varying degrees of severity. During development, the neural tube that closes to form the brain, spinal cord, and/or meninges does not fully develop or close. Although it can occur anywhere along the tube, it most commonly occurs in the region of the lumbar spine or sacrum. The condition has often been referred to as myelomeningocele or myelodysplasia. However, spina bifida has been the most widely accepted term in the literature [66, 67]. The overall U.S. hospital cost for treating a baby with spina bifida in the first year of life ranges from $21,000 to $1.4 million and $791,900 is the overall estimated lifetime direct cost [68, 69].

There are four types of spina bifida: occulta, closed neural tube defects, meningocele, and myelomeningocele. Occulta is the most common and mildest form where one or more vertebrae are malformed. The name occulta means hidden, implying that the malformation is covered by the skin and not visible to the human eye. This form rarely causes disability or symptoms, is present in 10 to 20% of the general population and is more common among males [70]. With closed neural tube defects, the spinal cord has malformations of bone, meninges, or fatty tissue. In many cases symptoms are absent or mild. However, in some cases it causes incomplete paralysis in conjunction with bowel and bladder problems. With meningocele, an abnormal vertebral opening exists where the meninges and spinal fluid protrude through. The malformation or bulge does not include neural elements and may or may not be covered by skin. Individuals with meningocele can have few to no symptoms or may experience complete paralysis with bowel and bladder dysfunction. The most severe form of spina bifida is myelomeningocele (MMC) where the spinal cord and neural tissue are exposed through a malformation or opening in the spine. This typically results in partial or complete paralysis of the body below the level of the malformation. Symptoms may be so severe that the individual is unable to ambulate, may have complete loss of bowel and bladder function, and may suffer from hydrocephalus or excess fluid on the brain [71]. In children with MMC, the absence or presence of hydrocephalus appears to be more significantly associated with functional independence than the actual neurologic level of the defect or lesion [72].

Rehabilitation Aim and Orthotic Considerations

It is important for healthcare professionals to consider the presence of hydrocephalus in children with spina bifida and the potential impact on achieving functional improvement and independence. The interdisciplinary team should consider utilizing the International Classification of Function model as a useful, comprehensive framework in helping children with spina bifida achieve maximal independence [72].

The two main reasons to consider orthotics for children with spina bifida are to improve independent function and prevent or correct deformities (i.e. clubfoot). Beliefs and protocols vary widely regarding best practices and timing of intervention. However, orthotic intervention commonly begins a few years after birth. The most common orthoses utilized for children with MMC who present with gait and foot alignment issues are custom ankle foot orthoses (AFOs) [66, 73]. PT services should focus on interventions that promote establishing or restoring functional independence. The orthotist, physician, PT, and interdisciplinary team should work together closely to ensure progress towards functional goals and optimize patient-centered outcomes.

Idiopathic Toe Walking

Epidemiology, Etiology, and Cost

Children who walk on their toes have a characteristic gait where the heel does not touch or minimally touches the ground, most notably at initial contact or during the stance phase of gait. This is commonly described as "toe-walking" or "tip-toe-walking." These children may have a "springy" or "bouncy" gait where the heel is in minimal contact with the ground at any point during the gait cycle, if at all. Toe walking can be unilateral or bilateral, depending on etiology. In the absence of any known cause, the condition is considered idiopathic toe walking (ITW). Toe walking has been considered to be a normal, temporary, variant in many children, but should be investigated if persistent beyond age 2 [74, 75]. A thorough clinical exam and history should be used to differentiate between different types of toe walking and determine the most appropriate treatment for each individual child [76].

There are many causes of toe walking in children and the condition is not uncommon. The prevalence of toe walking at age 5.5 years is approximately 2% in normally developing children and over 40% in children with a neuropsychiatric diagnosis or developmental delay [76]. The overall cost burden is unknown [77]. Some conditions where toe walking is commonly seen are: congenitally short calcaneal tendon(s), cerebral palsy, muscular dystrophy, encephalopathy, brain injury, transient focal dystonia, spinal cord injury or conditions, developmental disorders or conditions, and autism spectrum disorders [78]. These conditions all manifest with separate and distinct signs and symptoms (i.e. orthopedic/anatomic anomaly, equinovarus contracture, spasticity, hypertonicity, clonus, seizure activity or history, speech delays, low muscle tone, or other pronounced developmental delay, etc.).

The diagnosis of ITW is made by exclusion and in the absence of any of the above-mentioned signs or symptoms. These cases typically present as bilateral and symmetrical, intermittent, toe walking. There is evidence to suggest a familial association and a possible sensory processing or organization component [79]. Due to the many different causes and the possible marker for other developmental problems, it is always prudent to ensure children or adolescents who present with ITW be thoroughly evaluated and or referred to the appropriate provider(s) for a comprehensive developmental assessment [77, 80]. Many cases of ITW resolve on their own after a period of time and the long-term effects and sequelae of ITW into adulthood are unknown. However, it should not be assumed that children will simply outgrow ITW or that it should not be treated. Parents and patients often seek out treatment for ITW due solely to cosmetic and social concerns which, in and of themselves, can justify treatment. If neither parent nor child has concerns about the toe walking and the condition is not painful or limiting function, the provider should question whether treatment is indicated [81]. Any treatment or corrective efforts considered should be justifiable and reinforced by a prudent clinical rationale that is supported by evidence.

Rehabilitation Aim and Orthotic Considerations

When devising a plan of care for patients with ITW, the age, underlying cause, patient and parental concerns, amount of time spent toe walking, and the severity of any tendon contractures present should all be considered. Some common treatments for mild to moderate ITW include ankle casting or serial casting, night splints, AFOs, PT, and lower leg botulinum toxin type A injections. Severe cases are sometimes treated with denervation or surgical lengthening procedures of the heel cord or Achilles tendon. A combination of these interventions is recommended based upon clinical presentation and assessment [75, 76, 80]. However, a consensus about optimal medical management and best practice has not yet been established.

When the decision is made to treat conservatively, physical therapy should be an integral part of treatment for ITW. PT should focus on functional goals and include: a thorough evaluation, therapeutic activities, stretching, strengthening, sensory input, and recommendations for bracing [77]. Any pain or functional limitations should also be a major focus of treatment efforts. The PT should work closely with the orthotist and medical team to establish the most appropriate bracing and course of treatment. For severe cases that do not respond favorably to conservative management, surgery for Achilles tendon or heel cord lengthening is a corrective option [75, 76]. However, surgical intervention is not without risk and procedures are costly.

SUMMARY

This chapter provided a brief overview of selected pathologies that may result in multidisciplinary management including orthotic services. As the body of medical knowledge increases and rehabilitation advances, it is more evident than ever that the best practices in healthcare require providers to work closely together to optimize patient outcomes. Healthcare teams must adapt to changing organizational values and provide new and updated modes of service delivery that have become increasingly more reliant upon interdisciplinary care [63]. Nurses, physical therapists, physicians, prosthetists, orthotists, and other healthcare providers should communicate openly and work synchronously with one unified objective to provide the best medical, rehabilitation, orthotic, and prosthetic care possible. The overarching theme with many conditions requiring rehabilitation and orthotic care is to pursue the most conservative therapeutic measures first, before progressing to more aggressive interventions—as these typically carry greater risk of harm to the patient. A conservative-minded, unified team of caring providers, working in a patient-centered approach, can positively affect the lives of many patients and their families [64].

REFERENCES

[1] American Stroke Association. About Stroke | American Stroke Association. Accessed July 30, 2024. https://www.stroke.org/en/about-stroke.

[2] Mozaffarian D, Benjamin EJ, Go AS, et al. Heart disease and stroke statistics—2015 update: a report from the American Heart Association. *Circulation*. 2015;e29–e322.

[3] Langhorne P, Stott DJ, Robertson L, et al. Medical complications after stroke: a multicenter study. *Stroke.* 2000;31:1223–1229.

[4] Koton S, Schneider A, Rosamond W, et al. Stroke incidence and mortality trends in US communities, 1987 to 2011. *JAMA.* 2014;312(3):259–268.

[5] Accardo PJ, ed. *Caputo and Accardo's Neurodevelopmental Disabilities in Infancy and Childhood,* 2008. 3rd edition, p. 17. Paul H. Brookes Publishing, Baltimore, MD.

[6] Winstein CJ, Stein J, Arena R, et al; on behalf of the American Heart Association Stroke Council, Council on Cardiovascular and Stroke Nursing, Council on Clinical Cardiology, and Council on Quality of Care and Outcomes Research. Guidelines for adult stroke rehabilitation and recovery: a guideline for healthcare professionals from the American Heart Association/American Stroke Association. *Stroke.* 2016;47:6; e98–e169–72.

[7] Bruno RL. Paralytic vs. "non-paralytic" polio: distinction without a difference? *Am J Phys Med Rehabil.* 2000;79:4–12.

[8] March of Dimes. Post-polio syndrome: identifying best practices in diagnosis and care, 2001. March of Dimes Birth Defects Foundation, White Plains, NY.

[9] Weichers DO, Hubbell SI. Late changes in the motor unit after acute poliomyelitis. *Muscle Nerve.* 1981;4:524–528.

[10] Halstead LS, Gawne AC, Pham BT. National rehabilitation hospital limb classification for exercise, research, and clinical trials in post-polio patients. *Ann NY Acad Sci.* 1995;753:343–353.

[11] National Spinal Cord Injury Statistical Center. Spinal cord injury facts and figures at a glance. *J Spinal Cord Med.* 2014 May;37(3):355–356.

[12] Delaney K, Fairfull A. SCI traumatic part one: disease/disorder and essentials of assessment. December 1, 2011; updated November 1, 2023. In: *Rehabilitation of Central Nervous System Disorders.* PM&R Knowledge now. American Academy of Physical Medicine & Rehabilitation. Accessed July 30, 2024. https://now.aapmr.org/sci-traumatic-part-1-diseasedisorder-essentials-of-assessment/.

[13] American Spinal Injury Association. *International Standards for Neurological and Functional Classification of Spinal Cord Injury—Revised 2011.* ASIA, Atlanta, GA.

[14] Marino RJ, Burns S, Graves DE. Upper- and lower-extremity motor recovery after traumatic cervical spinal cord injury: an update from the National Spinal Cord Injury Database. *Arch Phys Med Rehabil.* 2011;92:368–375.

[15] Christopher & Dana Reeve Foundation. Functional electrical stimulation. Accessed August 1, 2024. https://www.christopherreeve.org/todays-care/living-with-paralysis/rehabilitation/functional-electrical-stimulation/.

[16] He Y, Xu Y, Hai M, et al. Exoskeleton-assisted rehabilitation and neuroplasticity in spinal cord injury. *World Neurosurg.* 2024;185:45–54.

[17] Mekki M, Delgado AD, Fry A, et al. Robotic rehabilitation and spinal cord injury: a narrative review. *Neurotherapeutics.* 2018;15(3):604–617.

[18] Matney C, Bowman, K, Berwick D, eds. *Traumatic Brain Injury: A Roadmap for Accelerating Progress,* February 1, 2022. National Academies of Sciences, Engineering, and Medicine; Health and Medicine Division; Board on Health Care Services; Board on Health Sciences Policy; Committee on Accelerating Progress in Traumatic Brain Injury Research and Care; National Academies Press (US), Washington, D.C.

[19] *VA/DoD Clinical Practice Guideline for the Management of Concussion/Mild Traumatic Brain Injury,* V2.0, 2016. Department of Veterans Affairs, Department of Defense. Accessed August 5, 2024. https://www.healthquality.va.gov/guidelines/rehab/mtbi/mtbicpgfullcpg50821816.pdf.

[20] Faul M, Xu L, Wald MM, Coronado VG. *Traumatic Brain Injury in the United States: Emergency Department Visits, Hospitalizations and Deaths 2002, 2006, 2010.* Centers for Disease Control and Prevention, National Center for Injury Prevention and Control, Atlanta, GA.

[21] Champion HR, Holcomb JB, Young LA. Injuries from explosions. *J Trauma.* 2009;66:1468–1476.

[22] Coronado VG, Xu L, Basavaraju SV, et al. Surveillance for brain injury related deaths—United States 1997–2007. *CDC Morbidity & Mortality Weekly Report. Surveillance Summaries.* 2011 May 6;60(SS05):1–32. Accessed August 5, 2024. https://www.cdc.gov/mmwr/preview/mmwrhtml/ss6005a1.htm.

[23] Wright, J. *The Functional Assessment Measure,* 2000. The Center for Outcome Measurement in Brain Injury. Accessed August 5, 2024. https://www.tbims.org/combi/FAM/.

[24] U.S. Bone and Joint Initiative. *The Burden of Musculoskeletal Diseases in the United States.* 4th edition. Accessed August 5, 2024. https://www.boneandjointburden.org/print/book/export/html/965.

[25] Thomas E, Peat G, Harris L, et al. The prevalence of pain and pain interference in a general population of older adults: cross-sectional findings from the North Staffordshire Osteoarthritis Project (NorStOP). *Pain.* 2004;110:361–368.

[26] Woolf AD, Pfleger B. Burden of major musculoskeletal conditions. *Bull World Health Organ.* 2003;81:646–656.

[27] McCormick A, Fleming D, Charlton J. *Morbidity Statistics from General Practice: Fourth National Study 1991–1992,* 1995. HMSO, London.

[28] Palmer K, Goodson N. Ageing, musculoskeletal health and work. *Best Pract Res Clin Rheumatol.* 2015;29(3):391–404.

[29] Palmer KT. Occupational activities and osteoarthritis of the knee. *Brit Med Bull.* 2012;102:147–170.

[30] Patel RA, Wilson RF, Patel PA, Palmer RM. The effect of smoking on bone healing: a systematic review. *Bone Joint Res.* 2013;2(6):102–111.

[31] Washington State Department of Labor and Industries. Work-related carpal tunnel syndrome diagnosis and treatment guideline 2017. Washington State Department of Labor and Industries, Olympia, WA. Accessed August 5, 2024. https://www.lni.wa.gov/patient-care/treating-patients/treatment-guidelines-and-resources/_docs/CTSGuideline2017.pdf.

[32] Polytrauma System of Care. VHA Directive 1172.01. April 18, 2024. U.S. Department of Veterans Affairs. Veterans Health Administration, Washington, D.C.

[33] Sayer SA, Chiros CE, Sigford B, et al. Characteristics and rehabilitation outcomes among patients with blast and other injuries sustained during the Global War on Terror. *Arch Phys Med Rehabil.* 2008;89:163–170.

[34] DiMaggio CJ, Avraham JB, Lee DC, et al. The epidemiology of emergency department trauma discharges in the United States. *Acad Emerg Med.* 2017 Oct;24(10):1244–1256.

[35] Keel M, Trentz O. Pathophysiology of polytrauma. *Injury.* 2005;36:691–709.

[36] Highsmith MJ, Nelson LM, Carbone NT, et al. Outcomes associated with the Intrepid Dynamic Exoskeletal Orthosis (IDEO): a systematic review of the literature. *Mil Med.* 2016 Nov;181(S4):69–76.

[37] American Diabetes Association. Statistics about diabetes. Accessed August 5, 2024. https://diabetes.org/about-diabetes/statistics/about-diabetes.

[38] Boyko EJ, Monteiro-Soares M, Wheeler SGB. Peripheral arterial disease, foot ulcers, lower extremity amputations, and diabetes. In: Cowie CC, Casagrande SS, Menke A, et al., eds. *Diabetes in America,* 2018. 3rd edition. National Institute of Diabetes and Digestive and Kidney Diseases, Bethesda, MD.

[39] Reiber GE, Boyko EJ, Smith DG. Lower extremity foot ulcers and amputations in diabetes. In: Harris M, Cowie CC, Stearn

MP, eds. *Diabetes in America*, 1995. 2nd edition, pp. 409–428. National Diabetes Data Group of the National Institute of Diabetes and Digestive and Kidney Diseases, National Institutes of Health, Bethesda, MD.

[40] Castelli G, Desai KM, Cantone RE. Peripheral neuropathy: evaluation and differential diagnosis. *Am Fam Physician*. 2020; 102(12):732–739.

[41] Singer MA, Vernino SA, Wolfe GI. Idiopathic neuropathy: new paradigms, new promise. *J Peripher Nerv Syst*. 2012 May;Supp 2:43–49.

[42] Richardson JK, Hurvitz EA. Peripheral neuropathy: a risk factor for falls. *J Gerontol*. 1995;50(4):211–215.

[43] Bril V, England JD, Franklin GM, et al. Evidence-based guideline: treatment of painful diabetic neuropathy—report of the American Association of Neuromuscular and Electrodiagnostic Medicine, The American Academy of Physical Medicine & Rehabilitation. *Muscle Nerve*. 2011;43:910–917.

[44] Lam L, Copeland R, Yan G, Husu EN. Inflammatory arthritides. PM&R Knowledge Now. Medical Rehabilitation. Originally published November 10, 2011. Updated May 18, 2023. Accessed August 6, 2024. https://now.aapmr.org/inflammatory-arthritides/.

[45] Hsu H, Siwiec, RM. Knee osteoarthritis. *StatPearls*. Updated June 26, 2023. https://www.statpearls.com/point-of-care/41509.

[46] Osteoarthritis Action Alliance. OA prevalence and burden. Accessed August 6, 2024. https://oaaction.unc.edu/oa-module/oa-prevalence-and-burden/.

[47] American College of Rheumatology. Diseases and conditions. Lupus, spondyloarthritis, psoriatic arthritis. Accessed August 6, 2024. https://rheumatology.org/patients/diseases-and-conditions.

[48] Ringold S, Singer NG. Measures of disease activity in rheumatoid arthritis: a clinician's guide. *Curt Rheumatol Rev*. 2008;4:259–265, 259.

[49] Escalante A, Haas RW, Rincon I, et al. Measurement of global functional performance in patients with rheumatoid arthritis using rheumatology function tests. *Arthritis Res Ther*. 2004;6(4):R315–R325.

[50] Cosman F, de Beur SJ, LeBoff MS, et al. Clinician's guide to prevention and treatment of osteoporosis. *Osteoporos Int*. 2014;25(10):2359–2381.

[51] World Health Organization. *Prevention and Management of Osteoporosis*. Report of a WHO Scientific Group. WHO Technical Report Series. Accessed August 6, 2024. https://iris.who.int/bitstream/handle/10665/42841/WHO_TRS_921.pdf.

[52] International Osteoporosis Foundation. Osteoporosis—about. Accessed August 6, 2024. https://www.osteoporosis.foundation/health-professionals/about-osteoporosis.

[53] Abrahamsen B, van Staa T, Ariely R, et al. Excess mortality following hip fracture: a systematic epidemiological review. *Osteoporos Int*. 2009 Oct;20(10):1633–1650.

[54] Diaz-Curiel M. Effects of exercise on osteoporosis. *J Osteopor Phys Act*. 2013;1(1). Available online at https://www.longdom.org/open-access-pdfs/effects-of-exercise-on-osteoporosis-2329-9509.1000e104.pdf.

[55] Christensen D, Van Naarden Braun K, Doernberg N. Prevalence of cerebral palsy, co-occurring autism spectrum disorders, and motor functioning—Autism and Developmental Disabilities Monitoring Network, U.S.A., 2008. *Dev Med Child Neurol*. 2014 Jan;56(1):59–65.

[56] Centers for Disease Control and Prevention (CDC). Economic costs associated with mental retardation, cerebral palsy, hearing loss, and vision impairment—United States, 2003. *MMWR Morb Mortal Wkly Rep*. 2004 Jan 30;53(3):57–59.

[57] Anttila H, Autti-Rämö I, Suoranta J, et al. Effectiveness of physical therapy interventions for children with cerebral palsy: a systematic review. *BMC Pediatr*. 2008;24(8):14.

[58] Novacheck TF, Kroll G, Rasmussen A. Orthoses for cerebral palsy. In: Webster JB, Murphy DP, eds. *Atlas of Orthoses and Assistive Devices*, 2019. 5th edition, pp. 337–349. Elsevier, Philadelphia, PA.

[59] Begnoche DM, Chiarello LA, Palisano RJ, et al. Predictors of independent walking in young children with cerebral palsy. *Phys Ther*. 2016;96(2):183–192.

[60] NINDS. Muscular dystrophy. National Institute of Neurological Disorders and Stroke. Accessed August 6, 2024. https://www.ninds.nih.gov/health-information/disorders/muscular-dystrophy.

[61] Liew WKM, Kang PB. Recent developments in the treatment of Duchenne muscular dystrophy and spinal muscular atrophy. *Ther Adv Neurol Disord*. 2013;6(3):147–160.

[62] Landfeldt E, Lindgren P, Bell CF, et al. The burden of Duchenne muscular dystrophy: an international, cross-sectional study. *Neurology*. 2014;83(6):529–536.

[63] Bushby K, Finkel R, Birnkrant DJ, et al. Diagnosis and management of Duchenne muscular dystrophy, part 1: diagnosis, and pharmacological and psychosocial management. *Lancet Neurol*. 2010;9(1):77–93.

[64] Birnkrant DJ, Bushby K, Bann CM, et al. Diagnosis and management of Duchenne muscular dystrophy, part 2: respiratory, cardiac, bone health, and orthopaedic management. *Lancet Neurol*. 2018;17(4):347–361.

[65] Stevens PM. Lower limb orthotic management of Duchenne muscular dystrophy: a literature review. *J Prosthet Orthot*, 2006;18(4):111–119.

[66] Lunsford CL, Abel MF, King KM. Orthoses for myelomeningocele. In: Webster JB, Murphy DP, eds. *Atlas of Orthoses and Assistive Devices*, 2019. 5th edition, pp. 350–359. Elsevier, Philadelphia, PA.

[67] CDC. About spina bifida. Centers for Disease Control. Accessed August 6, 2024. https://www.cdc.gov/spina-bifida/about/index.html.

[68] Grosse SD, Berry RJ, Tilford JM, et al. retrospective assessment of cost savings from prevention. folic acid fortification and spina bifida in the US. *Am J Prev Med*. 2016 May;50(5 Suppl 1):S74–S80. Published online January 11, 2016.

[69] Spina Bifida Association. 2021 State fact sheets. Accessed August 6, 2024. https://www.spinabifidaassociation.org/wp-content/uploads/2021State-Fact-Sheet-with-Jump-Links-2-1.pdf.

[70] Eubanks JD, Cheruvu V. Prevalence of sacral spina bifida occulta and its relationship to age, sex, race, and the sacral table angle: an anatomic, osteologic study of three thousand one hundred specimens. *Spine*. 2009;34(15):1539–1543.

[71] Roach JW, Short BF, Saltzman HM. Adult consequences of spina bifida: a cohort study. *Clin Orthop Relat Res*. 2011 May;469(5):1246–1252.

[72] Steinhart S, Kornitzer E, Baron AB, et al. Independence in self-care activities in children with myelomeningocele: exploring factors based on the International Classification of Function model. *Disabil Rehabil*. 2018 Jan;40(1):62–68. Published online November 10, 2016.

[73] Polliack A, Elliot S, Landsberger S, et al. Lower extremity orthoses for children with myelomeningocele: user and orthotist perspectives. *J Prosthet Orthot*. 2001;13(4):123–129.

[74] Engelbert R, Willem J, Uiterwaal C, et al. Idiopathic toe-walking in children, adolescents and young adults: a matter of local or generalised stiffness? *BMC Musculoskelet Disord*. 2011;12:61.

[75] Edinger J, Sinha A, Fisher M. Congenital and acquired disorders. In: Webster JB, Murphy DP, eds. *Atlas of Orthoses and Assistive Devices*, 2019. 5th edition, pp. 303–312. Elsevier, Philadelphia, PA.

[76] Ruzbarsky JJ, Scher D, Dodwell E. Toe walking: causes, epidemiology, assessment, and treatment. *Curr Opin Pediatr*. 2016;28(1):40–46.

[77] Hoppestad B. Toe walking in children: a benign phase of youth, or harmful condition requiring treatment? *Advance Healthcare Network for Physical Therapy and Rehab Medicine.* 2013;24(22):16–28.

[78] Newman CJ, Ziegler AL, Jeannet PY, et al. Transient dystonic toe-walking: differentiation from cerebral palsy and a rare explanation for some unexplained cases of idiopathic toe-walking. *Dev Med Child Neurol.* 2006;48(2):96–102.

[79] Williams CM, Tinley P, Curtin M. Idiopathic toe walking and sensory processing dysfunction. *J Foot Ankle Res.* 2010;3:16.

[80] Zimbler S. Idiopathic toe walking: current evaluation and management. *OJHMS.* 2007;9:98–100. 2007. Accessed August 7, 2024. https://www.orthojournalhms.org/volume9/manuscripts/ms10.pdf.

[81] Dietz F, Khunsree S. Idiopathic toe walking: to treat or not to treat, that is the question. *Iowa Orthop J.* 2012;32:184–188.

CHAPTER 13

Lower Limb Orthotic Management
Orthoses Below the Knee

Jill Seale and Phil M. Stevens

OBJECTIVES

Upon completion of this chapter, the reader will be able to:

1. Define basic orthotic classification and nomenclature for lower limb orthoses.
2. Identify the general activity and participation level limitations which warrant lower limb orthotic intervention.
3. Identify the interdisciplinary team involved in lower limb orthoses.
4. Define the biomechanical components of each lower limb orthoses by segment.
5. Identify the biomechanical goals/intended outcomes of the most commonly prescribed lower limb orthoses.
6. Describe the appropriate pre- and post-orthotic examination and evaluation by the physical therapist.
7. Identify, by segment, the biomechanical pathology which indicates orthotic management.
8. Synthesize biomechanical pathology with the appropriate biomechanical components in the orthotic intervention.
9. Identify current best practice recommendations related to lower limb orthoses.
10. Demonstrate the appropriate prescription process for lower limb orthoses.
11. Formulate strategy for assessing effectiveness of lower limb orthoses.
12. Develop the appropriate post-orthotic plan of care.

INTRODUCTION

Physical therapists have a large role in the management of lower limb dysfunction: examination and evaluation, diagnosis of movement dysfunction, and recommending appropriate intervention. Appropriate intervention may include orthotic management. Orthotic management should be a collaborative effort among the patient and the healthcare team. Evidence indicates that effective orthotic management can contribute to improved patient outcomes

DOI: 10.4324/9781003526025-15

from impairment to patient participation. But what makes up effective lower limb orthotic management? In this chapter the stated objectives will provide the necessary background, evidence, and tools for effective lower limb orthotic management.

The lower limb orthosis is defined as an "externally applied device used to modify the structural and functional characteristics of the neuromuscular and skeletal systems" of the lower limb, which includes the foot, lower leg, thigh, and pelvic girdle [1]. Lower extremity orthoses can range from shoes to orthotic devices which encompass the trunk, pelvis, and entire lower limb. Orthoses are commonly named by the joints they encompass and the type of motion control they provide. Foot orthoses (FOs) are applied to the foot and generally placed inside the shoe. Ankle foot orthoses (AFOs) are applied to the foot and ankle, terminating distal to the knee. They can be applied to the shoe or, more commonly, worn inside the shoe. While there are additional lower limb orthoses that extend proximal to the knee, this chapter presents the most frequently prescribed lower limb orthoses that terminate distal to the knee.

Lower limb orthoses can serve many functions and address several goals in persons with musculoskeletal and neuromuscular dysfunctions. General goals include prevention of deformity, provision of stability, and facilitation of function. Although improved gait activity seems an obvious goal of lower limb orthotic interventions, they may also be utilized to improve transfers, facilitate safe therapeutic standing activities, improve static alignment in sitting and supine, and prevent and/or manage spasticity and contractures.

social worker/case management. A primary care provider oversees the overall health and well-being of the patient and is well positioned to determine how the patient's broader health may be influenced by an orthotic intervention. Notably, their signature is required for orthotic prescription. The PT is responsible for the examination and evaluation that leads to the diagnosis of a movement dysfunction that would be appropriate for orthotic intervention and should contribute to the development of an orthotic recommendation based on these findings. This process should ideally happen in collaboration with the orthotist. The orthotist stays abreast of developing advancements in materials and components and works with the physician and PT to design, fabricate, and fit a device that will meet the desired functional objectives.

Among the ancillary team members, an OT can provide valuable collaboration in training the donning/doffing of the lower limb orthotic device, as well as incorporation of the device into activities of daily living. Particularly in inpatient or assisted living scenarios, nurses and nursing assistants may support this process by ensuring the patient's utilization of the device at appropriate times and monitoring for adverse events such as skin breakdown. In certain scenarios, social work and/or case management can facilitate evaluation of caregiver support and provide the critical link to the patient's payor source.

It is worth noting that the only members of the healthcare team required by regulations to contribute to the orthotic prescription are the primary care provider and the orthotist. However, interdisciplinary collaboration can help ensure maximal success of the lower limb orthotic intervention.

THE INTERDISCIPLINARY TEAM IN ORTHOTIC MANAGEMENT

A collaborative team approach is essential to effective lower limb orthotic management. Before discussing the healthcare professionals who comprise this team, it is imperative to understand that the patient and the patient's caregiver(s) are the central component of this team. Importantly, Evidence Based Practice is an integration of three central tenets: scientific evidence, clinical expertise, and patient/caregiver values and perspectives [2]. Therefore, while evidentiary support and clinical expertise may indicate the appropriateness of an orthotic prescription, without the patient and caregiver's acceptance, support, and commitment, the ultimate success of any orthotic intervention will likely be undermined.

Other core members of the interdisciplinary team generally include the primary care provider (physician, physician assistant, nurse practitioner), orthotist, and physical therapist (PT). Ancillary members to this team may include an occupational therapist (OT), nurse, and

REVIEW OF LOWER LIMB BIOMECHANICS

While an in-depth review of lower extremity kinetics and kinematics during quiet standing and gait is beyond the scope of this text, a general overview is warranted. Passive stability during quiet standing is obtained through maintenance of the body's ground reaction force relative to major joints of the lower extremity. When this force passes just posterior to the hip joint and anterior to the knee joint, the ligamentous tension on the flexor side of these joints stabilizes the lower extremity against gravity without muscular contraction (Figure 13.1).

Deviation from this strategy of passive stability is observed at the ankle joint where considerable joint mobility occurs into both plantarflexion and dorsiflexion away from a neutral alignment. As such, adequate ligamentous tension is not normally observed in standing at this joint. Rather, the ground reaction force normally passes through the center of the longitudinal length of the foot, approximately 5 cm anterior to the ankle joint. Given this requiring lower limb orthoses may present with contracture or weakness of the muscles of the lower extremities that compromise basic standing stability. Lower limb orthoses may be used to correct or accommodate these aberrant alignments.

With regard to ambulation, gait analysis is customarily broken down into the familiar phases of initial contact, loading response, mid stance, terminal stance, pre-swing, initial swing, mid swing, and terminal swing [3]. The derivation of the most appropriate lower extremity orthosis design requires a working knowledge of the lower extremity kinetics and kinematics associated with each major joint segment throughout these various phases. Observational gait analysis should be used to identify all gait deviations and the specific phases in which those deviations occur. This will be described in further detail later in this chapter.

The sagittal movements of the ankle can be reduced to four distinct sub-phases (Figure 13.2) [4]. Controlled plantarflexion occurs through the first half of loading response as eccentric activity of the dorsiflexors controls the rate of ankle plantarflexion from neutral to about 8° of plantarflexion. This is followed by a protracted period of controlled dorsiflexion that begins in the middle of loading response and persists through mid and terminal stance. During this sub-phase, the plantarflexors regulate the progressive dorsiflexion of the ankle from 8° of plantarflexion to roughly 10° of dorsiflexion. At the conclusion of terminal stance, the ankle begins a phase of powered plantarflexion that reasonably approximates the pre-swing phase of gait. During this period, a propulsive power burst from the plantarflexors moves the ankle through roughly 30° from 10° of dorsiflexion to 20° of plantarflexion. After this propulsive event, the ankle enters a period of swing dorsiflexion in which active concentric dorsiflexion brings the ankle from 20° of plantarflexion into a neutral alignment to assist with swing phase clearance and prepare for

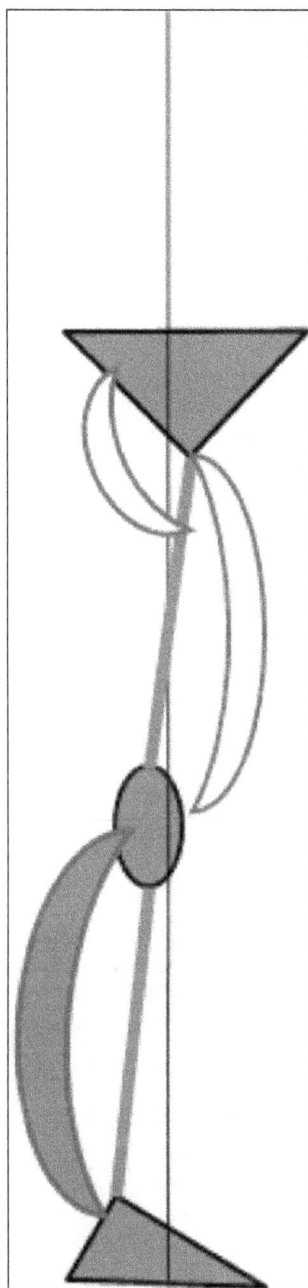

Figure 13.1. Passive stability at the hip and knee with active stabilization from active plantarflexors.

alignment, modest activity of the plantarflexors is generally required to maintain standing stability.

Two predominant strategies are used to maintain the desired relationship between the ground reaction force and the joints of the lower extremity. Within the top-down "hip strategy," sagittal movements across the hip joint position the collective mass of the head, arms, and trunk in the desired orientation relative to the lower extremities. Within the bottom-up "ankle strategy," controlled movements across the ankle joints manipulate the distal location of the ground reaction force as well its sagittal relationship to the hip and knee.

These stabilizing principles and strategies are relevant within this chapter as many of those individuals

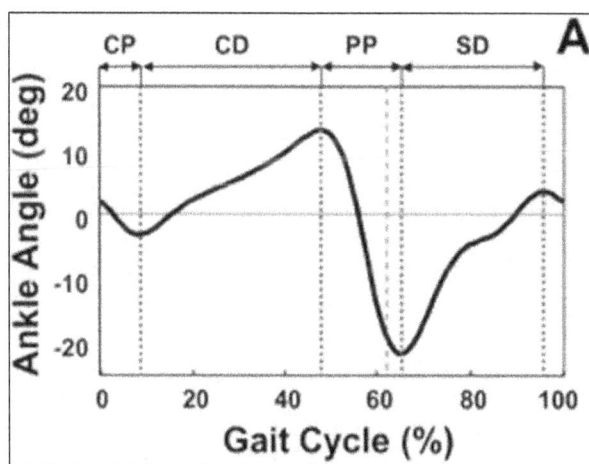

Figure 13.2. Four sub-phases of sagittal movements/motion observed at the ankle where controlled plantarflexion (CP), controlled dorsiflexion (CD), powered plantarflexion (PP), and swing phase dorsiflesion (SD) [3].

the next controlled plantarflexion event that will occur with the next step.

As with static balance, compromise to the strength, motor control, and mobility of the muscles and/or soft tissues of the ankle joint, commonly observed in patients referred for lower limb orthoses, will often undermine one or more of the sub-phases identified for the ankle above.

Lower Limb Orthoses

In general, lower limb orthoses are used to permit, assist, resist, or block movement around the joints of the lower limb. These functions can be used to facilitate real time biomechanical benefits during standing and ambulation. Additionally, sustained usage can discourage the development of progressive joint contracture or, in the opposite extreme, hypermobility. In addition to their immediate and sustained effects on joint mobility, lower limb orthoses can be used to correct flexible aberrant limb alignments, accommodate rigid aberrant limb alignments, and reduce limb pain.

Many lower limb orthoses can be provided as both off-the-shelf non-custom versions or as custom devices uniquely molded to the individual's lower limb anatomy. In general, off-the-shelf options are intended for short term applications (less than 6 months) when corrective forces are needed only in a single anatomic plane (typically sagittal plane deviations). Applications where long-term use is anticipated, where deviations are occurring in two or more anatomic planes or when there are bony or soft-tissue contractures or deformities, are often best managed with custom devices. Increasingly, documentation to support the need for a custom device has become the responsibility of all treating team members.

Foot Orthoses

Foot orthoses (FOs) can be broadly classified as accommodative or functional. The most common application of the former is to protect the dysvascular foot with rigid deformities from the development of pressure ulcers and subsequent infection. In this application, the FO is intended to accommodate and cushion these noncorrectable deformities. As such, softer materials are preferred and regular replacement is necessary.

With functional (also described as biomechanical) FOs, corrective forces are applied through the plantar surface of the foot to optimize the alignment of the subtalar joint, often in the presence of bony malalignments of the hindfoot and/or forefoot. As these patients are generally otherwise healthy with protective sensation, rigid, more durable materials are generally preferred.

Functional FOs can facilitate improved subtalar alignment through accommodative or corrective support. For example, in the presence of an untreated rigid hindfoot

varus deformity, the subtalar joint will pronate rapidly in early stance to bring the medial aspect of the calcaneus in contact with the floor. These destructive forces can be mitigated through a functional FO with an accommodative medial hindfoot post (medial wedge) that preloads the medial aspect of the calcaneus and precludes the need for excessive subtalar pronation (Figure 13.3).

In an alternate example of an untreated, flexible first ray deformity, the flexibility of the medial column of the forefoot is unable to resist weight-bearing forces during terminal stance. The resultant forefoot varus creates a destructive subtalar pronation in late stance and compromises the body's toe lever in late stance. By preloading the medial column of the foot with a corrective medial forefoot post (medial wedge), the need for accommodative subtalar pronation is mitigated and the body's late stance toe lever is preserved (Figure 13.4).

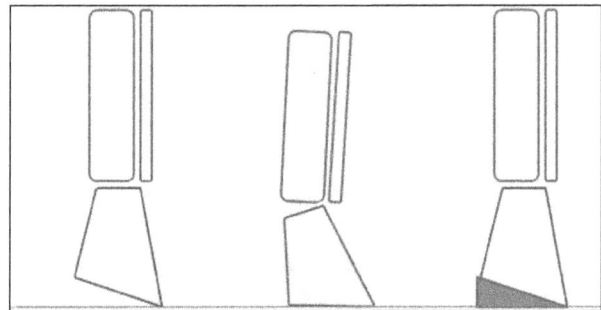

Figure 13.3. Diagram of the posterior view of A. right hindfoot varus deformity; B. untreated with resultant hindfoot valgus alignment and pronation; and C. treated with an accommodative medial wedge to maintain appropriate alignment of the subtalar joint.

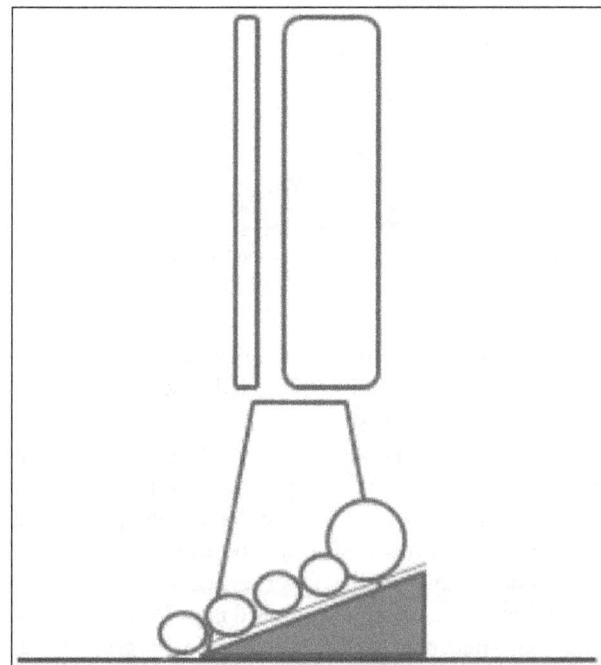

Figure 13.4. Depiction of a corrective medial forefoot wedge used to preload a flexible first ray deformity, preserving the alignment and architecture of the midfoot.

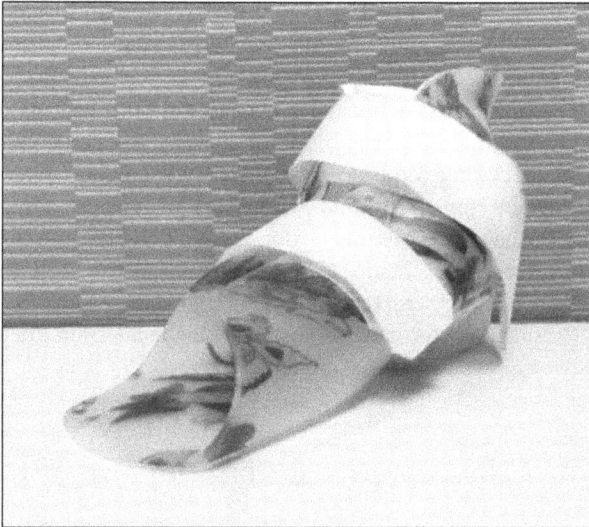

Figure 13.5. Supramalleolar orthosis (SMO).

Supramalleolar Orthosis

The supramalleolar orthosis (SMO) is a semi-rigid orthosis that wraps around the instep of the foot and ankle and extends proximally just beyond the vertical height of the malleoli (Figure 13.5). Its primary effect is to stabilize the coronal alignment of the foot and ankle. Common applications include presentations of mild to moderate valgus instability, commonly associated with a hypotonic pes plano valgus foot and mild varus instabilities associated with mild hypertonicity. Its efficacy is limited to coronal instabilities and the device is inadequate to control any substantial ankle deviations in the sagittal plane or affect knee joint biomechanics.

Solid AFO

The Solid AFO is a non-articulated orthosis that extends from the plantar surface of the foot to a proximal height often extending beyond the apex of the muscle belly of the calf and approximating the proximal head of the fibula (Figure 13.6). At the instep and along the longitudinal length of the orthosis the plastic extends anterior to the malleoli, thus restricting both plantarflexion and dorsiflexion at the ankle joint. Its primary effect is to effectively immobilize the ankle joint, with secondary effects on the biomechanics of the knee joint. Given the unyielding nature of this device, careful consideration must be given to the ankle angle with regard to available range of motion at the ankle and knee and the anticipated heel height of the shoe.

Considerable attention has been devoted to the resultant shank angle, produced by the combination of the AFO alignment ankle and the heel height of the shoe [5–8]. Wearing a shoe with a higher or lower heel height than was used during the planning, fabrication and fitting of the AFO can result in a suboptimal shank angle with associated deficits to balance and functional ambulation.

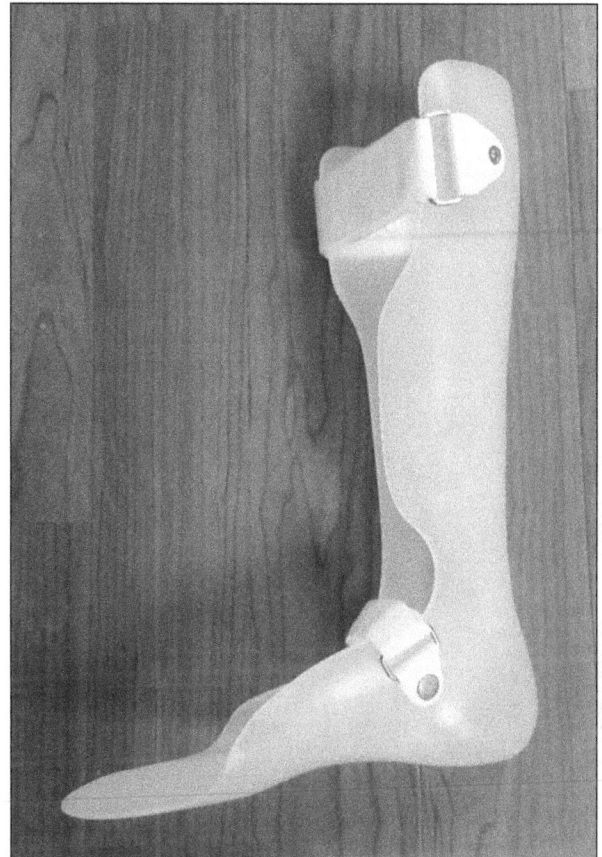

Figure 13.6. Solid ankle foot orthosis.

Posterior Leaf Spring AFO

When the trimlines of a plastic AFO are trimmed posterior to the malleoli the device is no longer able to immobilize the sagittal movements of the ankle. Such devices are referred to as posterior leaf spring (PLS) AFOs (Figure 13.7). The amount of mobility afforded by these devices is dependent upon the height, weight, and activity level of the patient in conjunction with such material considerations as the thickness of the plastic, the posterior radius of the plastic, and the posterior distance from the malleoli to the sagittal trimlines of the device [9].

The PLS is typically indicated for the management of flaccid swing phase deviations. That is, while their relative ankle stiffness may be adequate to support the weight of a flaccid foot during swing phase to assist with clearance, it is generally inadequate to affect stance phase kinematics at the ankle or knee.

Articulated AFOs

A range of orthotic ankle joints have been developed for use in AFOs. These joints can serve to allow unrestricted motion, to assist a desired motion, to resist an undesired motion, or to block motion within a desired range of motion. Thus, an articulated AFO often requires

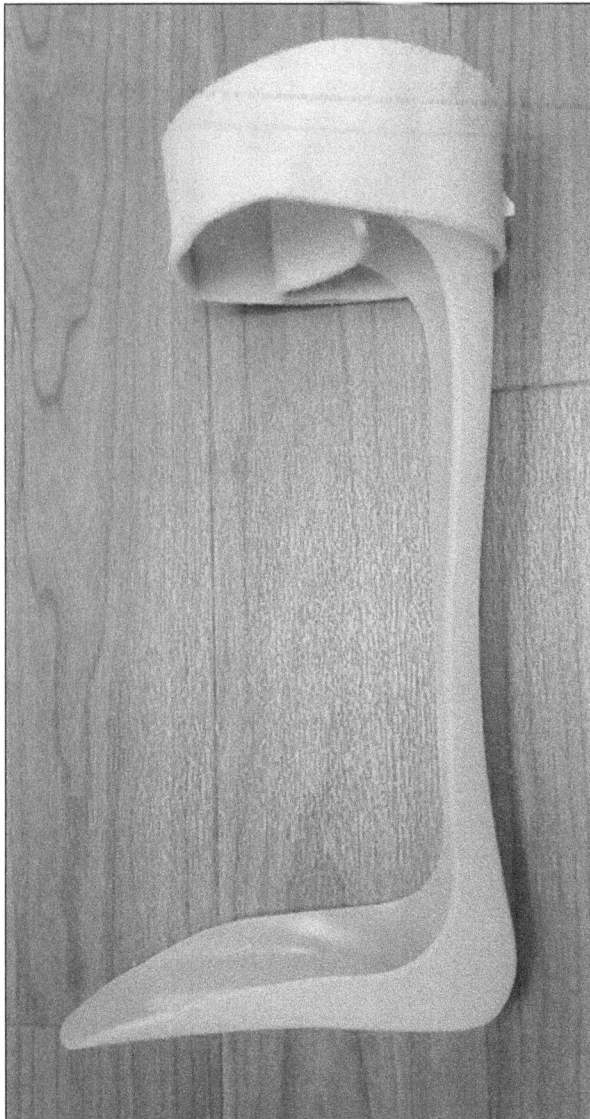

Figure 13.7. Posterior leaf spring (PLS) ankle foot orthosis.

additional narrative to describe fully its design and function. Qualifying terms such as "free motion," "dorsiflexion assist," and "plantarflexion stop" provide a clearer description of such devices (Figure 13.8).

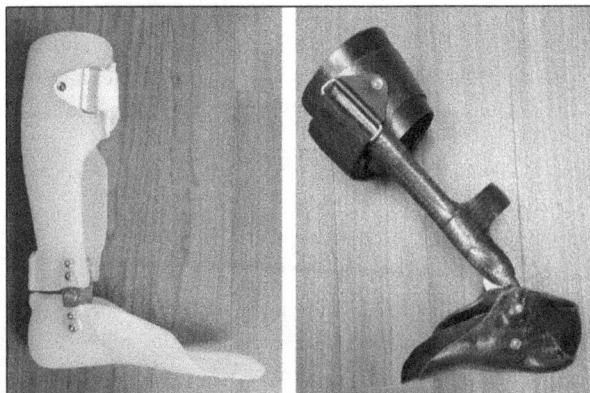

Figure 13.8. Articulated ankle foot orthoses. A. Posterior plantarflexion stop. B. Dorsiflexion assist ankle joints.

Articulated AFOs are indicated when the affected anatomic ankle joint presents with current or anticipated range of motion. When possible, the use of articulated AFOs can preserve normal kinematics at both the ankle and the knee. Importantly, joint stops at the ankle can also affect knee joint biomechanics. For example, a plantarflexion stop that limits plantarflexion during loading response will increase the flexion moment acting upon the knee during early stance (Figure 13.9). It can also serve to reduce knee hyperextension during mid stance. Similarly, a dorsiflexion stop may serve to reduce the aberrant knee flexion associated with a crouch gait.

Floor Reaction AFO

The terms "floor reaction" and "ground reaction" are synonyms that refer to the structural design of the AFO. While standard AFOs are comprised of a posterior shell over the lower limb, a floor reaction AFO features an anterior shell extending proximally to a height approximating the tibial tubercle (Figure 13.10). A floor reaction AFO can be further qualified as being solid or articulated. Importantly, the efficacy of the floor reaction design requires some mechanism of stopping or resisting ankle dorsiflexion. The anterior panel of these designs can be viewed as an extended lever arm of any dorsiflexion resistance provided by the AFO.

Floor reaction AFOs are indicated for cases where resistance to stance phase ankle dorsiflexion and/or knee

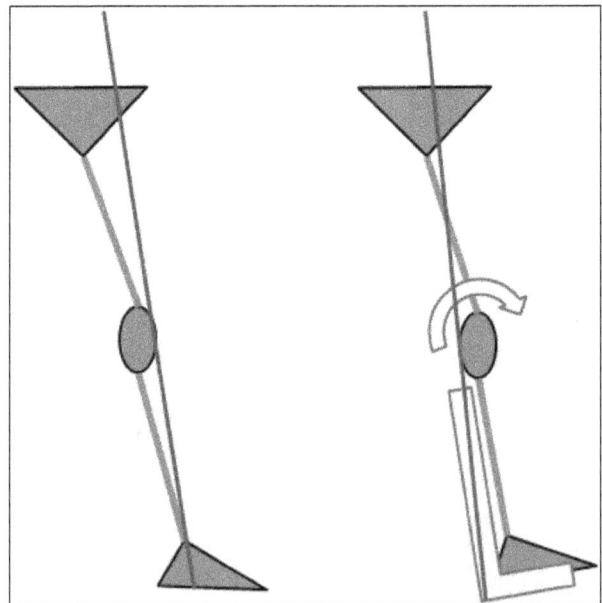

Figure 13.9. During loading response, A. plantarflexion allows anterior translation of the ground reaction force, reducing the external flexion moment acting upon the knee; B. the presence of a plantarflexion stop retains a posterior ground reaction force that now passes posterior to the knee joint and increases the external flexion moment acting upon this joint.

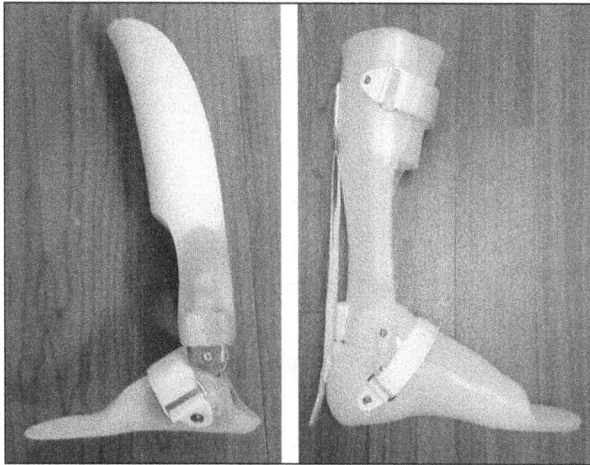

Figure 13.10. Ground reaction ankle foot orthoses. A. Anterior shell with a dorsiflexion stop ankle joint. B. Posterior shell with and anterior panel and posterior dorsiflexion restraint strap.

flexion is desired. The ankle angle of these devices must be carefully considered as excessive plantarflexion can create hyperextension forces at the knee.

Composite AFOs

Recent years have seen a tremendous increase in the use of carbon fiber and other composite materials in the fabrication and manufacture of both off-the-shelf and custom AFOs. In contrast to the more frequently encountered thermoformable plastics used in AFO fabrication, carbon fiber allows increased material stiffness, often at a reduced weight of the device. All of the AFO types described to this point can be constructed out of carbon fiber.

In one application, composite materials allow for comparable material stiffness with reduced size and tissue coverage relative to the thermoplastic equivalent (Figure 13.11). These principles are observed in a number of off-the-shelf composite AFOs that are often preferred by patients because of their reduced size, bulk, and weight.

In a separate application, carbon fiber struts can be used to store and release energy during ambulation. AFO designs like the Otto Bock Carbon Ankle Seven and the IDEO AFO are two examples where carbon fiber is used to store energy through stance phase and release it in late stance to mimic the push-off observed in normal locomotion (Figure 13.12).

Leather Ankle Gauntlet

Another frequently encountered AFO variant is the leather ankle gauntlet (Figure 13.13). The intimate fit of the compliant leather provides aggressive stabilization of the subtalar joint. This device is commonly applied in cases of

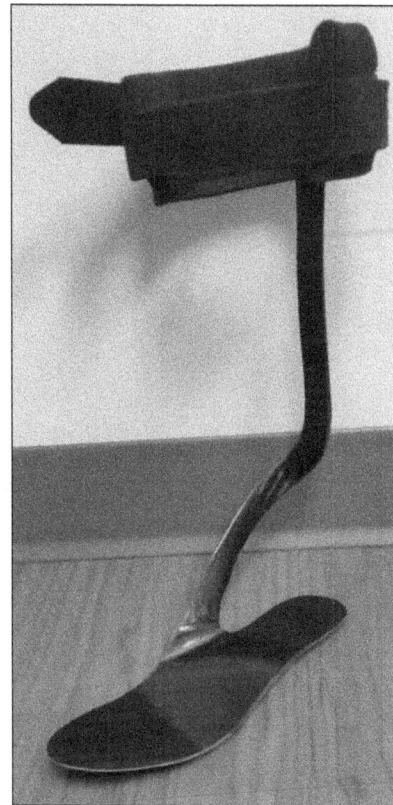

Figure 13.11. Lightweight carbon fiber ankle foot orthosis.

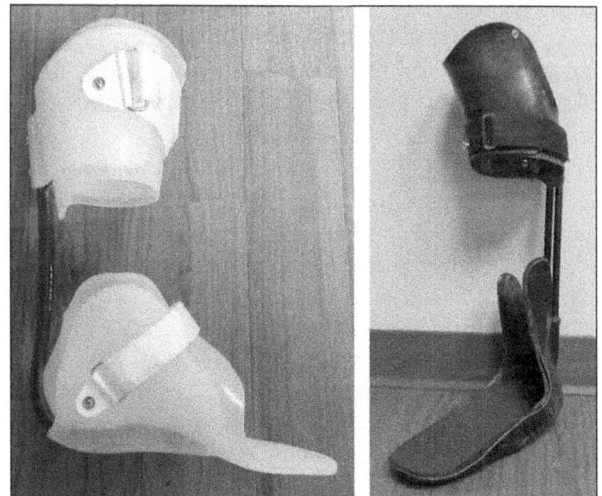

Figure 13.12. AFOs with composite struts designed to store energy during deflection and release that energy during dynamic activity.

ankle osteoarthritis and posterior tibial tendon dysfunction where mid and hindfoot stabilization are needed.

Functional Electrical Stimulation

Recent years have seen the introduction of single channel functional electrical stimulation (FES) systems

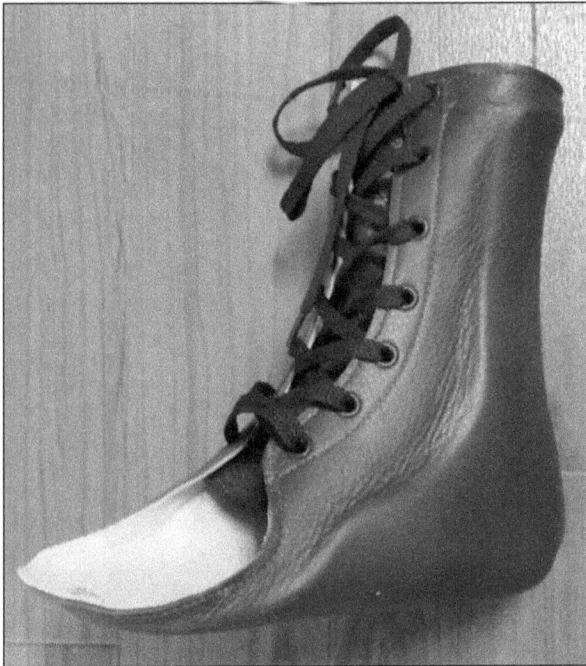

Figure 13.13. Leather ankle gauntlet.

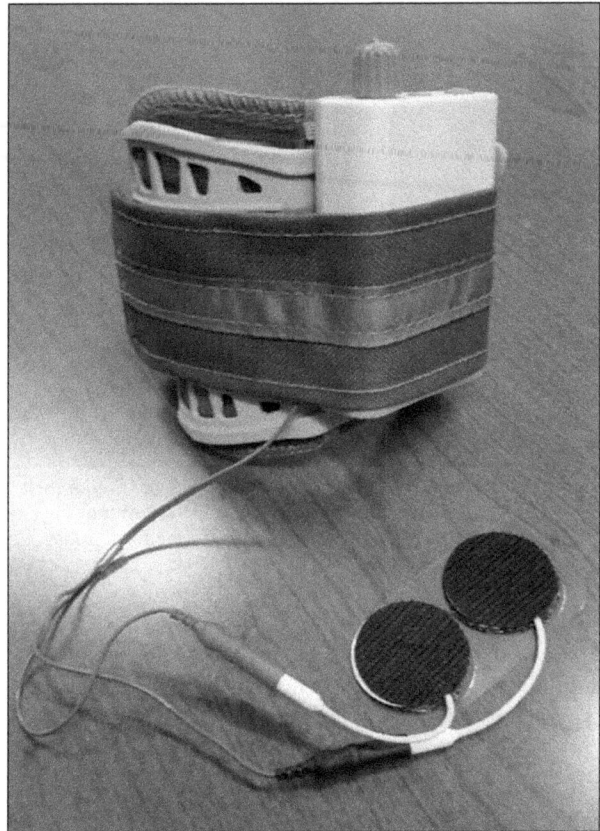

Figure 13.14. One example of a functional electrical stimulation unit.

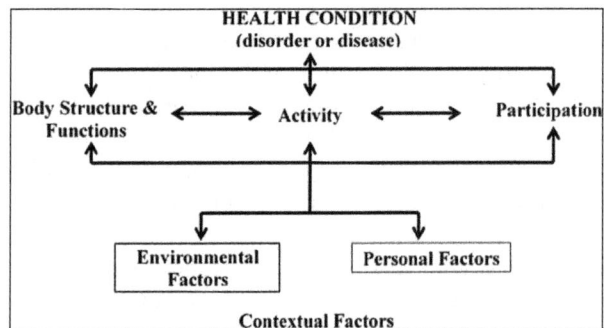

Figure 13.15. The ICF model facilitates consideration of the health condition in terms of its impact on Body Structure & Functions, Activity, and Participation.

in which targeted stimulation of the peroneal nerve elicits active dorsiflexion of the affected extremity to assist with swing phase clearance. The BioNESS L300, WalkAide, and Odstock Dropped Foot Stimulator represent the three most common commercially available applications of this technology (Figure 13.14). Depending upon the FES technology, the cyclical stimulations can be triggered by the relative advancement of the tibia or the relative position of the affected heel against the floor.

Candidacy for FES is limited to those patients presenting with upper motor neuron injuries such as stroke, multiple sclerosis, and incomplete spinal cord injuries, in which the peripheral nervous system of the affected lower extremity is intact. As the dynamic stimulation can only elicit movement through the patient's available range of motion, plantarflexion contracture represents a contraindication to FES. As single-channel FES is only effective in addressing swing phase dorsiflexion, it does not address stance phase gait deviations such as knee hyperextension.

THE EXAMINATION AND EVALUATION

Once a PT has determined that there is a neuromuscular and/or musculoskeletal movement dysfunction for which an orthotic intervention is appropriate, an accurate, objective examination is necessary to generate the most appropriate orthotic prescription possible. The examination should include all domains of the International Classification of Functioning (ICF) (Figure 13.15) [10]. The ICF model defines *Function* as the physiological and psychological functions of body's systems and structure; *Activity* as the execution of a task or action by an individual; and *Participation* as an individual's involvement in a life situation.

As with all PT examinations, this process starts with a systems review, both at the impairment level and at the level of the functional task (activity level). Cognition and memory assessment are necessary to determine the patient's capacity to participate and follow-through with the orthotic intervention. If memory and/or cognition are impaired, a caregiver who can assist with the orthosis use must be identified. A thorough examination of the integumentary system for the lower limb is crucial to determine not only if an orthotic intervention is possible, but also to identify any risk factors for integumentary dysfunction which may impact orthotic use. The cardiopulmonary system evaluation should include attention to any conditions which might cause lower limb volume fluctuations, as well as baseline vital signs.

For those patients with orthotic goals related to gait, structured observational gait analysis (OGA) is the starting point for further examination. The OGA should provide clear delineation of gait deviations in both limbs in all phases of the gait cycle. All methods of improving accuracy and reliability of the OGA should be utilized including video recording of gait from standardized viewpoints and use of OGA tools. Some validated OGA tools include the Gait Assessment and Intervention Tool (GAIT) [11] for persons with stroke, Rancho Observational Gait Analysis [12], the Edinburgh Gait Score [13] for pediatrics, and the Spinal Cord Injury Functional Ambulation Inventory [14]. At this point, a hypothesis-driven examination of the musculoskeletal and neuromuscular systems can occur. For each major gait deviation identified in the OGA, hypotheses regarding the causative factors are generated. These can be identified and confirmed or ruled out.

The following is a summary of the key musculoskeletal and neuromuscular impairment components of the lower limb orthotic examination and evaluation.

Musculoskeletal:
- Accurate passive range of motion (PROM) exam of all joints impacted by orthosis, with special attention to the flexibility of those muscles which cross multiple joints. For AFO or KAFO prescription, it is imperative to assess the gastrocnemius length (ankle dorsiflexion with knee extension).
- Accurate Manual Muscle Test (MMT) of all lower limb muscles which contribute to functional activity goals or that will be impacted by the orthotic intervention. A careful assessment of strength, eliminating any compensatory movements and attending to accurate testing positions, is important.

Neuromuscular:
- Muscle tone of lower limb muscles impacted by orthosis. The Modified Tardieu Scale or the Modified Ashworth Scale [15–16] can be utilized to determine the presence of velocity dependent resistance to passive movement and to differentiate altered muscle tone from muscle tightness/contracture.
- Sensory function of the lower limb. Superficial sensation testing of all skin that will be contacted by the orthosis is necessary. Superficial sensation and kinesthesia testing of the entire limb will be useful in determining the orthotic prescription. Impaired or absent sensation is not a contraindication for orthotic wear, but is a precaution and may impact choices of materials and components, as well as post-orthotic plan of care.

A review of systems at the level of the task will be determined by the specific activity and participation goals of the orthotic intervention. For those patients whose goals relate to functional mobility such as transfers and general locomotion, the Functional Independence Measure (FIM) [17] or Functional Ambulation Categories [18] can be utilized. For goals related to gait, a detailed OGA as described above should be completed in conjunction with appropriate objective outcome measures. These could include measures of gait speed, gait endurance, and/or balance. The 10-meter walk test is the highly valid and reliable across all diagnoses for assessment of gait speed [19]. For endurance, the 6-minute walk test has strong psychometric properties across diagnoses [20]. For assessment of balance, the timed up and go (TUG) [21] was recommended by the American Academy of Orthotists and Prosthetists' State-of-the-Science Conference on "The Effects of Ankle Foot Orthoses on Balance" as the balance measure of choice for research investigating the effects of AFOs on balance [22]. Outcome measures which capture the participation domain should also be included, and these might include the Activities-specific Balance Confidence Scale [23], Goal Attainment Scaling [24], or other diagnosis specific measures of quality of life and participation.

A comprehensive examination and evaluation will be necessary to diagnose the specific movement dysfunction, and from this the most appropriate orthotic prescription can be generated. This examination will then be repeated, once the orthosis has been provided, in order to determine effectiveness of the intervention.

COMMONLY ENCOUNTERED DEVIATIONS

While an exhaustive narrative of every conceivable deviation observed in physical rehabilitation is beyond the scope of this chapter, there are a number of commonly encountered deviations that can be effectively managed through the provision of an appropriately designed lower limb orthosis.

Swing Phase Equinus (Foot Drop)

Swing phase equinus (often simplistically referred to as "foot drop") refers to a failure of the affected limb to attain the swing dorsiflexion described above. In addition to undermining the ability of the limb to attain adequate clearance through swing phase, swing phase equinus compromises the normal biomechanics of loading response, forcing patients to initiate floor contact with either the forefoot or midfoot rather than with the heel.

Swing phase equinus can be broadly classified as either flaccid or hypertonic. This represents an important distinction as the two presentations are managed very differently. When equinus is flaccid and the patient's presentation is confined to isolated weakness of the dorsiflexors, the resultant deviation is confined to swing phase and orthotic management may be limited to a PLS AFO (Figure 13.7) or an articulated AFO with dorsiflexion assist ankle joints (Figure 13.8B). These designs provide adequate resistance to prevent excessive plantarflexion during swing phase, but are flexible enough that their impacts on stance phase kinematics are minimal.

By contrast, swing phase equinus that is hypertonic in its etiology and presentation requires stiffness beyond that associated with a PLS AFO. The active plantarflexion associated with this presentation will generally overpower the PLS AFO, compromising its efficacy in this scenario. Rather, a rigid plantarflexion stop, in the form of a solid AFO (Figure 13.6) or as a design element in an articulated AFO (Figure 13.8A), is warranted.

Unfortunately, limitations in today's technology do not allow for the application of a plantarflexion stop in swing phase that releases or disengages in stance phase. As a result, the desirable application of a plantarflexion stop in swing phase is coupled with the less desirable application of this joint stop in loading response, eliminating the availability of controlled plantarflexion in loading response (Figure 13.9). While this can be partially mitigated through a cambered shoe heel, the absence of this event necessarily increases the external flexion moment acting upon the knee during early stance. Thus, a clinical assessment of the functional strength of the knee extensors and plantarflexors of the affected limb is warranted prior to the application of any AFO that restricts plantarflexion.

Hyperextension of the Knee or Knee Extensor Thrust

As indicated above, the closed-chain kinematics of the ankle and knee joints are such that restrictions to ankle motion can often affect the behavior of the anatomic knee joint. In cases where mild to moderate hyperextension of the knee or a knee extensor thrust is observed in mid stance, it can often be managed with the provision of a plantarflexion stop as part of a solid AFO (Figure 13.6) or as a design element in an articulated AFO (Figure 13.8A). As described earlier, the desirable application of a plantarflexion stop in mid stance to prevent hyperextension of the knee necessitates the less desirable application of the joint stop in loading response, eliminating controlled plantarflexion that would normally occur and increasing the knee flexion moment experienced during this phase of gait. However, the beneficial effects of sparing the integrity of the knee joint outweigh the detriment to loading response kinematics, provided the patient has adequate knee extensor strength to prevent anterior buckling of the knee.

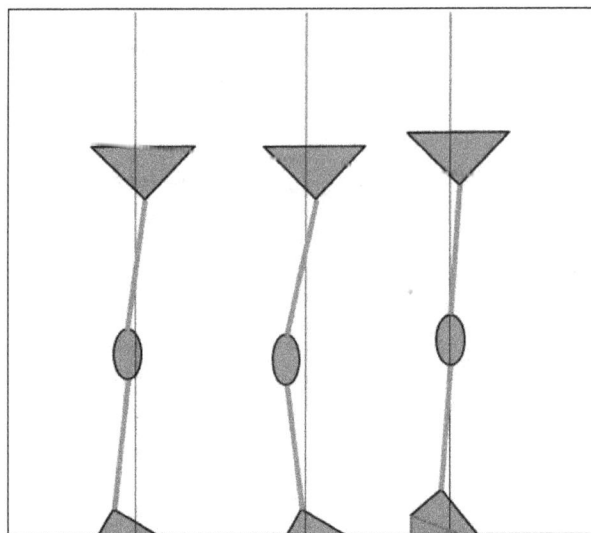

Figure 13.16. The effect of ankle alignment on knee alignment. A. normal ankle mobility; B. plantarflexion contracture creating knee hyperextension; and C. normalized knee alignment observed when a compensatory heel lift is used to accommodate a plantarflexion contracture.

When observed earlier in gait, knee hyperextension is generally a product of quadriceps weakness and is best managed by an orthosis that extends proximal to the knee, an application that is beyond the scope of this chapter. Knee hyperextension can also occur as a result of plantarflexion contracture, precluding normal tibial advancement. In such cases, an accommodative heel lift is often indicated to permit the anterior translation of the tibia in both quiet standing and through gait (Figure 13.16).

In most cases of acquired hemiplegia such as acute stroke, knee hyperextension occurs as an accommodation for weak plantarflexors immediately following the stroke. In the absence of functional plantarflexors, the individual is unable to consistently and constantly perform the controlled dorsiflexion that should characterize mid and late stance. Rather, they adopt a pattern of knee hyperextension to ensure their stability in stance. If such cases are identified before this gait deviation is fully adopted, the provision of an articulated AFO with a dorsiflexion stop (Figure 13.10A) can reestablish a consistent controlled dorsiflexion, eliminating the need for the compensatory hyperextension of the knee. The coupling of a dorsiflexion stop with dorsiflexion assist, along with attentive physical therapy can collectively assist swing dorsiflexion, permit controlled plantarflexion, and retrain controlled dorsiflexion following acquired hemiplegia for those patients with adequate motor control.

Crouch

Crouch gait is generally a manifestation of weak plantarflexors, commonly observed in patients with lower lumber myelomenigocele or spinal cord injury and in some patients with diplegic cerebral palsy. It can also be observed unilaterally in patients who have sustained a stroke, particularly during the acute phase of their recovery. In the absence of functional plantarflexors the controlled dorsiflexion of mid and terminal stance that permits the controlled anterior translation of the body's ground reaction force from the heel to the forefoot does not occur. Rather, this force vector remains through the heel throughout stance phase, described as a calcaneal gait.

Such cases are best managed through the provision of a dorsiflexion stop, either within a solid AFO (Figure 13.6) or as a design element of an articulated AFO (Figure 13.10). This joint restriction mimics the function of the compromised plantarflexors by restraining the amount of dorsiflexion observed during late stance. This mechanical restraint is often supplemented by extending and expanding the lever arm of the AFO through a ground reaction design as described earlier.

The angle of this dorsiflexion stop must take into account the available range of motion of the knee and hip joints of the affected extremity. Flexion contractures at either of these joints preclude the use of a dorsiflexion stop set to mimic the modest dorsiflexion observed in normal human locomotion. If such proximal joint contractures are not accommodated by the allowance of additional dorsiflexion at the ankle or accommodative heel lifts, the closed-chain kinematics of the affected extremity will result in posterior instability.

In addition to the rigid dorsiflexion stops that have been traditionally utilized in thermoplastic AFOs there are a number of non-custom and custom carbon fiber AFOs and AFO design elements that mimic the progressively increasing stiffness associated with controlled dorsiflexion (Figure 13.12). In addition to enhancing the smoothness of gait through terminal stance, these elements can provide a measure of propulsion at the ankle as the material deformation that occurs through the controlled dorsiflexion of late stance is released during pre-swing to mimic a modest powered plantarflexion. This principle has been used to restore athletic pursuits in patients lacking adequate plantarflexor strength and function to perform powered plantarflexion.

Anterior Knee Instability

While crouch gait, knee hyperextension, and knee extensor thrust patterns are readily observed in clinical settings, anterior knee instability is a more subtle phenomenon. These patients will either experience a sudden buckling of the lower limb into knee flexion or limit their activity because of their fear of falling. They often complain of falls, stating that their knee simply "gave out." Patients experiencing this instability, generally due to weakness or fatigue of the knee extensors, plantarflexors, or both muscle groups, will often compensate by manipulating their

ground reaction force to ensure that it passes anterior to their knee joint providing sagittal stability. As with crouch gait, these deficits can often be managed by the provision of resistance to dorsiflexion through either thermoplastic or carbon fiber AFOs with appropriate design elements. However, in cases of extreme quadriceps weakness, coupled with compounding weakness in the plantarflexors and hip extensors, an intervention extending proximal to the knee joint may be indicated.

THE PRESCRIPTION PROCESS

Orthotic prescriptions vary greatly depending on the healthcare professional generating the prescription. A primary care provider or therapist may simply prescribe a "left foot orthosis" or "right AFO" with no greater detail, and this is the starting point for the patient and the orthotist. This approach places all examination, evaluation, and decision making in the hands of the orthotist. While orthotists are trained in examination and evaluation of the lower limb and have the decision-making capacity to recommend and provide an appropriate orthosis in collaboration with the patient/caregiver, doing so in isolation may undermine any treatment goals that the therapist may have established with the patient. As mentioned previously, a collaborative approach between the patient and the interdisciplinary team is optimal in the lower limb prescription process.

The lower limb orthotic prescription is a clinical decision-making process. The process initiates with the identification of a neuromuscular and/or musculoskeletal dysfunction for which a lower limb orthosis would provide benefit towards the patient/caregiver's identified goals. At this point, initiating collaboration with an orthotist would be ideal. This will likely involve collaboration with social work/case management to identify an appropriate orthotic provider for the patient given their payor source. At this juncture, it is also essential to ascertain the patient/caregiver's support for an orthotic intervention. The PT should explain the findings of the examination, along with their evaluation of the orthotic options which would benefit them in reaching their identified goals. Adequate information including benefits, risks, costs, commitment (wearing, training), and cosmesis should be provided PRIOR to committing time and resources in moving forward with the prescription process.

The PT should conduct a thorough pre-orthotic examination and evaluation as described previously. The PT should identify the specific impairments, activity, and participation limitations to be addressed with the orthotic intervention and define the specific goals for the orthosis such as control dorsiflexion in mid and terminal stance to provide stance stability, restrict plantarflexion in swing to facilitate swing limb clearance, or provide medial/lateral stability of the rear and hindfoot during weight bearing.

The PT may be more prescriptive, specifying the type of orthosis, components, and materials. However, this degree of prescriptive input is not usually necessary when strong collaborative relationships exist between the PT and the orthotist.

In addition, the PT is responsible for justification of the lower limb orthotic device being prescribed. Justification can be made at the levels of body functions and structure, activity, and participation (Figure 13.15). Focus should be given to how the orthosis will not only increase function, but how the device will benefit the patient's overall health. How might this device decrease the risk for future episodes of care? Examples might include decrease of risk for adverse events such as falls, skin breakdown, or improved capacity of activity.

THE POST-ORTHOTIC PLAN OF CARE

During orthotic fitting, the overall fit and function of the orthosis is evaluated, and any necessary modifications to the device are made. Once these modifications are complete, fit and function will be re-assessed, and assuming all is satisfactory, training in the device can begin with the orthotist during this session. The device should be fully functional, comfortable, and meet the goals and specifications outlined in the prescription at the completion of the delivery appointment with the orthotist. When feasible, it is beneficial for the PT to be present for this fitting appointment.

The PT, whether collaboratively with the orthotist or during the patient's subsequent PT sessions, should provide a thorough examination of the device, its fit on the patient, and the patient's function with the device. The patient's skin should be thoroughly evaluated and any issues documented. Any initial problems with fit or function should be reported to the orthotist immediately, and the patient should not wear the device until issues are corrected. Assuming the fit and function are appropriate, the PT should ensure that the patient has a wearing schedule for the device. This is typically provided by the orthotist, and reinforced by the PT. However, if no wearing schedule is in place, the PT needs to provide one. The amount of initial wearing is fairly patient specific depending on the patient's risk for skin breakdown, the type of device, and the activities that will be conducted while in the device. A conservative starting schedule might be on 30 minutes, 3 times daily, progressing by adding 10–15 minutes to each wear time daily. If the patient is only supine or sitting during most of the day, wearing times might be progressed more quickly. For those patients who do longer periods of standing and walking, wear times may be progressed more slowly. It is crucial to educate the patient and/or caregiver on appropriate skin inspection which occurs before and after each wearing of the device. Skin inspection can be reinforced in OT as well, and any necessary tools such as mirrors can be procured for the patient/caregiver.

An often-overlooked component of initial orthotic training is donning and doffing the device. Improper donning of the device can lead to skin breakdown and poor function. It is therefore imperative that the patient and/or their caregiver be able to effectively don and doff the device easily. For some of the more complex devices, this may require a good amount of practice, and again, collaboration with OT can be invaluable in helping problem solve strategies for success for the patient/caregiver. Devices that require too much effort to don and doff, or that the patient can't don/doff independently, may be rejected or under-utilized.

Another aspect of the post-orthotic plan that is specific to AFOs is AFO tuning. This involves making small dimension changes at the foot and ankle to improve biomechanical alignment and function at the hip and knee. In an articulated AFO, small changes to the restrictions at the ankle angle, via changes to plantarflexion stops and or dorsiflexion restraints, can impact knee flexion and extension moments. In a solid AFO, shoe modifications, often in the form of heel lifts, are used to manipulate the resultant angle of tibial advancement. Specifically, in the latter application, ankle foot orthosis and footwear combination (AFO-FC) tuning has been described as an essential component of the AFO prescription [5–7]. AFO-FC tuning was described by Owen [8] as the process of making fine adjustments to the foot–shank angle design of the AFO-FC in order to optimize biomechanics.

It is also important to assess how leg length may be impacted by the orthotic device. Adding a lower limb orthosis increases the length of the limb. Depending on materials utilized and design of the orthosis, the leg length increase may range from negligible to an amount that impacts function. Especially in those with significant unilateral weakness, such as stroke, the slight increase in leg length on the hemiparetic side may significantly increase difficulty of initiating swing. Solutions to minor leg length differences could be to remove the shoe insert on the orthotic side and/or add small lifts on the contralateral side. Both tuning and adjusting for leg length discrepancies should occur before the patient is provided the definitive device by the orthotist, but these need to be evaluated by the PT as part of the orthotic training procedure. Any modifications are best made in collaboration with the orthotist.

Training in the orthotic device is necessary to maximize effectiveness. Simply providing an appropriate orthosis and placing it on the patient does not ensure that the patient will be able to use the device and extract the full potential for improved function. It is important for the PT to provide task specific and appropriately intensive training with the orthosis. For those patients with an orthotic goal related to standing and gait, this may entail a progression from static standing to weight shifts in standing (lateral and anterior/posterior), stepping in all directions, and finally to gait over all surfaces. Training in transitional movements such as sit to stand, stand to sit, and transfers is also necessary, as is training in obstacle and stair management. The goal of an orthotic intervention is to promote normal biomechanical alignment and kinematics, so training should strive to abolish any abnormal patterns the patients may have adopted prior to the orthotic intervention, and promote utilization of the orthosis to normalize alignment and movement. For patients who are utilizing a device to promote stance limb stability, it is critical to re-train normal weight-shifting over the involved limb, allowing the orthosis to provide the stability and restriction of motion it was designed for. Likewise, in persons using a lower limb orthosis to provide swing limb clearance, training must include elimination of compensatory strategies such as hip hiking, excessive hip/knee flexion, vaulting, or trunk lean.

The final component of the post-orthotic intervention is to determine the effectiveness of the orthotic device. For this, one must return to the orthotic goals and determine if they have been met or not met. Re-examination across the ICF, with a focus on the orthosis's impact on the patient's activity as well as satisfaction and quality of life, will determine overall effectiveness of the intervention.

A comprehensive post-orthotic plan is paramount to successful acceptance and utilization of the lower limb orthosis. An orthosis should be seen as an investment for the patient, and warrants the time and effort of education and training in order to ensure maximum benefit.

Best Practice in Lower Limb Orthotic Management

The value of lower limb orthoses in reducing overall healthcare costs has been confirmed in a review of Medicare Healthcare Utilization Data [25]. In this analysis the authors identified a large cohort of individuals with non-traumatic joint disorders, osteoarthritis, stroke, paralysis, multiple sclerosis, and spinal cord injury who had received a lower limb orthosis as part of care. In addition to the cost of the orthoses, the authors examined the next 18 months of healthcare utilization and costs associated with inpatient and outpatient hospital visits, long-term care hospitalization, skilled nursing facilities, inpatient rehabilitation facilities, home health agencies, and hospice and physician visits. Using propensity score matching techniques, these individuals were retrospectively paired to a similar peer based on such considerations as diagnosis, comorbid health conditions, historical healthcare utilization, gender, race, and age. For these

matched controls, 18-month healthcare utilization and its associated costs were also tracked. The subsequent analysis observed that healthcare spending was reduced by an average of 10% among those individuals who received lower limb orthoses.

The 2016 Guidelines for Adult Stroke Rehabilitation and Recovery [26] found IB level evidence (evidence for and/or general agreement that treatment is useful and effective, derived from single randomized trial or nonrandomized studies) supporting the use of AFOs for ankle instability or dorsiflexor weakness in persons with stroke and found that use of AFOs was an effective method of compensating for lower limb motor impairments. The review found IA level evidence (evidence for and/or general agreement that treatment is useful and effective, derived from multiple randomized clinical trials or meta-analyses) for recommending an AFO after stroke for individuals with "remediable gait impairments (e.g., foot drop) to compensate for the foot drop and to improve mobility and paretic ankle and knee kinematics, kinetics, and energy cost of walking."

A systematic review of 60 publications reporting AFO interventions on gait and functional mobility in persons with stroke or cerebral palsy concluded that most studies demonstrated improvement in walking speed and ankle dorsiflexion, but effects on knee stability were unclear [27]. A systematic review in 2008 of literature on the efficacy of AFOs on gait in children with cerebral palsy found that available research "suggest positive effects of the use of AFOs on the passive and active ankle ROM, gait kinetics and kinematics, as well as on functional activities related to mobility of children with CP [cerebral palsy]," but cited poor quality of evidence and limited ability to draw strong conclusions [28]. More recent studies are continuing to report similar improvements in function and ambulation [29, 30].

Despite the compelling evidence in favor of AFO utilization following a stroke, in a qualitative study of PTs treating patients with post-stroke hemiplegia, the majority of subjects expressed a reluctance (or complete opposition) to utilization of orthotics. Participants expressed a perception that orthotics impeded recovery and prevented strengthening of muscles [31]. Time and again, participants stated this desire to maximize recovery, and intimated that orthotic use somehow hampered motor recovery. However, multiple studies have presented electromyography data that indicate that there is no clear evidence that use of orthotic devices decrease muscle activation or cause long-term detriment to muscle activity [32–42].

The use of FES for ambulation in persons with stroke has been found to be effective in increasing walking speeds, increasing walking distance, and improving activity levels when compared with no intervention or walking training alone [43–45]. When compared with an ankle foot orthosis, a study utilizing the Odstock Dropped-Foot Stimulator declared the AFO and ODFS to be comparable in their effect on functional ambulation, as well as finding a preference for the ODFS by patients [46]. However, another publication found that while participants preferred FES, they frequently supplemented FES with use of some type of orthosis in specific situations [47]. And a study by Bethoux et al. [48] concluded the FES was equivalent to AFOs at 12 months post intervention. However, it is important to note that in all these studies, the AFOs designs were not standardized and the only requirement was that the device alleviate foot drop. Limited or arguably any AFO/FES comparison studies to date have analyzed lower limb kinematics or any factors related to stance stability [49–51]. In most of these studies, stability may be inferred based on outcomes such as stance duration, gait velocity or other factors.

SUMMARY

Lower limb orthoses may be utilized to meet a variety of goals in many neuromuscular and musculoskeletal diagnoses. The evidence is largely supportive of the efficacy of lower limb orthoses. However, more rigorous research is warranted, especially to investigate various designs of orthoses and to compare the effectiveness of various orthotic types, as well as comparisons of orthoses to other interventions. An ideal orthotic intervention is a collaborative process among several healthcare professionals (including the patient and/or caregiver), and requires thorough examination, post-orthotic training, and evaluation of orthotic effectiveness.

REFERENCES

[1] Schuch CM, Pritham CH. International standards organization terminology: application to prosthetics and orthotics. *JPO*. 1994;6:29–33.

[2] Masic I, Miokovic M, Muhamedagic B. Evidence based medicine—new approaches and challenges. *Acta Inform Med*. 2008;16(4):219–225.

[3] Perry J, Burnfield JM. *Gait Analysis. Normal and Pathological Function*, 2010. 2nd edition. Slack Inc., Thorofare, NJ.

[4] Mavroidis C, Ranky RG, Sivak ML, et al. Patient specific ankle-foot orthoses using rapid prototyping. *J Neuoroeng Rehabil*. 2011;8:1.

[5] Bowers R, Ross K. A review of the effectiveness of lower limb orthoses used in cerebral palsy. In: Morris C and Condie D, eds. *Recent Developments in Healthcare for Cerebral Palsy: Implications and Opportunities for Orthotics*, 2009. International Society for Prosthetics and Orthotics, Copenhagen, pp. 235–297.

[6] Owen E, Bowers RJ, Meadows CB, eds. Tuning of AFO-footwear combinations for neurological disorders. Invited presentation at the Symposium of the 11th World Congress of the International Society for Prosthetics and Orthotics (IPSO), Hong Kong, August 1–6, 2004.

[7] Bowers R, Ross K. Development of a best practice statement on the use of ankle-foot orthoses following stroke in Scotland. *Prosthet Orthot Int*. 2010;34(3):245–253.

[8] Owen E. The importance of being earnest about shank and thigh kinematics especially when using ankle-foot orthoses. *Prosthet Orthot Int*. 2010;34(3):254–269.

[9] Ramsey JA. Development of a method for fabricating polypropylene non-articulated dorsiflexion assist ankle foot orthoses with predetermined stiffness. *Prosthet Orthot Int*. 2011;35(1):54–69.

[10] WHO. *International Classification of Functioning, Disability, and Health: ICF*, 2001. World Health Organization, Geneva, Switzerland.

[11] Daly JJ, Nethery J, McCabe JP, et al. Development and testing of the Gait Assessment and Intervention Tool (G.A.I.T.): a measure of coordinated gait components. *J Neurosci Methods*. 2009;178:334–339.

[12] Perry J. *Gait Analysis: Normal and Pathological Function*, 1992. Slack, Thorofare, NJ.

[13] Read HS, Hazlewood ME, Hillman SJ, et al. Edinburgh visual gait score for use in cerebral palsy. *J Pediatr Orthop*. 2003; 23(3):296–301.

[14] Field-Fote EC, Fluet GG, Schafer SD, et al. The Spinal Cord Injury Functional Ambulation Inventory (SCI-FAI). *J Rehabil Med*. 2001;33:177–181.

[15] Bohannon RW, Smith MB. Interrater reliability of a modified Ashworth scale of muscle spasticity. *Phys Ther*. 1987;67:206–207.

[16] Boyd RN, Barwood SA, Ballieu CE, Granham HK. Validity of a clinical measure of spasticity in children with cerebral palsy in a double-blinded randomized controlled clinical trial, abstract. *Dev Med Child Neurol*. 1998;40(Suppl 78):7.

[17] Hamilton BB, Laughlin JA, Fielder RC, Granger CV. Interrater reliability of the 7-level functional independence measure (FIM). *Scand J Rehabil Med*. 1994;26:115–119.

[18] Holden MK, Gill KM, Magliozzi MR, et al. Clinical gait assessment in the neurologically impaired. Reliability and meaningfulness. *Phys Ther*. 1984;64:35–40.

[19] Wade DT. *Measurement in Neurological Rehabilitation*, 1992. Oxford University Press, Oxford.

[20] American Thoracic Society. ATS statement: guidelines for the six-minute walk test. *Am J Respir Crit Care Med*. 2002;166:111–117.

[21] Mathias S, Nayak U, Isaacs B. Balance in elderly patients: the "get-up and go" test. *Arch Phys Med Rehabil*. 1986;67:387–389.

[22] Seale J. Valid and reliable instruments for the clinical assessment of the effect of ankle-foot orthoses on balance. *J Orthot Prosth*. 2010;10:P38–P45.

[23] Powell LE, Myers AM. The Activities-specific Balance Confidence (ABC) scale. *J Gerontol. A: Biol Sci Med Sci*. 1995;50:M28–M34.

[24] Turner-Stokes L. Goal attainment scaling (GAS) in rehabilitation: a practical guide. *Clin Rehabil*. 2009;23:362–370.

[25] Dobson A, El-Gamil A, Shimer M, DaVanzo JE. Economic value of prosthetic services among Medicare beneficiaries: a claims-based retrospective cohort study. *Mil Med*. 2016;181:18–24.

[26] Winstein CJ, Stein J, Arena R, et al; on behalf of the American Heart Association Stroke Council, Council on Cardiovascular and Stroke Nursing, Council on Clinical Cardiology, and Council on Quality of Care and Outcomes Research. Guidelines for adult stroke rehabilitation and recovery: a guideline for healthcare professionals from the American Heart Association/American Stroke Association. *Stroke*. 2016;47:6; e98-e169.

[27] Chisholm AE, Perry SD. Ankle-foot orthotic management in neuromuscular disorders: recommendations for future research. *Disabil Rehabil: Assist Tech*. 2010;7:437–449.

[28] Figueiredo EM, Ferreira GB, Moreira RCM, et al. Efficacy of ankle-foot orthoses on gait of children with cerebral palsy: systematic review of literature. *Pediatr Phys Ther*. 2008;20:207–223.

[29] van Duijnhoven E, Koopman FS, Ploeger HE, et al. Effects of specialist care lower limb orthoses on personal goal attainment

and walking ability in adults with neuromuscular disorders. *PLOS One.* 2023 Jan 18;18(1):e0279292.

[30] Tomioka K, Matsumoto S, Ikeda K, et al. Short-term effects of physiotherapy combining repetitive facilitation exercises and orthotic treatment in chronic post-stroke patients. *J Phys Ther Sci.* 2017 Feb;29(2):212–215.

[31] Seale J, Utsey C. Physical therapist's clinical reasoning in patients with gait impairments from hemiplegia: a qualitative study. Poster presented at: American Physical Therapy Association Combined Sections Meeting, February 19, 2016, Anaheim, California.

[32] Lairamore C, Garrison MK, Bandy W, Zabel R. Comparison of tibialis anterior muscle electromyography, ankle angle, and velocity when individuals post stroke walk with different orthoses. *Prosthet Orthot Int.* 2011 Dec;35(4):402–410.

[33] Ohata K, Yasui T, Tsuboyama T, Ichihashi N. Effects of an ankle-foot orthosis with oil damper on muscle activity in adults after stroke. *Gait Posture.* 2011 Jan;33(1):102–107.

[34] Mulroy SJ, Eberly VJ, Gronely JK, et al. Effect of AFO design on walking after stroke: Impact of ankle plantar flexion contracture. *Prosthet Orthot Int.* 2010 Sep;34(3):277–292.

[35] Hesse S, Werner C, Matthias K, et al. Non-velocity-related effects of a rigid double-stopped ankle-foot orthosis on gait and lower limb muscle activity of hemiparetic subjects with an equinovarus deformity. *Stroke.* 1999 Sep;30(9):1855–1861.

[36] Romkes J, Hell AK, Brunner R. Changes in muscle activity in children with hemiplegic cerebral palsy while walking with and without ankle-foot orthoses. *Gait Posture.* 2006 Dec;24(4):467–474.

[37] Lam WK, Leong JC, Li YH, et al. Biomechanical and electromyographic evaluation of ankle foot orthosis and dynamic ankle foot orthosis in spastic cerebral palsy. *Gait Posture.* 2005 Nov;22(3):189–197.

[38] Radtka SA, Skinner SR, Johanson ME. A comparison of gait with solid and hinged ankle-foot orthoses in children with spastic diplegic cerebral palsy. *Gait Posture.* 2005 Apr;21(3):303–310.

[39] Rethlefsen S, Kay R, Dennis S, et al. The effects of fixed and articulated ankle-foot orthoses on gait patterns in subjects with cerebral palsy. *J Pediatr Orthop.* 1999 Jul–Aug;19(4):470–474.

[40] Radtka SA, Skinner SR, Dixon DM, Johanson ME. A comparison of gait with solid, dynamic, and no ankle-foot orthoses in children with spastic cerebral palsy. *Phys Ther.* 1997 Apr;77(4):395–409.

[41] Beekman C, Perry J, Boyd LA, et al. The effects of a dorsiflexion-stopped ankle-foot orthosis on walking in individuals with incomplete spinal cord injury. *Topics in Spinal Cord Injury Rehabilitation.* 2000 Jan;5(4):8.

[42] Geboers JF, Wetzelaer WL, Seelen HA, et al. Ankle-foot orthosis has limited effect on walking test parameters among patients with peripheral ankle dorsiflexor paresis. *J Rehabil Med.* 2002 Mar;34(2):80–85.

[43] Robbins SM, Houghton PE, Woodbury MG, Brown JL. The therapeutic effect of functional and transcutaneous electric stimulation on improving gait speed in stroke patients: a meta-analysis. *Arch Phys Med Rehabil.* 2006;87:853–859.

[44] Pereira S, Mehta S, McIntyre A, et al. Functional electrical stimulation for improving gait in persons with chronic stroke. *Top Stroke Rehabil.* 2012;19:491–498.

[45] Howlett OA, Lannin NA, Ada L, McKinstry C. Functional electrical stimulation improves activity after stroke: a systematic review with meta-analysis. *Arch Phys Med Rehabil.* 2015;96:934–943.

[46] Sheffler LR, Hennessey MT, Naples GG, Chae J. Peroneal nerve stimulation versus an ankle foot orthosis for correction of foot-drop in stroke: impact on functional ambulation. *Neurorehabil Neural Repair.* 2006;20:355–360.

[47] Bulley C, Shiels J, Wilkie K, Salisbury L. User experiences, preferences and choices relating to functional electrical stimulation and ankle foot orthoses for foot-drop after stroke. *Physiother.* 2011;97:226–233.

[48] Bethoux F, Rogers HL, Nolan KR, et al. Long-term follow-up to a randomized controlled trial comparing peroneal nerve functional electrical stimulation to an ankle foot orthosis for patients with chronic stroke. *Neurorehabil Neural Repair.* 2015;29:911–922.

[49] Skigen JT, Koller CA, Nigro L, et al. Customized passive-dynamic ankle-foot orthoses can improve walking economy and speed for many individuals post-stroke. *J Neuroeng Rehabil.* 2024 Jul 29;21(1):126.

[50] Vistamehr A, Neptune RR, Conroy CL. Articulated ankle-foot-orthosis improves inter-limb propulsion symmetry during walking adaptability task post-stroke. *Clin Biomech (Bristol, Avon).* 2024 Jun;116:106268.

[51] Ohtsuka K, Mukaino M, Yamada J. Effects of ankle-foot orthosis on gait pattern and spatiotemporal indices during treadmill walking in hemiparetic stroke. *Int J Rehabil Res.* 2023 Dec 1;46(4):316–324.

CHAPTER 14

Lower Limb Orthotic Management
Orthoses Above the Knee

Phil M. Stevens, Cheryl Costa, Eric Weber, and M. Jason Highsmith

OBJECTIVES

Upon completion of this chapter, the reader will be able to:

1. Recall common orthotic configurations and componentry for patients who may benefit from orthoses that directly influence the knee and hip.
2. Recall therapeutic considerations related to patients who may benefit from orthoses that directly influence the knee and hip.
3. Recall selected pathologies that commonly result in impairment that may benefit from orthoses that directly influence the knee and hip.

INTRODUCTION

Orthotic interventions that extend proximal to the knee joint are less commonly prescribed and provided than other levels of orthoses. In a recent practice analysis by the American Board for Certification in Orthotics, Prosthetics & Pedorthics, Inc. (ABC), it was reported that knee-ankle-foot-orthoses (KAFOs) account for less than 4% of the practice time of certified orthotists [1]. Hip-knee-ankle-foot-orthoses (HKAFOs) are even less common, accounting for less than 1% of an ABC-certified orthotist's time [1].

Historically, many physical therapists (PTs) have been taught to avoid the use of lower extremity orthoses, when possible, particularly with devices extending proximal to

the knee. Over-bracing has been a consistent concern, and the use of KAFOs or HKAFOs has often been seen as a last resort. Further, in an acute and subacute rehabilitation setting it is often difficult to make a definitive decision about bracing as there is often a changing patient profile. Unfortunately, because of this, bracing decisions may be avoided and ultimately neglected, potentially leaving the patient with less-than-optimal outcomes and no follow-up.

The PT is often the healthcare professional responsible for initiating orthotic intervention. In doing so, important patient considerations include their anticipated daily function, recent fall history, long term alignment and associated joint protection, neuroplasticity and the potential benefits associated with early ambulation, and new advancements in orthotic technology. Based on

DOI: 10.4324/9781003526025-16

these factors, in collaboration with the prescribing physician and treating orthotist, the PT can contribute to the decision of which lower extremity orthoses will best fit the patient profile.

The purpose of this chapter is to introduce the range of currently available orthotic designs extending proximal to the knee, present those patient populations most frequently managed with KAFOs and HKAFOs, provide general considerations relative to prescription recommendations, discuss benefits and drawbacks associated with these interventions, and introduce relevant training considerations. Hip and knee orthoses will also be discussed within the context of their more common applications.

AVAILABLE ORTHOTIC SOLUTIONS

Contrasting AFOs and KAFOs

Determining the appropriate level of bracing for a patient can be challenging. Generally, KAFOs should not be prescribed unless adequate stability cannot be provided by a less obtrusive intervention such as an ankle-foot-orthosis (AFO). In many instances, an AFO that restricts the relative dorsiflexion or plantarflexion of the affected extremity can control either anterior knee instability or knee hyperextension, respectively. However, if there is a need for increased knee stability which cannot be achieved by restricting ankle movement with an AFO, such as might be seen with significant anterior knee instability, genu recurvatum, varum, or valgum, a KAFO should be considered.

KAFOs

The KAFO, commonly called the "long leg brace," can be a valuable tool for the PT and orthotist. Typically, it is recommended for individuals with profound knee weakness, or knee joint instabilities including varus, valgus, and recurvatum. These devices are commonly reserved for those individuals with biomechanical deficits profound enough to justify their bulk and inconvenience and are generally considered only when adequate stability cannot be provided by an AFO. KAFOs cover a great deal of surface area, creating the potential of heat retention and skin irritation. These devices are inherently bulky, time-consuming to don, and tend to wear away any clothing that drapes over their knee hinges. These limitations notwithstanding, recent years have seen several advancements in available knee joint technologies and for many patients, their associated benefits outweigh their stated drawbacks.

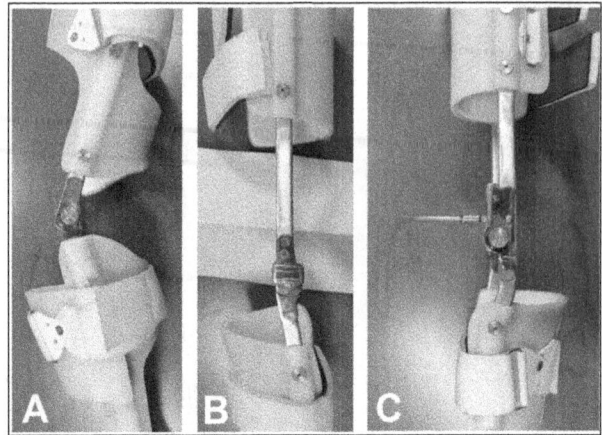

Figure 14.1. A. Single axis, free swinging knee joint; B. single axis, drop lock knee joint; and C. bail lock knee joint.

Single Axis, Free Swinging Knee Joint

The single axis, free swinging knee joint is a simple hinge that, when used in concert with a well-fitted orthosis, provides coronal stability against both varus and valgus forces acting upon the knee and prevents hyperextension of the knee joint (Figure 14.1A). As a free knee, it has no locking feature and is inappropriate for patients who lack the means of stabilizing their knee against anterior instability (i.e., knee buckling events).

Single Axis, Locking Knee Joint

Frequently, profound weakness of the knee extensors necessitates a knee joint that locks into extension and precludes any knee flexion until released. Several locking mechanisms are available, ranging from simple to more complex designs.

Drop Lock: Commonly encountered and chosen for its robust simplicity, the drop lock is a metallic ring that falls into place over the fully extended knee joints of a KAFO, locking out knee motion (Figure 14.1B). It is generally used bilaterally, on both the lateral and medial uprights of the device, to enhance its efficacy in stabilizing the limb. While drop locks can engage during sit to stand transfers simply due to gravity, patients should verify their locked status prior to dynamic or prolonged weight-bearing tasks. The locks remain engaged during weight bearing and ambulation and must be manually raised to permit flexion of the KAFO uprights at their mechanical knee joint axes. Spring-loaded *ball retainers* can be designed into the uprights, immediately proximal to the knee joints. These retainers prevent drop locks from falling into position over the joint when the patient wants to unlock the knee, such as while preparing to sit. When these are present, the patient must manually push the drop locks distally, past the *ball retainers* to allow them to engage over the knee joints.

Automatic Spring Lever Lock: As the name implies, in automatic spring lever locks a small spring-loaded lever extends posteriorly from the knee that locks the joint when it reaches full extension. The joint remains locked until a superiorly directed force raises the lever to release it. The lever locks can be manually raised, similar to the releasing of drop locks, or integrated into bail or trigger lock variations.

Bail Lock: In the bail variation, a U-shaped rod connects to the posterior aspect of both lever locks (Figure 14.1C). A superiorly directed force against the bail raises both lever locks, simultaneously releasing the medial and lateral knee joints. This concept allows the more adept user to release the knee joints by backing against the desired sitting surface. However, the bail can also be released unintentionally if adequately bumped. This could result in a fall.

Trigger Release: In the trigger release variation, cabling is attached to the posterior aspect of the locking lever and routed superiorly where it runs through cable housing positioned against the body of the KAFO. Exiting the housing, the cable terminates within a release lever, typically mounted on the lateral aspect of the KAFO's thigh section. Pulling on the release lever creates excursion on the cabling, drawing the locking levers superiorly and releasing the joint.

Offset Knee Joint

Offset knee joints are typically free motion joints in which the joint axis is offset posteriorly from the long axis of the uprights (Figure 14.2). This posterior offset allows the weight line to pass anterior to the knee joint more readily, increasing the stability of the KAFO as the joint will not flex until the weight line passes posterior to the knee joint. Importantly, during swing phase the knee joint swings freely.

Variable Position Knee Joint

Designed to accommodate contractures of the knee flexors, variable position knee joints are combined with drop locks and can be set to engage the locks across a range of available flexion angles. These joints are highly adjustable, allowing iterative changes to the locking angle of the joints if improvements in passive range of motion (ROM) are anticipated.

Stance Control Knee Joints

Unfortunately, for those that lack the knee extensor strength to use a free motion knee joint, the locked knee

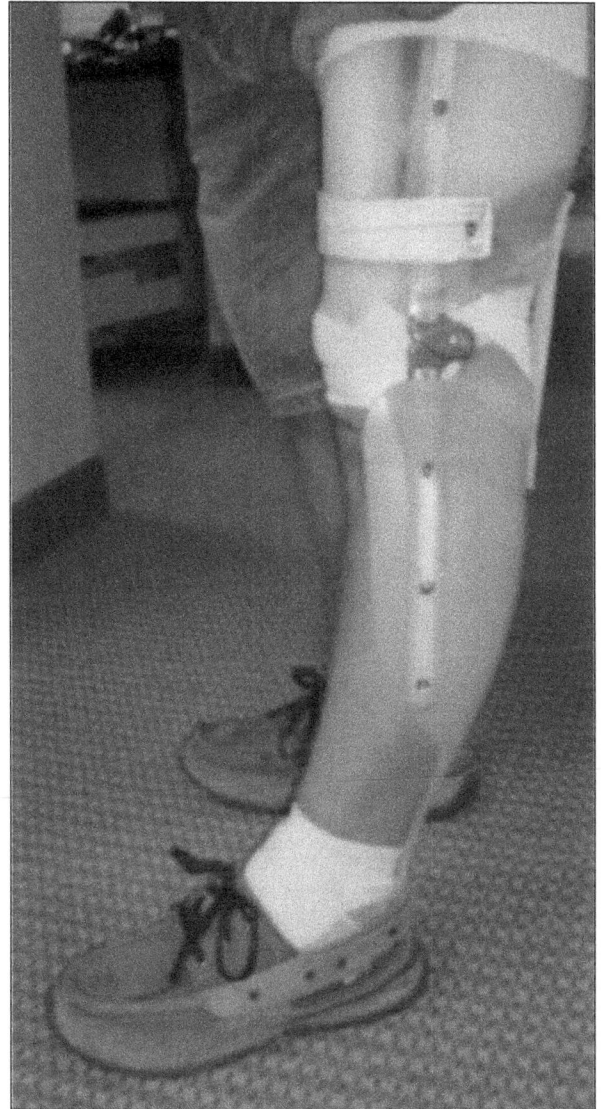

Figure 14.2. Posterior offset knee joint.

creates a physiologically longer leg. This leads to hip hiking or circumduction of the affected extremity to assist with limb progression and ground clearance during swing phase. The resultant pelvic obliquity is often coupled with pronounced plantarflexion of the sound foot and ankle during stance phase, or contralateral vaulting, to further aide with swing phase clearance [2].

Recognition of these deficits has led to the development of a relatively recent class of KAFO, the stance control orthoses (SCOs), that facilitate near normal knee flexion during swing with locked knee extension in stance. Studies suggest that the utilization of SCOs restore a more physiological gait pattern, reduce compensatory movements of pelvic obliquity and contralateral vaulting, increase walking speed, reduce energy consumption, and improve patient satisfaction [2].

The SCOs are designed to utilize ankle motion, hip motion, or weight bearing to alternate the characteristics of the knee joint between the swing and stance phases of gait. The knee locks during mid stance to create stability, and then releases for swing phase. This technology requires matching the correct SCO components with a specific patient profile. Once selected, gait retraining is frequently indicated, leading to close collaboration between the orthotist and the PT. The therapist must recognize the type of SCO technology being utilized as the triggers that alternate the condition of the knee joint vary by KAFO design.

Ankle-Activated SCO: Ankle-activated (AA) SCOs transition to a locked knee at the conclusion of swing phase, activated by full knee extension in terminal swing and a dorsiflexion moment at initial contact. The unlocking of the knee for swing phase of gait is activated during terminal stance through weight bearing, dorsiflexion, and knee extension.

Given these parameters, a functional range of ankle motion into relative dorsiflexion during terminal stance, and a functional range of motion into full knee extension during terminal swing and terminal stance are required. The use of AA SCOs is precluded by any presentation that compromises the triggers described above. This includes ankle fusion or contracture, frequent changes in stride length, lack of reciprocal gait, spasticity, or frequent exposure to extreme environmental obstacles like stairs and ramps.

Gait training with AA SCOs will focus on releasing the knee into flexion at the end of stance and attaining a locked knee at the conclusion of swing and the transition into stance. The former entails training the patient to roll over the toe of the affected extremity in terminal stance to obtain the necessary ankle dorsiflexion while positioning the knee in full extension. The latter requires that the patient attain full extension in terminal swing and initiate their step with their heel, creating the requisite dorsiflexion moment about the ankle.

Hip-Activated SCO: Hip-activated (HA) SCOs provide a locked knee at mid stance which is activated by full knee extension at initial contact. The swing phase of gait is activated by hip extension combined with full knee extension at terminal stance and pre-swing.

Given these parameters, there are no specific requirements at the ankle joint to activate this class of SCO. However, a functional range of motion into full knee extension during terminal stance is required to trigger the release of the knee joint into flexion, and again at initial contact to activate the stance lock of the unit. In addition, the hip joint must be capable of extension during terminal stance to trigger the knee release. The use of HA SCOs is precluded by any presentation that compromises the triggers described above. This includes contractures of the hip or knee flexors, hamstring spasticity, inconsistent knee extension during terminal swing, or frequent exposure to extreme environmental obstacles likes stairs and ramps.

Gait training with HA SCOs will focus on releasing the knee into flexion at the end of stance by ensuring active hip extension coupled with closed-chain knee extension. In addition, the patient must be trained to attain full extension in terminal swing.

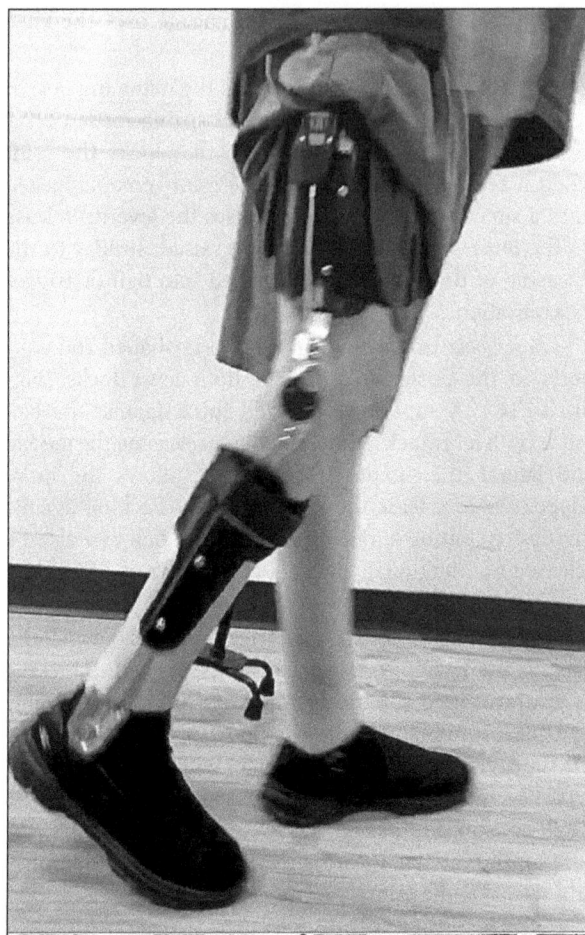

Figure 14.3. Patient walking in a weight-activated stance control orthosis (WA SCO).

Weight-Activated SCO: Weight-activated (WA) SCOs (Figure 14.3) provide a locked knee at mid stance which is activated by weight bearing at initial contact. The swing phase of gait is activated by unweighting the orthosis with the knee extended during terminal stance.

Given these parameters, there are no specific requirements at the ankle joint to activate this class of SCO. However, a functional range of motion into full knee extension during terminal stance is required to trigger the release of the knee joint into flexion once the limb is unweighted. The use of WA SCOs is precluded by any presentation that compromises the activation triggers described above. This includes contractures of the knee flexors.

Gait training with WA SCOs will focus on releasing the knee into flexion at the end of stance by ensuring full knee extension as the orthosis is unweighted.

Orthotronic Mobility System (C Brace®)

Recognized by its more familiar name, the C-Brace®, the Orthotronic Mobility System is not an SCO as the knee joint never locks during gait. Rather, it is controlled by hydraulic resistance. The C-Brace® is a recent advancement in KAFO technology designed around the successful prosthetic component, the C-Leg. As such, it is engineered with a microprocessor-controlled hydraulic knee joint system that allows selective control of knee resistance during both swing and stance phases of gait. This is done according to measured inputs from additional sensors in the KAFO which relay information on the knee angle and ankle movements to on-board microprocessors [3]. In contrast to SCOs, this brace allows functional and safe walking on all terrains and ramps, and allows for descending stairs step over step.

This device requires physical therapy for gait training as well as teaching the various modes of the device and their functional use. This is currently the most technologically advanced system and maximizing its use with training is essential. A recent study reported the C-Brace® reduced falls, and improved balance, mobility, and quality of life in a sample of 102 participants who relied on KAFOs [4].

HKAFOs

The term hip-knee-ankle-foot orthosis, or HKAFO, as it is broadly understood, contains several different classes of devices. The term is often used to include devices that not only cross the hip joint, but extend further superiorly to support the trunk. Two such classes of devices are more accurately termed reciprocating gait orthoses (RGOs) and trunk-hip-knee-ankle-foot orthoses (THKAFOs). The latter may also be referred to using the nomenclature of spinal orthotics, referencing a thoraco-lumbo-sacral-hip-knee-ankle-foot orthosis (TLS-HKAFO).

True HKAFOs are limited to orthoses that cross the hip joint and terminate on a pelvic band worn about the waist. Such devices are generally confined to controlling the alignment of the lower limb in the coronal and transverse planes, as sagittal stabilization of weak or absent hip musculature often requires the extended lever arms associated with trunk stabilization.

Two common HKAFO variants include derotation straps and torsion orthoses. Derotation straps represent a low-profile, lightweight solution to modest internal and external rotation presentations (Figures 14.4A and 14.4B) [5]. Elastic or non-stretch straps are attached proximally to a pelvic band and then wrapped circumferentially down the leg, with the direction of the wrap dependent on the presentation and desired line of pull. In the more common presentation of internal rotation, the straps begin posteriorly at midline on the pelvic band, pass over the greater trochanter and proceed to wrap anteriorly toward the medial aspect of the lower thigh. This wrap direction continues until it terminates distally, either at the patient's shoe or attaching to an AFO.

While this produces a modest corrective external rotation force, the generalized nature of this force cannot

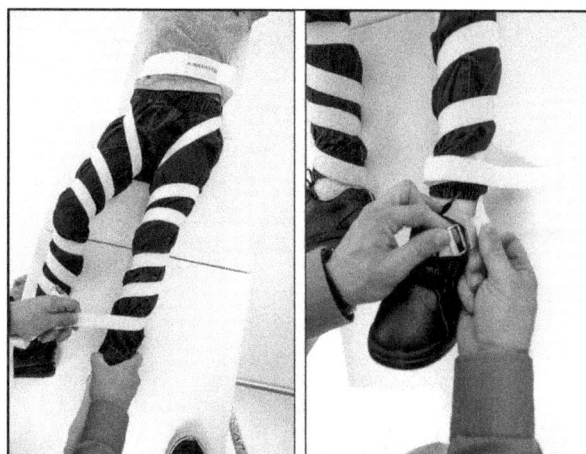

Figure 14.4. Derotation straps attached to a pelvic band.

be targeted to cross a specific segment. Further, because the elastic crosses posterior to the knee, this approach can create undesirable knee flexion forces.

In contrast, torsion orthoses are both heavier and bulkier, but are capable of providing localized derotation forces. This system is comprised of a rigid pelvic band, free motion joints positioned over the hip, knee, and ankle, torsion cables available in different durometers and in certain variations including rigid uprights. Torsion cables provide the desired rotational forces while rigid uprights translate these forces.

THKAFOs

Controlling sagittal alignment across flail hip joints generally requires additional support, extending superiorly to the trunk (Figure 14.5A, B, C). Depending upon the height and weight of the patient, THKAFOs may consist of either bilateral KAFOs or bilateral AFOs connected by lateral uprights to a posterior molded thoracolumbar shell. Locks at the hip and knee stabilize those two joints, but can be released to permit sitting in the orthosis (Figure 14.5C). The corrective hip extension force is a product of the anteriorly directed corrective force over the gluteal area, complemented by a posterior counter force in the form of an anterior strap and pad, generally positioned over the sternum. Ambulation with such devices, if it occurs, is accomplished with upper extremity assistive devices in a swing through fashion.

RGOs

In contrast to THKAFOs, where the hip joints are generally locked to provide static stability, in RGOs (Figure 14.6) the hip joints are connected in such a way that flexion of one hip creates extension of the contralateral hip. While the use of SCOs has been described in conjunction with RGO pelvic sections [6], RGOs are generally a combination of the reciprocating hip mechanism and bilateral KAFOs with locked knee joints.

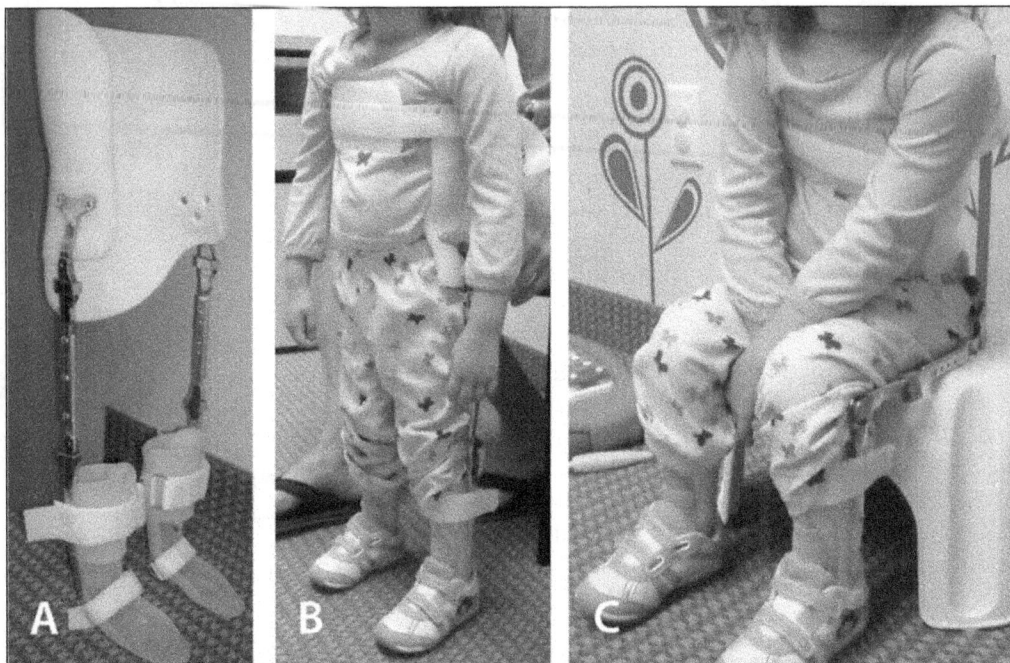

Figure 14.5. THKAFO with molded posterior trunk and pelvic section and locking hip and knee joints. A. undonned, B. locked in standing, and C. locks released to allow sitting.

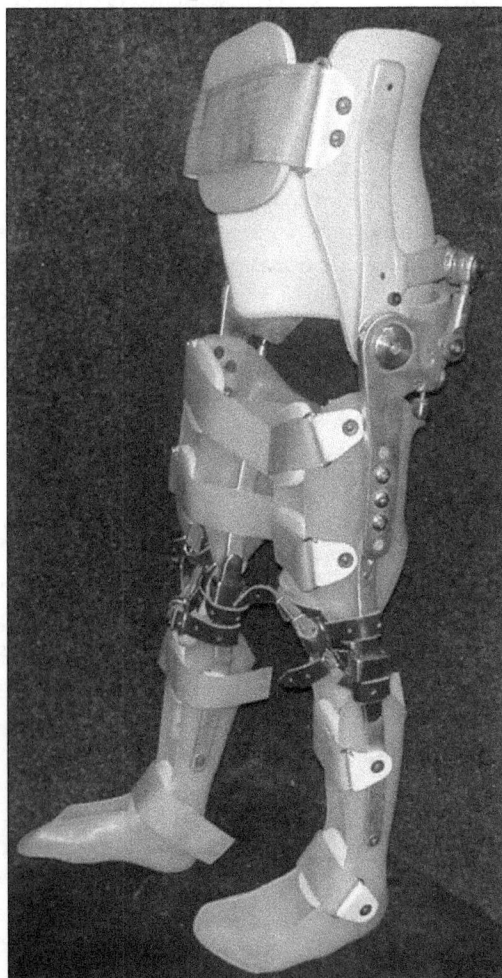

Figure 14.6. RGO with posterior pelvic section, reciprocating hip joint mechanism, drop lock knee joints, and solid ankle.

Patients with active hip flexors can ambulate with these devices by alternately flexing their hips, creating reciprocal contralateral hip extension to provide forward propulsion. However, even patients devoid of hip flexor strength can attain limited ambulation by shifting their trunks posteriorly and side to side, creating the extension movement at alternating hip joints to induce reciprocal hip flexion.

Standing Frames

A number of various standing supports that stabilize the knees and hips have been developed. The parapodium

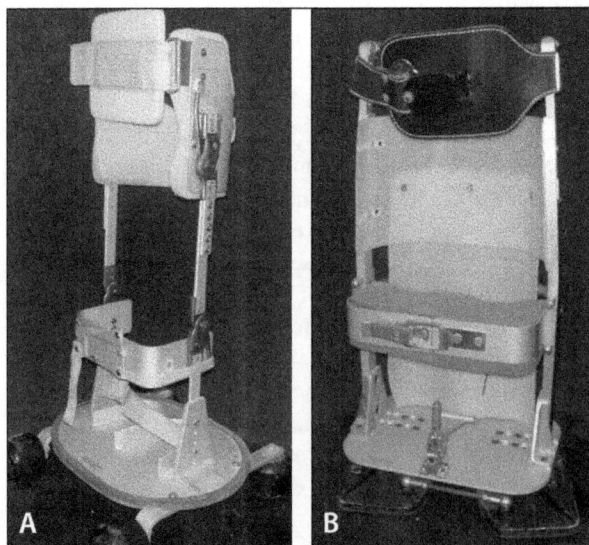

Figure 14.7. A. Parapodium and B. Swivel walker.

is a reasonably lightweight device inclusive of a stable standing base, an anterior bar restraining knee flexion and a pelvic section that provides posterior support against the gluteal area and an anterior support at the sternum (Figure 14.7A). Releases at hip and knee joints permit flexion to allow seating within the device.

The swivel walker is another type of standing support. The stabilizing forces are very similar to those described for the parapodium. However, the construct of the swivel walker does not permit hip or knee flexion (Figure 14.7B). Beneath the standing base is a pair of canted plates connected by a metal rod. The two plates can swivel at their superior attachment point. By shifting their weight from side to side, and generating sagittal propulsion through aggressive arm swinging, users can alternately load the foot plates, swiveling each in their turn and producing a form of reciprocal locomotion.

GENERAL PHYSICAL EXAMINATION CONSIDERATIONS

In addition to population specific considerations (described below), there are a number of general physical examination considerations that apply across the spectrum of impairment presentations and are key to appropriate orthotic design choices and subsequent training.

Strength and Range of Motion

Many advanced lower limb orthoses available today require specific combinations of patient strength and ROM to maximize function. If a patient's physical capabilities do not match the requirements of the orthotic technology, the patient will likely be unable to experience its full benefits regarding function and outcomes. For example, certain SCOs are described as "hip activated," requiring active hip extension to initiate swing phase. If a candidate fit with this technology has a 20° hip flexion contracture, there will be insufficient hip extension for the wearer to initiate swing phase. Lower limb range of motion, including contractures, must be assessed, considered, and accommodated. Moreover, the addition of a strength assessment can assist in determining static standing stability and appropriateness in all KAFO and HKAFO applications.

Postural Assessment

Current and desired posture in both static and dynamic states are important to consider. The patient's posture and postural control will help determine the most appropriate type of orthotic device and the patient's ability to utilize certain technologies. Postural and alignment

considerations will likely guide future therapy and training goals and priorities.

Regarding the contents of this chapter, the most immediate alignment considerations are observed at the knees. Commonly observed deviations include genu varum, genu valgum, genu recurvatum, knee extensor thrust, knee flexion contractures, or anterior knee instability. Additional standing alignment considerations include any observed joint contractures in the lower extremities as well as basic spinal curvature, the presence of scoliosis, leg length discrepancies, pelvic obliquity, postural hip rotations, and internal or external rotational deviations in the lower limb. The postural assessment can assist in determining the optimal goals and intervention options from all domains including medical, therapeutic and orthotic.

Sensation

Sensation encompasses a range of considerations. These include the patient's awareness of light surface touch as well as deep pressure localization. These may have implications for skin and tissue health. Such considerations are especially important in populations such as spinal cord injury and myelomeningocele, where sensory awareness is often compromised or completely absent.

Additional considerations include the patient's proprioception and kinesthetic awareness. From the standpoint of therapy and training, it is important for the PT to understand the extent to which their patient knows the relative position of their lower extremities and can sense movement correctly. Implications may be observed in standing and movement stability and efficiency. Moreover, optimal interventions may be selected when proprioception and kinesthetic awareness are understood.

Tone

In its most simplistic definition, tone can be thought of as a muscle's resistance to passive stretch [7]. The Modified Ashworth Scale for measurement of hypo or hypertonicity is a universally accepted tool and one that allows multidisciplinary communication among practitioners. Within the contents of this chapter, tone is a significant consideration as most SCOs are contraindicated in the presence of significant lower extremity tone.

Balance

Situations leading to the need for lower extremity orthotic use, orthotic management and training can have a considerable impact on balance and balance confidence. Thus, it is important to assess baseline static and dynamic balance with an initial evaluation and monitor improvements with appropriate outcome measures. For example, the Berg Balance Scale, Timed Up and Go, Tinetti Balance

Assessment Tool, or Mini-BESTest can all be used. However, balance and balance confidence should also be subjectively assessed.

Gait

The clinical gait assessment often represents a culmination of the above findings. The use of lower extremity orthoses can make gait safer and more efficient, decrease energy expenditure, improve balance, improve kinetic chain alignment, and provide long-term joint protection. Observational gait analysis should be performed prior to the recommendation of any ambulatory orthosis and should be revisited throughout the associated fitting, training, and follow-up with the device. Gait deviations and compensations should be identified and managed within the limitations and resources of the end user.

Upper Extremity Function

The donning and doffing of KAFOs and HKAFOs can be challenging and requires an acceptable degree of upper extremity strength and dexterity to complete. Hence, upper extremity function should be considered prior to definitive orthotic recommendations. Beyond an assessment of donning and doffing, barriers within the environment could complicate orthotic use. For example, the home should be evaluated for inordinately challenging barriers such as rough or steep yard barriers, tight passageways, slippery flooring, and others. Patients' means to alter their environmental barriers will vary greatly and must be considered when determining the optimal device.

Assistance and the Living Environment

For some patients, independent donning and doffing of KAFOs and HKAFOs is simply an unreasonable expectation. Such patients may still benefit from lower limb orthoses if their living environment includes individuals who are willing and able to assist with this process. Absent such assistance, compliant use with such devices may not be an attainable goal.

Cognition

Many orthotic devices with advanced technology require training to utilize their function. If a patient's cognition is inadequate, the treating therapist will have a difficult time with training and outcomes may not be maximized. General cognitive screening is an important starting point. Referral may be required for more complex cases.

Short- and Long-Term Goals

Patient goals should be the focus of therapy. Partnering with the patient to formulate and direct intervention toward achieving rehabilitation goals can assist with compliance and motivation as well as to help the patient find maximal relevance of the therapy. These are commonly divided into short- and long-term goals. Short-term goals may be achievable within a period of days to weeks whereas long-term goals may be achievable over months or integrated into the patient's activities into the future. Goals may be based on the patient's personal rehabilitation priorities and therapist's clinical assessment and reasonable expectations associated with appropriate orthotic management. An improved gait and exercise program incorporates many forms of exercise, gait, therapeutic, and functional activities related to rehabilitation and integration of the orthosis to optimize safety, function, and quality of life. The collaboratively established goals should play a considerable role in the selection of interventions. Utilization of this protocol provides a thorough, multidisciplinary orthotic rehabilitation approach.

PATIENT POPULATIONS

Adult Populations

Spinal Cord Injury

Bilateral locking KAFOs are frequently prescribed for patients who have experienced complete spinal cord injury in the thoracic or upper lumbar spine. For those patients presenting with flail lower limbs who retain adequate trunk strength, a stable standing alignment with locking KAFOs can be attained by immobilizing the knees and ankles in an alignment that draws the pelvis anterior to the patient's ground reaction force, which can be translated posteriorly by arching the lower back. If the ground reaction force passes behind the patient's hip joint, a stable, passive stance is obtained (Figure 14.8).

Ambulation for such individuals may be achieved using both reciprocal and swing through gait styles. In reciprocal gait, forearm crutches are used for both balance and anterior progression. Once the contralateral arm is advanced with its crutch, hiking the ipsilateral hip allows the hip to flex, responding to the tightness of the hip flexor elements. Once the patient transfers their weight to the leading lower extremity, the advancement of the contralateral arm with its crutch, along with unweighting and, where possible, contralateral hip hiking, allows contralateral hip flexion and contralateral extremity advancement. The cyclical arm swing, hip hiking, and weight shifting create a reciprocal gait pattern.

Swing through ambulation provides another means of forward mobility. Keeping the legs together, the patient these devices is such that, for many patients, the assisted ambulation is viewed as a form of therapy and exercise, and is accordingly limited.

Polio

Due to the aggressive vaccination efforts of the 1950s and 1960s, acute poliomyelitis is rarely encountered in current clinical practice. Polio was declared to be fully eradicated throughout the Americas in 1996 [6]. Globally, as of 2022 to 2023 only Afghanistan and Pakistan had not yet interrupted polio transmission [9]. However, while the management of acute cases is extremely unlikely, for adult survivors who contracted the disease in childhood, substantial physical limitations may persist. In addition, in the decades after the initial onset of the disease, patients may begin to experience new symptoms of muscle weakness in both initially affected and initially unaffected extremities. This increase in disability, experienced well after the initial onset of polio, has been termed post-polio syndrome (PPS). While there is tremendous variability in the physical presentations associated with PPS, the use of KAFOs in these patients has been shown to facilitate increased gait speed, cadence, and step length at reduced oxygen costs [10].

Patients with PPS often present clinically in one of two scenarios. Some present having never worn a lower extremity orthosis or having discontinued use of them in childhood. Now experiencing new weaknesses and limitations, these individuals must confront an illness and associated impairment(s) that they have long felt they had previously overcome. For such individuals, the suggestion of external bracing carries a substantial psychological burden that may initially undermine acceptance and compliance.

In the alternate presentation, individuals may have reached a level of orthosis-assisted function that represents a delicate balance between external stabilization and utilization of remaining muscle function. As this muscle function deteriorates with PPS, that legacy balance is compromised and a new balance must be attained. As with their peers described above, this transition is challenging, both physically and psychologically, and must be approached cautiously and thoughtfully.

Orthoses such as KAFOs may be appropriate for individuals who lack adequate knee extensor strength to control knee-buckling events. They may also be appropriate for individuals who experience knee hyperextension and those with genu varus and valgus deformities. For individuals lacking adequate knee extensor strength, some mechanism of locking the knee is generally indicated [10]. For those individuals presenting with established knee hyperextension, this is often an intended, established compensation for knee extensor weakness. For them, hyperextension provides a measure of sagittal knee stability and should, therefore, be preserved. The use of a KAFO with a

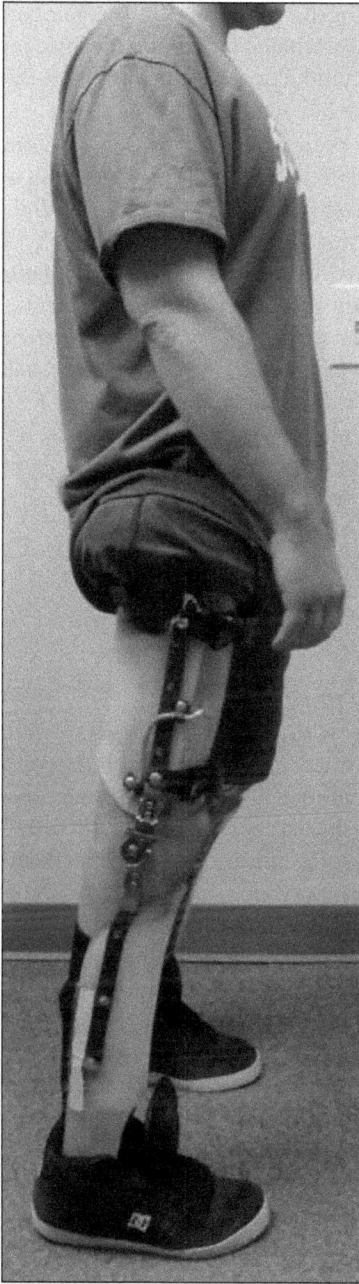

Figure 14.8. Patient with complete spinal cord injury demonstrates stable passive stance with bilateral KAFOs.

advances both crutches, planting them anterior to their feet. Transferring the entirety of their weight to their upper extremities, the patient's lower extremities swing through the body's center of mass, landing anterior to the crutch tips. Cyclical ambulation is attained through the alternating bilateral advancement of the legs and crutches.

Patients who lack trunk stability can be managed with RGOs. While these devices permit reciprocal gait via the mechanisms described earlier, they represent a bulky solution associated with high metabolic energy costs [8]. While sustained daily utilization of bilateral KAFOs and RGOs is possible, the high metabolic costs associated with posterior offset knee joint constructed with a carefully con-sidered sagittal knee angle will permit swing phase flexion while preventing end range hyperextension and associated damage to the posterior knee capsule. Varus and valgus deformities are often the result of intentional, established compensatory strategies. In such cases, a hip rotation pos-ture may allow the knee's collateral ligaments to stabilize it against a buckling event. For such cases, sagittal knee stability must be considered in subsequent KAFO design.

This population has also benefited from the spectrum of SCOs described earlier in the chapter, particularly in unilateral applications. For patients with extreme bilat-eral weakness, the principles of stability and ambulation described for spinal cord injury often apply. HKAFOs are rarely indicated with this pathology.

Stroke

Given the hemiparesis commonly observed post-stroke, the rehabilitation team must often consider the alignment and function of the joints of the affected lower extremity including the knee. Notably, the knee presen-tations most frequently observed following a stroke, a hyperextension thrust or crouched alignment, can often be managed by below-knee orthotic intervention. For example, an AFO that prevents plantarflexion will also dis-courage knee hyperextension in a closed chain alignment. Similarly, an AFO that blocks dorsiflexion of the ankle will stabilize the knee in the sagittal plane against a crouched alignment.

While above-knee solutions are uncommon in stroke rehabilitation, they have been advocated by some centers to address a small range of patient presentations [11]. When utilized in stroke management, KAFOs are largely limited to the acute or subacute stage of rehabilitation when knee extensor weakness is profound, and a patient is otherwise unable to stabilize the affected knee and ankle joint. KAFOs might also be indicated in cases of a domi-nant flexor synergy or genu recurvatum [11].

In contemplating the recommendation of a KAFO, the rehabilitation team should consider: whether or not rapid motor recovery is reasonably expected, the patient's ability to tolerate standing and ambulatory exercises, any substantial cognitive limitations, and the willingness of the patient and family to be compliant with an inherently bulky device [11]. Many patients who initially present with profound knee extensor weakness in the acute phase of their recovery will quickly experience sufficient motor return to obviate the need for a locked KAFO. In those occasions where a KAFO is prescribed, the thigh section and bilateral uprights can be removed later in the rehabili-tation process when an AFO will provide adequate lower extremity support.

Patients presenting with a flail lower extremity pre-disposed toward anterior knee instability may be managed

with a locking KAFO. However, the gait compensations frequently necessitated by locking the knee joint, hip hik-ing, and circumduction, may be prohibitively difficult for a patient with hemiparesis.

Patients presenting with genu recurvatum or a severe hyperextension thrust may be managed with a KAFO with posterior offset free motion knee joints. While this device can be manufactured to prevent knee hyperextension, before proceeding with such a recommendation, the reha-bilitation team should verify that the patient has adequate knee extensor strength to stabilize the extremity that can no longer hyperextend for passive stance stability. In the absence of such strength, constructing a KAFO in slight hyperextension to permit passive stance stability while preventing end range and destructive hyperextension, should be considered.

Pediatric Populations
Myelominigocele

Patients with myelomeningocele can be dichoto-mously classified into those presenting with and those presenting without functional knee extensors. For those with spinal defects approximating or distal to the 4th lumbar level, the knee extensors are likely functional. In such cases, orthotic management can generally be confined to interventions distal to the knee in the form of AFOs that restrict dorsiflexion and thus supplement sagittal knee stability [12]. Exceptions to this generaliza-tion may be encountered among patients who experience appreciable valgus thrust at the knee, a condition that appears to contribute to a high prevalence of knee pain later in life [13]. In such cases, KAFOs with free motion knee joints may be used to mitigate valgus forces acting upon the knee.

For those individuals lacking functional knee exten-sor strength, the level of their spinal lesion proximal to the 4th lumbar vertebra is such that hip extensor strength will also be severely compromised or absent entirely. For these individuals, some form of HKAFO may be utilized. For very young patients, standing frames, parapodiums, and swivel walkers may be used to encourage upright standing and facilitate a form of early ambulation. As children age, more efficient ambulation can be attained including recip-rocal gait with RGOs and swing through gait with THKA-FOs and forearm crutches. While a number of studies have compared these various approaches, there is still no clear consensus on whether anyone is more beneficial than the other [14]. Further, as most children affected at these proximal lesion levels will abandon ambulation during the second decade of life, some centers have chosen to focus on wheelchair-assisted mobility over the cost and effort associated with temporary orthosis-assisted ambulation.

Duchenne Muscular Dystrophy

Duchenne muscular dystrophy is a progressive disorder characterized by gradual increases in lower extremity muscle weakness and lower extremity joint contracture. As long as these young boys are ambulant, daytime bracing should generally be avoided [15]. However, progressive weakness of hip and knee extensors will eventually preclude independent ambulation. At this point, many centers have reported value in coupling surgical releases of hip, knee, and ankle plantarflexion contractures with the immediate introduction of lightweight KAFOs with locking knee joints [15]. If this approach is pursued, the timing of the surgeries and delivery of the orthoses must be closely orchestrated as any prolonged post-surgical immobility can dramatically undermine the success of this approach. Authors have reported that this stage of orthosis-assisted mobility can potentially add an additional 2–4 years of ambulation for affected boys [15].

OTHER HIP AND KNEE ORTHOSES

Hip Orthoses

A number of orthoses have been developed to manage various hip pathologies in both pediatric and adult pathologies. These include hip spica orthoses, generally used in unilateral applications, and hip abduction orthoses, frequently utilized in bilateral applications.

Hip Spica Orthosis

Several pathologies formerly managed with plaster hip spica casts are now frequently managed with hip spica orthoses. These devices are generally non-custom and inclusive of a thermoplastic pelvic module and thigh shell, connected by a lateral upright and hip joint. Hip joints are frequently designed with adjustable joint stops that allow clinicians to determine such considerations as flexion/extension range of motion and abduction angles.

A common application of unilateral hip spica orthoses is to preserve appropriate hip alignment following total hip joint replacement, particularly in cases of revision or complicated primary surgeries [16]. Hip dislocation in the early post-operative period is uncommon, with incidence rates between 2% and 7% [16]. However, the incidence has been observed to increase in revision arthroplasty, with rates between 11% and 14% [16]. The appropriate orthotic management is dependent upon the type of dislocation that the treating clinicians are trying to prevent.

Posterior dislocations occur 85% of the time and are associated with hip flexion, adduction, and internal rotation [16]. Activities commonly associated with posterior dislocations include sitting and reaching towards the uninvolved site, exiting a vehicle, retrieving an object from the floor, and leaning over to tie a shoelace [16]. When managing a hip at risk for posterior dislocation, the hip joint is typically set in 10°–20° of abduction with available hip flexion from 0° to 70°.

Anterior dislocations are much less common, and linked with external rotation and extension. Activities of some risk include reaching up to a high shelf or reaching behind the body in standing while donning a coat [16]. The flexion restrictions at the hip joint of an orthosis are set to allow hip flexion while preventing the final 20° to 40° toward hip extension.

In some cases of lumbosacral spinal instability, a hip spica component is attached to a lumbosacral orthosis to augment the efficacy of the orthosis in stabilizing the lumbosacral spine. However, the need for this hip spica component has been questioned [17].

Hip Abduction Orthoses

While adult-onset hip pathologies are generally managed with unilateral hip spica orthoses, in the pediatric presentation of congenital hip dysplasia, bilateral hip abduction is required. A range of hip abduction orthoses have been developed for these applications. For infants, the Pavlik harness may be used for example. This is a fabric harness that bilaterally cups the individual heel and lower leg, drawing them superiorly through anterior and posterior straps that rest over the shoulders, with a resultant alignment of hip flexion and abduction. For older infants and younger children, a number of hip abduction orthoses have been developed to hold the hips bilaterally in relative hip abduction. These include the Ilfeld hip abduction orthosis [18], the Frejka pillow [19], the Rhino cruiser orthosis, and other related variants.

The Pavlik harness is generally effective as the initial treatment for hip subluxation, dysplasia, and dislocation in infants during the first few months of life [20]. When this treatment fails, or if dysplasia is diagnosed later in infancy, hip abduction orthoses like those mentioned above have provided equivalent results to those observed with the more conventional approach of closed hip reduction and spica casting [18].

Knee Orthoses

The range of orthoses worn at the knee joint can largely be classified into one of three classes. Patella femoral orthoses are a class of relatively low-profile, flexible devices intended to maintain the appropriate alignment of the patellofemoral articulation. Ligament bracing orthoses contain a range of more rigid devices designed to support the architecture and alignment of the anterior cruciate ligament (ACL), posterior cruciate ligament (PCL), medial collateral ligament (MCL), and lateral collateral ligament (LCL). Finally, osteoarthritis knee orthoses are designed to manipulate the coronal alignment of the knee joint to unload either the medial or lateral meniscus.

Patellofemoral

The patellofemoral joint is comprised of the strong quadriceps muscle, acting across the extended lever arm of the femur and pulling through the sesamoid pulley of the patella. The patella, with its distinctive anatomy, articulates against the intercondylar groove of the distal femur, with the dynamic controlling elements of the vastus medialis and medial retinaculum opposing the lateral pull that arises from the Q-angle. Within the range of tracking dysfunctions that can occur, lateral patellar subluxation is the most common. Patellar tracking orthoses are designed to buttress the patella and maintain appropriate tracking at this joint.

Ligament Bracing

The collateral ligaments maintain the knee's coronal alignment, while the cruciate ligaments regulate sagittal translation. Ligament bracing knee orthoses (KOs) can be characterized as prophylactic, rehabilitative, and functional.

Prophylactic KOs remain controversial. Some athletes wear them to prevent injury, primarily to medial knee structures from laterally directed forces as well as hyperextension injuries. Their efficacy has been challenged [21–22] and their use has been associated with increases in foot, ankle and knee injuries, yet they are still used by many athletic programs.

Rehabilitative ligament KOs are off-the-shelf custom fitted orthoses applied to the knee in the immediate aftermath of orthopedic reconstruction procedures. They are not intended for either long term or heavy-duty use. These orthoses frequently feature some mechanism of adjusting available knee range of motion, allowing the surgeon to dictate the available range of motion of the knee immediately after surgery.

Functional post-operative KOs can be custom fitted off-the-shelf, or custom made. These are comparatively expensive, rigid devices designed for elevated activity levels. The intent of this category of KO is to prevent anterior translation of the tibia under the femur, control tibial rotation, and discourage hyperextension. While many end users report subjective improvements in stability and confidence, more objective reviews have been critical of their efficacy [23–24] with one review succinctly summarizing, "bracing after ACL reconstruction does not seem to help with pain, function, rehabilitation, and stability," and that, "the literature does not support the use of a postoperative brace following ACL reconstruction" [23].

Osteoarthritis Bracing

So called "unloader" KOs can be used to manage unicompartmental osteoarthritis (OA) of the knee. The more common presentation is medial OA as the majority of the loading forces occur through this compartment. By creating a corrective three-point pressure system across the knee joint, a KO can shift load-bearing forces to the less affected compartment and create space in the affected joint compartment.

Such orthoses can be generically classified as pre-stressed and thrust. Pre-stressed unloader KOs are frame-based orthoses with bilateral knee joints and uprights contoured to place the knee in relative varus or valgus according to the individual knee presentation. Thrust unloader KOs have a unilateral joint on the side of the knee affected by OA and a dynamic strap that crosses the knee on the contralateral side to create a corrective thrust that will open up the affected joint space. Systematic review has suggested the knee orthoses may be effective in decreasing osteoarthritis-related knee pain, joint stiffness, and drug dosage [25].

SUMMARY

While orthotic management across the knee and hip joints is inherently bulky, when appropriately indicated and properly designed, these devices can enhance the user's functionality. Orthotic management begins with a thorough evaluation, continues with appropriate design, fabrication, and fitting, and is completed with training and measurable outcomes. This process is best realized through multidisciplinary collaboration between the treating physical therapist and orthotist.

REFERENCES

[1]   ABC. *Practice Analysis for Certified Practitioners*, 2022. The American Board for Certification in the Disciplines of Orthotics and Prosthetics. Accessed September 12, 2024. http://www.abc-practitioner-practice-analysis-2022.pdf (abcop.org).

[2]   Zacharias B, Kannenberg A. Clinical benefits of stance control orthosis systems: an analysis of the scientific literature. *J Prosthet Orthot*. 2012;24:2–7.

[3]   DiBello TV, Kelley C, Vallbona C, Kaldis T. Orthoses for persons with postpolio sequalae. In: Hsu JD, Michael JW, Fisk JR, eds. *AAOS Atlas of Orthoses and Assistive Devices*, 2008. 4th edition, pp 419–432. Mosby Elsevier, Philadelphia, PA.

[4]   Ruetz A, DiBello T, Toelle C, et al. A microprocessor stance and swing control orthosis improves balance, risk of falling, mobility, function, and quality of life of individuals dependent on a knee-ankle-foot orthosis for ambulation. *Disabil Rehabil*. 2024 Aug;46(17):4019–4032. Epub September 26, 2023.

[5]   Nuzzo RM. Dynamic bracing: elastics for patients with cerebral palsy, muscular dystrophy and myelodysplasia. *Clin Orthop Relat Res*. 1980;148:263–273.

[6]   Rasmussen AA., Smith KM, Damiano DL. Biomechanical evaluation of the combination of bilateral stance-control knee-ankle-foot

orthoses and a reciprocating gait orthosis in an adult with a spinal cord injury. *J Prosthet Orthot.* 2007;19(2):422–427.

[7] Ganguly J, Kulshreshtha D, Almotiri M, Jog M. Muscle tone physiology and abnormalities. *Toxins* (Basel). 2021 Apr;13(4):282. Published online April 16, 2021.

[8] Arazpour M, Samadian M, Bahramizadeh M, et al. The efficiency of orthotic interventions on energy consumption in paraplegic patients: a literature review. *Spinal Cord.* 2015;53(3):168.

[9] Centers for Disease Control. Morbidity and Mortality Weekly Report (MMWR). Progress toward poliomyelitis eradication—worldwide, January 2022–December 2023 weekly. 2024 May 16;73(19):441–446. Accessed September 17, 2024. Progress Toward Poliomyelitis Eradication—Worldwide, January 2022–December 2023 | MMWR (cdc.gov).

[10] Hachisuka K, et al. Oxygen consumption, oxygen cost and physiological cost index in polio survivors: a comparison of walking without orthosis, with an ordinary or a carbon-fibre reinforced plastic knee-ankle-foot orthosis. *J Rehabil Med.* 2007;39(8):646–650.

[11] Yamanaka T, Akashi T, Ishii M. Stroke rehabilitation and long leg brace. *Top Stroke Rehabil.* 2004;11(3):6–8.

[12] Thomson JD, Ounpee S. Davis RB, DeLuca PA. The effects of ankle-foot orthoses on the ankle and knee in persons with myelomeningocele: an evaluation using three-dimensional gait analysis. *J Pediatr Orthop.* 1999;19(1):27–33.

[13] Williams JJ, Graham GP, Dunne KB, Menelaus MB. Late knee problems in myelomeningocele. *J Pediatr Orthop.* 1993; 13:701–703.

[14] Mazur JM, Kyle S. Efficacy of bracing the lower limbs and ambulation training in children with myelomeningocele. *Dev Med Child Neurol.* 2004;46(5):352–356.

[15] Stevens PM. Lower limb orthotic management of Duchenne muscular dystrophy: a literature review. *J Prosthet Orthot.* 2006;18(4):111–119.

[16] Lima D. Orthoses in total joint replacement. In: Hsu JD, Michael JW, Fisk JR, eds. *AAOS Atlas of Orthoses and Assistive Devices*, 2008. 4th edition, pp. 373–378. Mosby Elsevier, Philadelphia, PA.

[17] Axelsson, P, Johnsson R, Strömqvist B. Lumbar orthosis with unilateral hip immobilization: effect on intervertebral mobility determined by roentgen stereophotogrammetric analysis. *Spine.* 1993;18(7):876–879.

[18] Sankar WN, Nduaguba A, Flynn JM. Ilfeld abduction orthosis is an effective second-line treatment after failure of Pavlik harness for infants with developmental dysplasia of the hip. *J Bone Joint Surg Am.* 2015;97(4):292–297.

[19] Lempicki A, Wierusz-Kozlowska M, Kruczynski J. Abduction treatment in late diagnosed congenital dislocation of the hip: follow-up of 1,010 hips treated with the Frejka pillow 1967–76. *Acta Orthopaedica Scandinavica.* 1990;236:1–30.

[20] McClure SK, Tosi LL. Pediatric hip orthoses. In: Hsu JD, Michael JW, Fisk JR, eds. *AAOS Atlas of Orthoses and Assistive Devices*, 2008. 4th edition, pp. 465–479. Mosby Elsevier, Philadelphia, PA.

[21] Salata, MJ, Gibbs AE, Sekiya JK. The effectiveness of prophylactic knee bracing in American football: a systematic review. *Sports Health.* 2010;2(5):375–379.

[22] Pietrosimone BG, Grindstaff TL, Linens SW, et al. A systematic review of prophylactic braces in the prevention of knee ligament injuries in collegiate football players. *J Athl Train.* 2008;43(4):409–415.

[23] Rodríguez-Merchán, EC. Knee bracing after anterior cruciate ligament reconstruction. *Orthop.* 2016;39(4):e602–e609.

[24] Birmingham TB, et al. A randomized controlled trial comparing the effectiveness of functional knee brace and neoprene sleeve use after anterior cruciate ligament reconstruction. *Am J Sports Med.* 2008;36(4):648–655.

[25] Raja K, Dewan N. Efficacy of knee braces and foot orthoses in conservative management of knee osteoarthritis: a systematic review. *Am J Phys Med Rehabil.* 2011;90(3):247–262.

CHAPTER 15

Spinal Orthotics

C. Leigh Davis and Kristen Howell

OBJECTIVES

Upon completing this chapter, the reader should:
1. Understand common spinal pathologies necessitating orthotic treatment.
2. Recall basic indications, contraindications, and mechanics of spinal orthoses.
3. Recall therapeutic implications of spinal pathologies and orthotic usage.
4. Understand the role of chest orthoses for pectus carinatum.
5. Understand benefits from the partnership between orthotist and therapist for management success.

INTRODUCTION

Spinal bracing is typically utilized for one of three main goals: stabilization after fracture or surgery, prevention of worsening of scoliosis or kyphosis curvature, or pain management. Chest orthoses may be used to reduce chest deformity. Physical therapy (PT) is frequently prescribed in conjunction with bracing to facilitate compliance with bracing or further address the goals of bracing from a therapeutic exercise approach.

Spinal orthoses are named for the parts of the spine they cover. A cervical orthosis (CO) covers the cervical spine only, such as a cervical collar. CTOs, cervical thoracic orthoses, include an extension onto the chest. Examples of CTOs include the Minerva or SOMI (suboccipital mandibular orthoses). Most cervical collars can also have a thoracic extension added to extend coverage to the low cervical and upper thoracic spine. Thoracolumbar sacral orthoses (TLSOs) are the most typical "back brace." These extend from the sternal notch to the symphysis pubis anteriorly and from the mid-scapulae to mid-gluteal region posteriorly. The design varies greatly based on the goals. Scoliosis braces are considered TLSOs although the anterior trimline is at the xiphoid rather than the sternal notch. They extend higher lateral and posterior to affect the thoracic spine. For lower injuries and for low back pain, an LSO (lumbosacral orthosis) may be used. The superior trimline on an LSO is lower than a TLSO; LSOs terminate around the xiphoid anteriorly and inferior to the scapulae posteriorly.

DOI: 10.4324/9781003526025-17

Scoliosis Orthoses

Scoliosis is lateral curvature of the spine greater than 10° with rotation toward the convexity of the curve. Scoliosis is classified by cause and by age at diagnosis. Congenital scoliosis is caused by vertebral anomaly such as hemivertebra. Neuromuscular scoliosis is associated with pathology of the stabilizing muscles of the spine such as cerebral palsy or spinal cord injury [1]. The most common type is idiopathic scoliosis, where there is no known cause. Idiopathic scoliosis is further categorized by age groups. Onset before age 4 is classified as Infantile Scoliosis. Juvenile Scoliosis occurs between 4 and 9 years old. Adolescent Scoliosis develops at age 10 and older [2].

Scoliosis is measured via Cobb angle. The Cobb angle is the angle between a line drawn on the superior endplate of the most tilted, most superior vertebra and a line drawn on the inferior endplate of the most tilted, most inferior vertebra (Figure 15.1). When reviewing a scoliosis X-ray, decompensation and Risser sign should also be assessed. Decompensation, or frontal plane imbalance is the displacement of the C7 vertebra from the central sacral line. The Risser sign is a sign of skeletal maturity viewed by looking at the ossification of the iliac crests. Risser is from 0–5, with all young children being 0 and all adults being 5. During adolescence, the Risser sign progresses from lateral to medial from 1 to 4 and then fuses to become 5 (Figure 15.2).

Biomechanics of Scoliosis Braces

The goal of scoliosis bracing and PT for scoliosis is to prevent progression of the curvature in the growing child. When children grow, particularly during the rapid growth of the adolescent "growth spurt," spinal curvature tends to worsen. Factors associated with increased risk of progression include skeletal immaturity (measured by age, Risser sign, Sanders scale, and onset of menses in females), curve location, curve type, and curve magnitude. Still other considerations may include axial rotation, gender, and family history. Thoracic primary curves and double curves are more likely to progress than lumbar or thoracolumbar. Larger magnitude curves are more likely to progress than smaller. Management decisions are made based on assessment of the risk of progression for each individual. In general, for patients with growth remaining, the Scoliosis Research Society treatment recommendations are as follows [3]:

- Curve <20°: observation
- Curve 20–45°: bracing
- Curve >45°: surgery

PT can be prescribed for curves of any magnitude. PT intervention can be initiated prior to bracing in an effort to halt curve progression before it reaches 20°, in

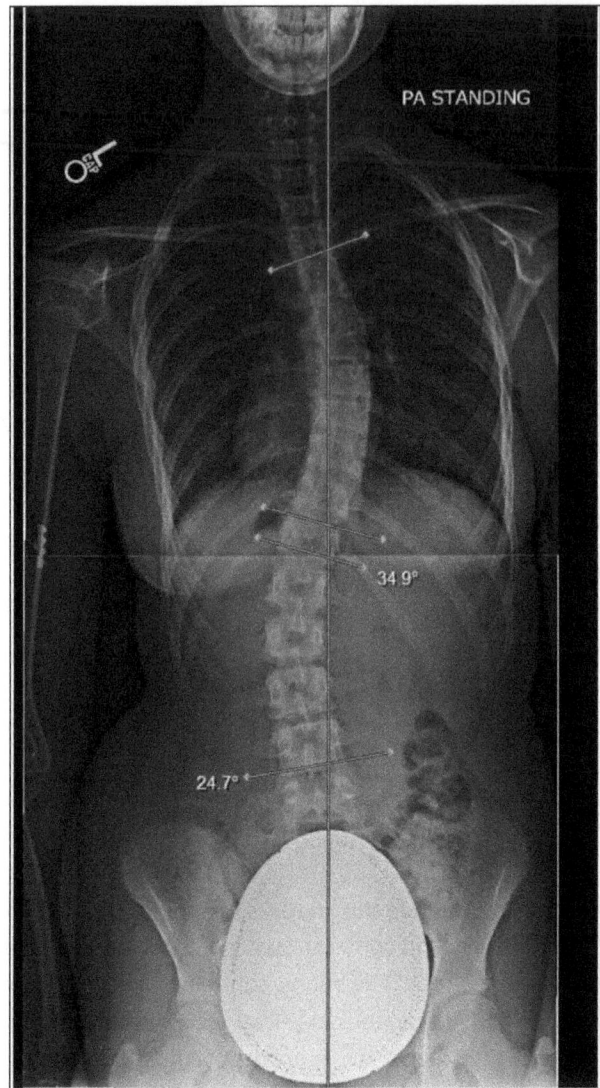

Figure 15.1. X-ray of scoliosis patient. The Cobb angle is the angle between the most superior most tilted vertebra and the most inferior most tilted vertebra.

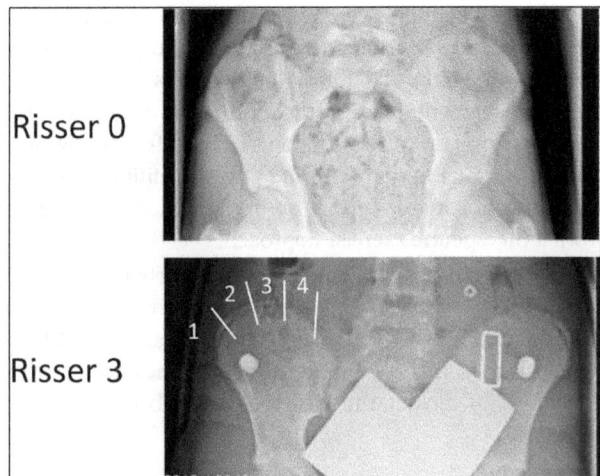

Figure 15.2. X-ray of iliac crests depicting Risser sign, a common indicator of skeletal maturity.

conjunction with bracing for curves between 20° and 45° to facilitate compliance with bracing and minimize curve progression, or to minimize the effect of associated impairments in curves greater than 45° if a patient cannot or chooses not to undergo surgical intervention. Traditional PT can be utilized to address symmetrical impairments in muscle strength, range of motion, or function. However, literature suggests that physiotherapeutic scoliosis-specific exercise (PSSE) may be more effective than traditional PT at addressing the specific (and often asymmetrical) impairments caused by scoliosis [4]. The International Scientific Society on Scoliosis Orthopaedic and Rehabilitation Treatment (SOSORT) has published guidelines for the conservative management of scoliosis and recommends that PT treatment for scoliosis include three-dimensional auto-correction, training in ADLs, stabilizing the corrected posture, and patient education [5]. They also recommend that PSSEs be used "as the first step to treat idiopathic scoliosis" to accomplish the aforementioned goals (Figure 15.3). The goal of bracing for scoliosis is to three-dimensionally correct the spine using a passive positioning approach. The goals of exercise are the same; however, here an active approach to correction of the curvature is used to strengthen the stabilizing muscles of the spine and prevent progression of the curvature.

There are many brace types that can be used for scoliosis management. All aim to reduce spinal curvature and misalignment while the brace is on (known as in-brace correction) with the overall goal of preventing worsening of the curve. Scoliosis is a tri-planar deformity, and brace corrective force systems are designed with this in mind. The focus and mechanism of correction varies with brace type, but generally speaking all spinal braces aim to reduce the following [6]:

1) lateral vertebral displacement from the central sacral line
2) vertebral rotation about the longitudinal axis
3) vertebral lateral tilt (Cobb)
4) abnormal curvature in the sagittal plane.

Three-point pressure systems and force couples are integrated into the orthosis to provide these corrective forces (Figures 15.4 and 15.5).

Due to variability among bracing studies, there was still dissention in the orthopedic community prior to 2013 about the efficacy of scoliosis bracing for preventing curve progression. In 2013 the results from the first randomized, controlled, multicenter trial for scoliosis treatment were

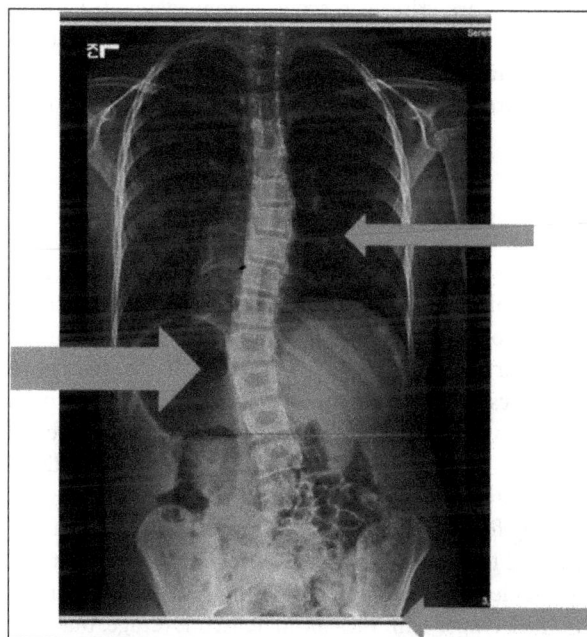

Figure 15.4. Free body diagram illustrating a TLSO three-point pressure system in the coronal plane.

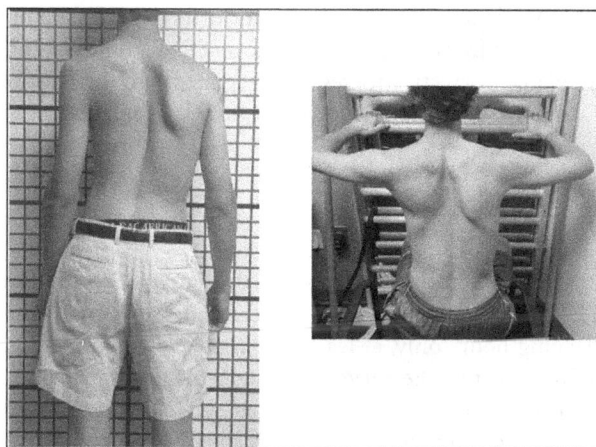

Figure 15.3. A. A 17-year-old patient with adolescent idiopathic scoliosis at his initial PT evaluation. He presented with a 48° right thoracic curvature. Surgery was recommended by his orthopedist but the family did not wish to pursue surgery and instead chose conservative management with bracing and PT at the time of his PT evaluation. B. Same patient while performing Schroth exercises, a type of physiotherapeutic scoliosis-specific exercise. This is an example of PT intervention for patients with idiopathic scoliosis.

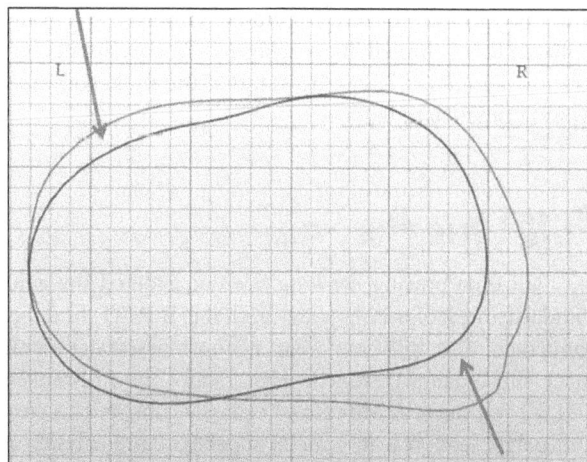

Figure 15.5. Free body diagram illustrating a TLSO force couple system in the transverse plane.

published convincingly showing that bracing changes the natural history of scoliosis. This study, known as the Bracing in Adolescent Idiopathic Scoliosis Trial (BrAIST) was a 25-site study of 242 subjects; 146 subjects received a brace. The brace type was left to the discretion of the treatment team, but all were full-time braces and all subjects were prescribed 18+ hours per day wear. Compliance with prescribed wear was monitored via an imbedded temperature sensor. Treatment success was defined as skeletal maturity without curve progression to 50° or more and without surgery. The trial was stopped early due to efficacy of bracing. Overall, 72% of patients who were braced had a successful outcome compared with 48% of patients observed. The temperature data also verified the dose-response of brace treatment, with more wear highly correlated to higher success. For patients who wore their braces more than 12.9 hours per day, success with treatment was 90–93% [7]. These data are critical to scoliosis management. Patients and families must understand that the most important factor affecting successful treatment is how many hours per day the brace is worn.

Scoliosis Brace Types

There are numerous types of scoliosis orthoses. They are typically named for the city where they were developed or for the developer. Although each has its nuances, the important thing is that all braces utilize sound spinal mechanics to address all aspects of the scoliosis deformity. The focus varies from brace to brace, between different orthotists, and is dependent on each patient's individual presentation. Full-time braces have the advantage of allowing for longer wear time during the day, but must be trimmed to allow comfortable sitting and movement and acceptable appearance under clothing. Night-time braces can have longer trimlines for increased leverage, but wear is limited to hours during sedentary activity (sleeping and homework/TV/computer time). Some patients can be treated with both a day brace optimized for upright wear and a night brace for sleeping hours. However, the availability of this is limited due to insurance and payment constraints. Discussed below are some of the most common types in practice today.

Full-Time Bracing

Full-time bracing has long been considered the gold standard for scoliosis bracing, and the BrAIST findings confirmed that full-time wear is most associated with successful bracing treatment. Historically, the Milwaukee CTLSO was used. A Milwaukee orthosis consists of a custom pelvic section with a metal superstructure extending up to the cervical spine. Corrective pads are affixed to the

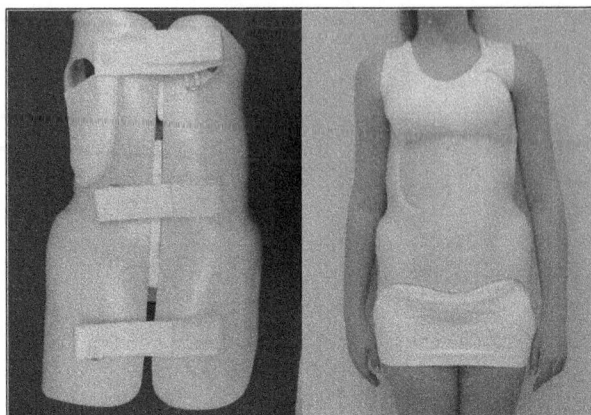

Figure 15.6. Posterior (A) and anterior (B) views of the Boston TLSO.

metal superstructure. With the cervical ring extending up out of the wearer's clothing, this brace is not well accepted by adolescents. In the 1970s, with the onset of thermoplastic usage in orthotics, the Boston TLSO was developed, and it remains the most commonly used full-time brace today (Figure 15.6). The Boston is a rigid plastic TLSO made from measurements, cast, or digital scan. Standard Boston TLSOs are made using the principles in the Boston handbook [8]. Measurements are taken and a symmetric model is created. The corrective forces are added via padding glued into the brace during the fitting process. The majority of the orthoses in the BrAIST study were Boston-style TLSOs. Many orthotists make their own version of a Boston TLSO blending the principles of the Boston brace handbook with knowledge of spinal mechanics and their own experience. Scanning and CAD/CAM technologies may also be used in shape capture and fabrication for the Boston Brace [9].

In recent years, European style asymmetric bracing has gained traction, particularly the Rigo-System Cheneau (RSC) orthosis. These are also plastic orthoses and are typically made from a digital scan. The opening is anterior and tri-planar corrective forces are integrated into the plastic. Corrective pads may be added for increased correction.

Night-time Braces

Night-time braces, such as the Providence (Figure 15.7) or Charleston TLSOs (Figure 15.8), are worn during sleeping hours only, at least 8 hours per night. They aim to hypercorrect the curve, taking advantage of the recumbent position. Night braces are assumed to have improved compliance and less impact on quality of life as the recommended wear time is significantly lower than full-time braces and does not include school hours. They are best indicated for small magnitude curves and for single curves. The treatment success rate for the Providence is up to 70% for curves under 35° and for lumbar or thoracolumbar curves [10–12]. There is limited literature to support the use of night braces for curves over 35° [10, 13].

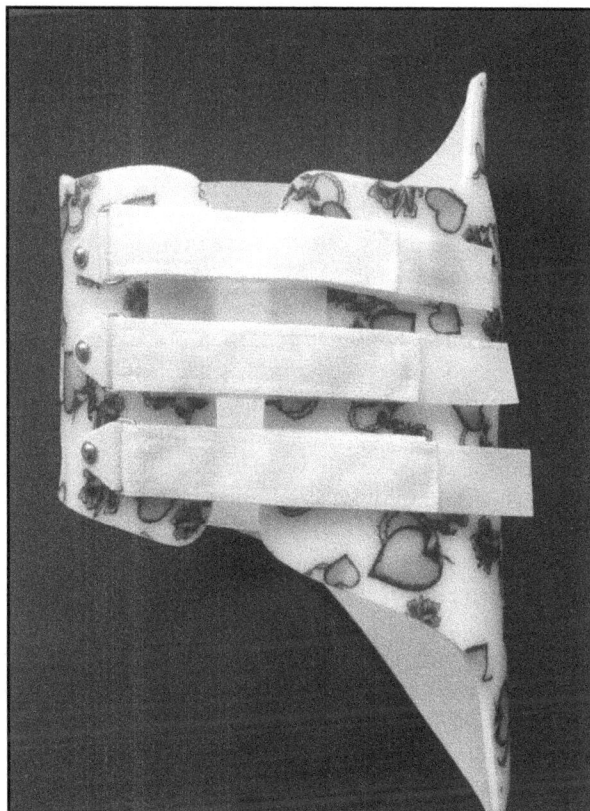

Figure 15.7. The Providence TLSO.

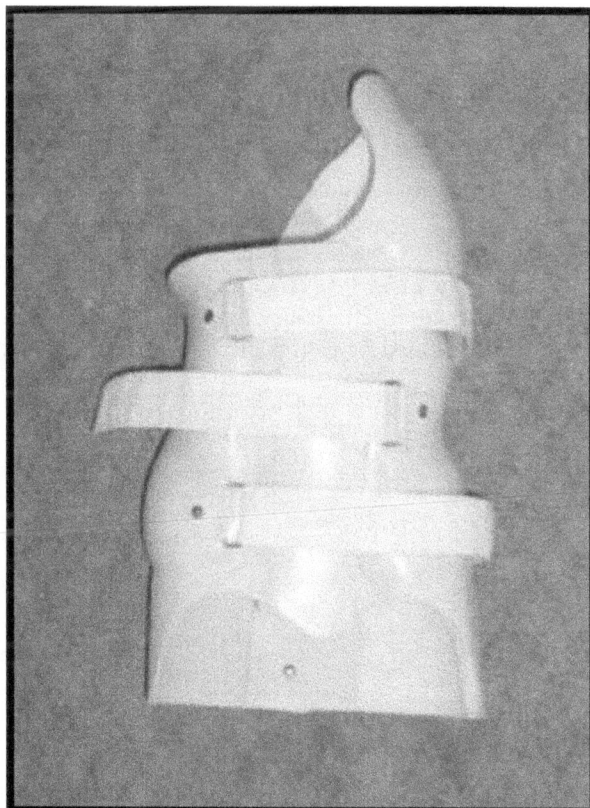

Figure 15.8. The Charleston TLSO.

KYPHOSIS ORTHOSES

Kyphosis of 20°–40° is the normal alignment of the thoracic spine in the sagittal plane. However, it can become excessive in cases of severe postural hyperkyphosis or Scheuermann's disease. Postural hyperkyphosis is frequently associated with shoulder/scapular protraction resulting in over-lengthening and muscle weakness in the back/scapular musculature as well as muscle restrictions/tightness in the anterior chest wall or pectoral musculature. Scheuermann's disease is a severe form of hyperkyphosis with no known cause in which structural changes accompany postural impairments. To be diagnosed as Scheuermann's, the kyphosis must measure >40° on a sagittal radiograph and there must be ≥5° wedging in three or more adjacent vertebrae (Figure 15.9). The Scoliosis Research Society recommends full-time bracing for kyphosis curves >60° of either etiology. PT should always accompany orthotic treatment of hyperkyphosis to address the associated physical impairments and potentially increase effectiveness/tolerance to bracing [14].

Kyphosis orthoses are TLSOs with an anterior corrective pad to apply a posteriorly directed force to reduce thoracic kyphosis. They are similar to Boston TLSOs in design and materials. The posterior trimline terminates just inferior to the apex of the kyphosis. The anterior corrective pad is over the sternum as high as possible, which is typically ½ inch inferior to the sternal notch (Figure 15.10). The molded plastic of the TLSO aims to reduce the patient's lumbar lordosis as well, as this tends to flatten the entire spine and is an indirect mechanism to reduce kyphosis. Full time wear, 16–20 hours per day, is thought to be necessary as the orthoses effect the most change in posture during upright wear [14]. Kyphosis naturally reduces when lying down. Patients must present for follow-up regularly, at which the anterior pad can be increased or angled posteriorly to static-progressively increase the correction. With compliance with wear time, these patients can have lasting correction in their curvature.

For less severe postural kyphosis, soft bracing may be considered. These are corset-style orthoses with delto-pectoral straps aimed to encourage a more upright posture. Although these orthoses can have an apparent improvement in standing posture, the lasting effects are questionable. Prolonged use of corset-style bracing can weaken core muscle strength. Therefore, this type of orthosis could worsen the problem over time. When significant postural kyphosis is associated with pain, a corset-type TLSO may be used for pain relief for a limited length of time. PT is especially important in this situation to address the pain and improve the patient's quality of life in addition to strengthening the core musculature to prevent the potential adverse effects of corset-style bracing.

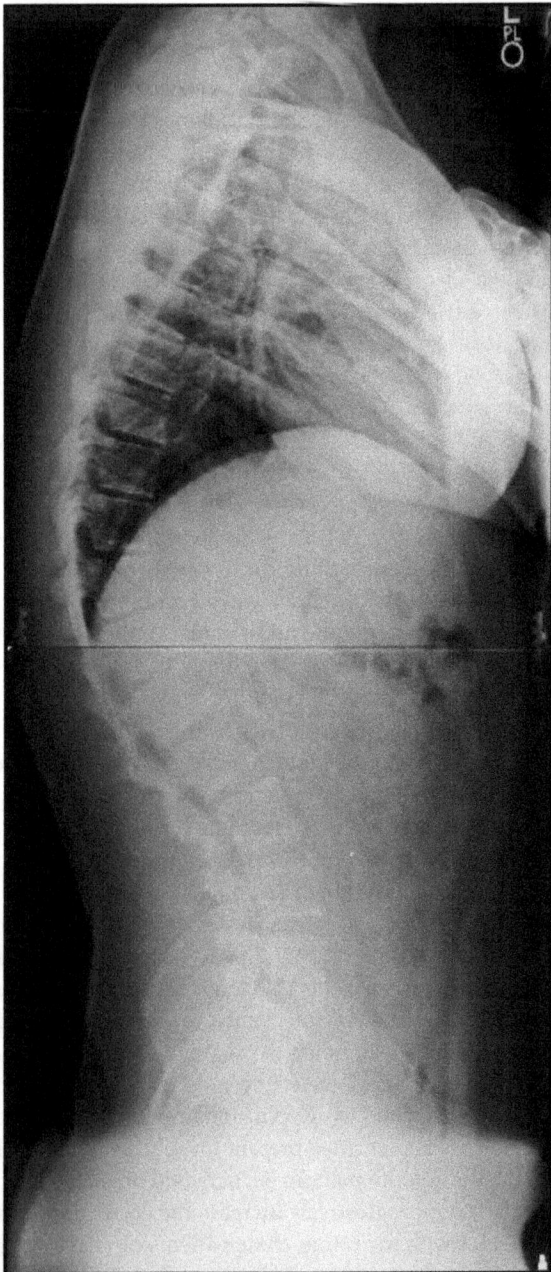

Figure 15.9. Radiograph showing hyperkyphosis.

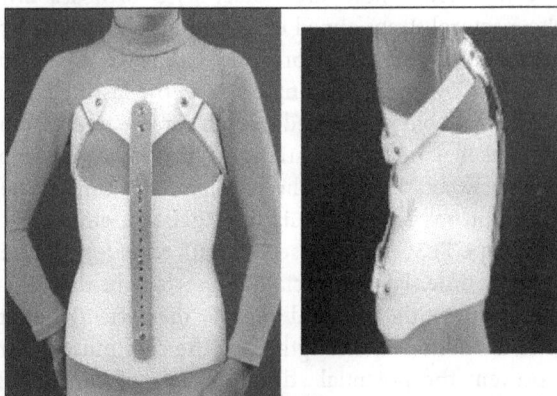

Figure 15.10. Kyphosis TLSO with corrective anterior chest pad (anterior and sagittal views).

Pectus Carinatum Orthoses

Pectus carinatum is a protrusion of the sternum most often seen in adolescent males. It can be idiopathic or may be associated with other skeletal conditions such as Marfan's disease. Many patients have no other symptoms with pectus carinatum, but some experience shortness of breath. If the deformity is flexible, meaning that external force can reduce the protrusion, then bracing treatment is recommended. Corrective forces are applied directly to the protrusion via plastic pads affixed to metal bars (Figure 15.11). The patient can tighten the corrective pad to their maximum tolerable force. In the absence of a study quantifying the minimum wear time necessary for change, most physicians and orthotists opt for a "more is better" approach. The wear time most commonly recommended in the literature is the Calgary protocol: 23 hours per day until flattening of the protrusion, then 8 hours per day maintenance until skeletal maturity [15]. Bracing and/or surgery are the preferred treatment for pectus carinatum deformities. If PT intervention is recommended for this patient population, it is typically aimed at improving postural impairments and respiratory capacity.

The goal of pectus carinatum bracing is lasting reduction of the deformity. The success with this is variable in the literature, but generally high at between 67% and 100% [16–18]. One article also found that self-esteem was increased with successful bracing treatment [18].

Spinal Injury Orthoses

Spinal injuries including fractures and ligamentous injuries reduce the stability of the spine and necessitate external support. Orthoses can be used pre-operatively, post-operatively, or in lieu of surgery depending on the severity and location of the injury. Even with stable injuries, orthoses may be used for pain management. If the orthotic

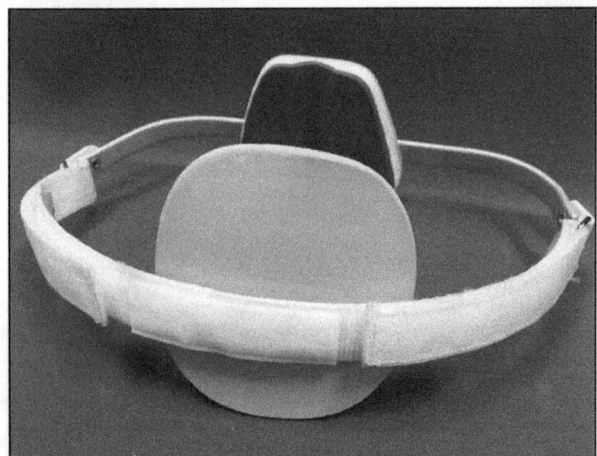

Figure 15.11. Pectus carinatum orthosis.

goal is pain management, softer foam or fabric solutions may be utilized. Injuries that are unstable or have a high risk of neurologic compromise require more rigid materials.

Cervical and Cervical Thoracic Orthoses

The neck is the most mobile area of the spine, and thus most prone to injury. Instability of the cervical spine is treated very cautiously due to the catastrophic effects of a spinal cord injury in the cervical spine.

Generally, longer and more rigid orthoses provide increasing range of motion restriction. Halo treatment provides the most control, eliminating 90–95% of the motion of the cervical spine [19]. However, halo treatment requires pins to be inserted through the skin into the skull, increasing the risk of complications such as pin site infection. Motion at the upper cervical spine including the atlanto-occiptal joint and down to C2 is best limited by halo treatment [20]. Rigid collars (Figure 15.12) are used for unstable cervical spine injuries C2–C5 [20]. Rigid cervical collars limit 65–75% of cervical flexion/extension and rotation, but may allow up to 65% of normal lateral bending. Collars are available off the shelf from a variety of manufactures. Correct sizing is important for proper ROM limitation. Soft foam collars are appropriate for pain relief only as they only restrict about 20% of normal range of motion [19]. For injuries C5–T7, thoracic extensions for cervical collars and CTOs such as Minerva orthoses provide increased leverage for ROM restriction in the cervical spine and upper thoracic spine [20]. The amount of restriction provided by these devices varies greatly across devices and is dependent on appropriate fitting and donning of the chest piece.

TLSOs

TLSOs are used for injuries T6–L3 [20]. They may be frame-type or total contact. Frame-type designs are off the shelf and used for single plane injuries. Compression fractures limited to the anterior column from T10 to T12 may be treated with extension frame TLSOs such as the Jewett (Figure 15.13) or cruciform anterior spinal hyperextension (CASH) orthoses [20]. These provide a simple three-point force system to extend the spine and unload the anterior structures. The corrective force is posterior near the level of the waist and counter forces are anterior near the

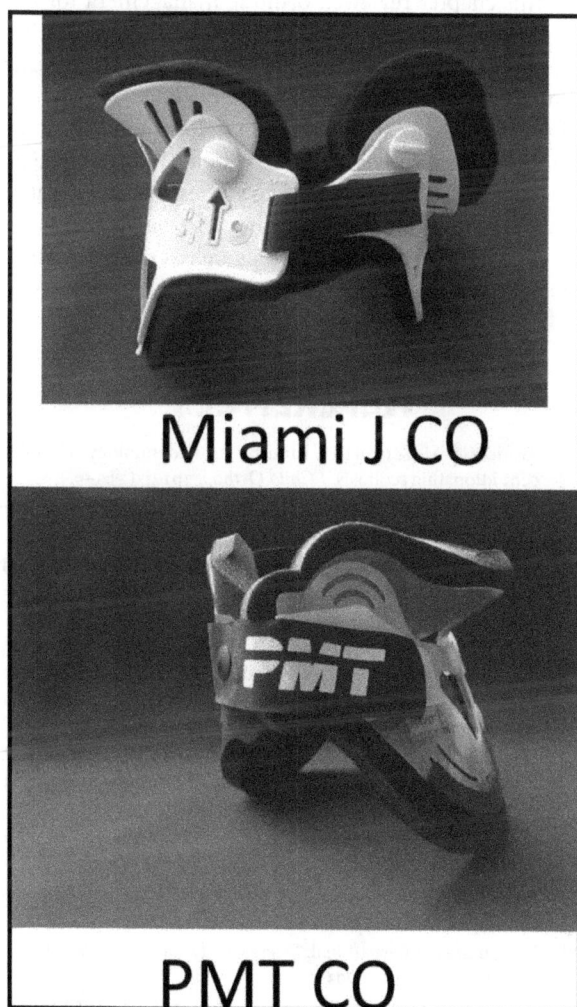

Figure 15.12. A. Miami J rigid cervical collar. B. PMT rigid cervical collar.

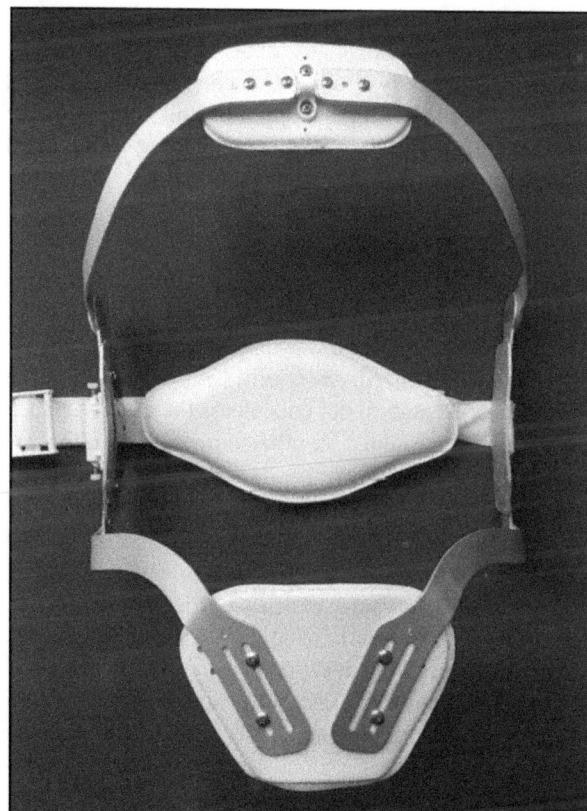

Figure 15.13. Jewett Hyperextension TLSO used primarily for anterior column compression fractures.

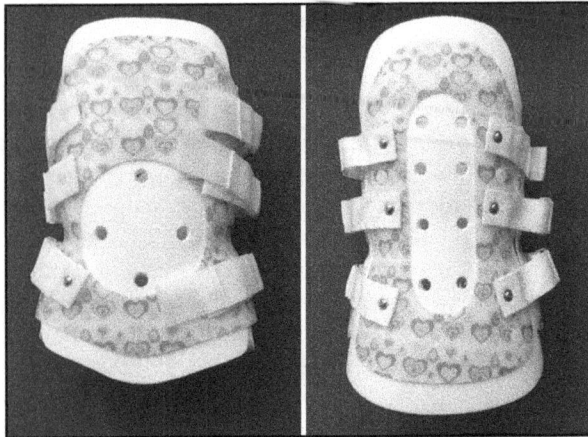

Figure 15.14. Anterior and posterior views of a total contact plastic and foam TLSO. This type of TLSO provides tri-planar control of the spine from T7 to L3. A hip extension could be added for control for L4–L5.

sternal notch and symphysis pubis. For multiplane fractures such as burst fractures or unstable injuries, a circumferential total contact plastic TLSO (Figure 15.14) provides increased ROM restriction in flexion/extension, lateral bending, and rotation. These are most often foam-lined and two pieces with lateral openings and Velcro® straps. These may be custom made to cast, scan, or measurement, or customized from pre-made models. Pre-made TLSOs have the advantages of being less costly and more rapidly fabricated, but can also be less comfortable. Patients with asymmetry from scoliosis or other spine deformity are not candidates for modular TLSOs. Pediatric patients almost always require custom-made TLSOs. Injuries above T7 require the addition of a cervical component (CTLSO). Injuries of the lower lumbar spine L4 and L5 require the addition of hip ROM restriction by adding a unilateral thigh cuff (TLSO with thigh extension) [20].

LSOs

For injuries isolated to the lumbar spine, lower profile devices may be utilized. Anteriorly, LSOs terminate at the xiphoid process and do not encompass the chest. Again, a thigh cuff must be added for restriction of ROM in the low lumbar levels.

Spondylolysis and spondylolisthesis are injuries of the pars interarticularis usually at the L4 or L5 levels. The mechanism of injury is repeated stress in extension and is commonly seen in young athletes, particularly gymnasts. Rest and PT as well as bracing are indicated treatments. For spondylolysis without slippage, a corset-type brace can be used. For spondylolisthesis with slippage, greater ROM restriction is achieved with an LSO. A Boston Overlap Brace (BOB) is a typical LSO for spondylolisthesis. This is an anterior opening circumferential brace made from semi-rigid plastic. The goal of bracing in spondylolysis and spondylolisthesis is to restrict extension ROM. LSOs are made in

reduced lumbar lordosis to reduce anterior pelvic tilt and offload the posterior aspects of the vertebrae for healing.

Corsets

Lumbar back pain is a very common complaint affecting nearly 80% of adults. It is a significant cause of disability and the leading contributor to missed workdays [21]. Corsets are often prescribed during periods of acute back pain for pain relief and kinesthetic reminder to reduce range of motion. They may increase intracavity pressure, offloading the spine, but this theory is not well confirmed. Again, as prolonged use of corsets may weaken the abdominal musculature, it is important that they are used for limited length of time and in conjunction with PT to address the underlying cause of pain [20]. Short-term usage does not reduce muscle strength [22].

SUMMARY

This chapter reviewed orthotic management for scoliosis, hyperkyphosis, spine injuries, and pectus carinatum. For all spinal pathologies, orthoses apply external corrective forces to reduce asymmetry or to provide stability. Adequate wear time is essential for either goal. PT techniques are aimed at teaching patients to reproduce the corrective forces actively and at addressing concomitant impairments. Optimal patient care relies on close collaboration between orthotist and PT, as well as the other members of the patient's care team.

REFERENCES

[1] Konieczny M, Senyurt H, Krauspe R. Epidemiology of adolescent idiopathic scoliosis. *J Child Orthop.* 2013;7(1):3–9.

[2] Scoliosis Research Society. Scoliosis, 2023. Accessed September 17, 2024. http://www.srs.org/patients/conditions/scoliosis.

[3] Rowe DE. *The Scoliosis Research Society Brace Manual,* 2003. Accessed January 12, 2019. http://www.srs.org/UserFiles/file/bracing-manual/section1.pdf.

[4] Negrini S, Zaina F, Romano M, et al. Specific exercises reduce brace prescription in adolescent idiopathic scoliosis: a prospective controlled cohort study with worst-case analysis. *J Rehabil Med.* 2008;40(6):451–455.

[5] Negrini S, Donzelli S, Aulisa AG, et al. 2016 SOSORT guidelines: orthopaedic and rehabilitation treatment of idiopathic scoliosis during growth. *Scoliosis Spinal Disord.* 2018;13(3).

[6] Carlson JM. Clinical biomechanics of orthotic treatment of idiopathic scoliosis. *J Prosthet Orthot.* 2003;15(4S):17–30.

[7] Weinstein S, Dolan L, Wright J. Effects of bracing in adolescents. *New Engl J Med.* 2013;369(16):1512–1521.

[8] Boston Brace International. *Reference Manual for the Boston Scoliosis Brace.* Boston, 2003.

[9] Boston Orthotics and Prosthetics. Boston Brace 3D Scoliosis Brace. Accessed September 17, 2024. https://www.bostonoandp.com/products/scoliosis-and-spine/boston-brace-3d/.

[10] D'Amato C, Griggs S, McCoy B. Nighttime bracing with the Providence brace in adolescent girls with idiopathic scoliosis. *Spine.* 2001;26(18):2006–2012.

[11] Yrjonen T, Ylikoski M, Schlenzka D, et al. Effectiveness of the Providence nighttime bracing in adolescent idiopathic scoliosis: a comparative study of 36 female patients. *Eur Spine J.* 2006;15:1139–1143.

[12] Janicki J, Poe-Kochert C, Armstrong DG, Thompson GH. A comparison of the thoracolumbosacral orthoses and Providence orthosis in the treatment of adolescent idiopathic scoliosis. *J Pediatr Orthop.* 2007;27(4):369–374.

[13] Katz DE, Richards BS, Browne RH, Herring JA. A comparison between the Boston Brace and the Charleston Bending Brace in adolescent idiopathic scoliosis. *Spine.* 1997;22(12):1302–1312.

[14] de Mauroy J, Weiss H, Aulisa A, et al. 7th SOSORT consensus paper: conservative treatment of idiopathic & Scheuermann's kyphosis. *Scoliosis.* 2010;5(9).

[15] Kravarusic D, Dicken B, Dewar R, et al. The Calgary protocol for bracing of pectus carinatum: a preliminary report. *J Pediatr Surg.* 2006;41(5):923–926.

[16] Cohee A, Lin J, Frantz F, Kelly R. Staged management of pectus carinatum. *J Pediatr Surg.* 2013;28(2):315–320.

[17] Martinez-Ferro M, Fraire C, Bernard S. Dynamic compression system for the correction of pectus carinatum. *Semin Pediatr Surg.* 2008;17(3):194–2008.

[18] Colozza S, Bütter A. Bracing in pediatric patients with pectus carinatum is effective and improves quality of life. *J Pediatr Surg.* 2013;48(5):1055–1059.

[19] Evans NR. A 3D motion analysis study comparing the effectiveness of cervical spine orthoses at restricting spinal motion through physiological ranges. *Eur Spine J.* 2013;22(Suppl 1): 10–15.

[20] Agabegi SS, Asghar F, Herkowitz H. Spinal orthoses. *J Am Acad Orthop Surg.* 2010;18(11):657–667.

[21] National Center for Complementary and Integrative Health. National Institutes of Health (NIH). U.S. Department of Health & Human Services (DHHS). U.S. National Survey Identifies Associations Between Chronic Severe Back Pain and Disability. Accessed September 17, 2024 at https://www.nccih.nih.gov/research/research-results/us-national-survey-identifies-associations-between-chronic-severe-back-pain-and-disability.

[22] Fayolle-Minon I, Calmels P. Effect of wearing a lumbar orthosis on trunk muscles: study of the muscle strength after 21 days of use on healthy subjects. *Joint Bone Spine.* 2008;75(1):58–63.

CHAPTER 16

Orthotic Management of Cranial Deformities and Associated Comorbidities

Phil M. Stevens and Mary L. Emerson

OBJECTIVES

Upon completing this material, the reader will be able to:
1. Recall the epidemiology and etiology of various presentations of cranial deformities.
2. Explain characteristics that distinguish between various presentations of cranial deformities along with means to determine severity.
3. Understand multidisciplinary management principles associated with cranial deformities.

INTRODUCTION

There are a number of deviations from the so-called "normocephaly," or an infant's typical cranial morphology with normal dimensions and proportions. These can be characterized as asymmetrical presentations, commonly referred to as *plagiocephaly*; as symmetrical presentations characterized by deviant ratios of cranial width to cranial length, referred to as *brachycephaly* and *scaphocephaly*; or as mixed presentations in which both symmetry and ratios are atypical.

Among infants with atypical head shapes, differential diagnosis must be performed to determine if the cranial morphology is the result of a premature fusion of one or more cranial sutures, described as a *craniosynostosis* or a *synostotic* deformity [1], or if the head shape is the product of environmental forces acting upon the head, described

as *positional* or *deformational* presentations. Craniosynostosis requires corrective surgical intervention that is often coupled with post-operative use of a cranial remolding orthosis. Deformational presentations can often be managed conservatively, through corrective repositioning efforts and stretching techniques, but may require the use of a cranial remolding orthosis in moderate to severe cases.

The most commonly encountered variant of normocephaly is deformational plagiocephaly, a condition that is frequently accompanied by concomitant torticollis and is often managed conservatively through physical therapy. Variations of plagiocephaly emerge from a host of reasons perinatally (e.g. prolonged vaginal delivery, use of forceps, etc.), postnatally (e.g. position of crib relative to stimulus, position of baby for sleep, preferentially breast feeding from one side relative to the other, etc.). and for other reasons such as the "Back to Sleep" campaign [2,

DOI: 10.4324/9781003526025-18

3]. As the prevalence of this presentation has increased, it has become increasingly important for physical therapists to recognize aberrant infant head shapes, treating those deformational cases that can be managed conservatively while referring potential synostotic cases to the appropriate craniofacial surgeons and moderate to advanced deformational cases to cranial orthotists.

CRANIOSYNOSTOSIS

Craniosynostosis is a rare presentation with prevalence rates approximating 1 per 2,000 births [4, 5]. It can be encountered in both simple and compound presentations [4]. Simple craniosynostoses are more common and often confined to a single cranial suture in children that are otherwise healthy [4]. Compound craniosynostoses involve multiple cranial sutures and are often observed in infants with complex syndromes and associated comorbid challenges such as Crouzon's disease, Apert's syndrome, and Pfeiffer's disease [4]. Such syndromic craniosynostoses account for approximately 20% of synostotic cranial presentations [4].

Nonsyndromic craniosynostosis occurs sporadically with unknown etiology and a wide range of potential risk factors. Familial nonsyndromic craniosynostosis is observed, but only in a minority of cases. The sagittal suture is the most commonly affected cranial suture in simple synostotic head shapes, accounting for roughly half of these presentations. This is followed in frequency by premature fusion of one or both coronal sutures, while premature fusion of the metopic suture is observed in less 10% of simple synostoses [4]. Unilateral lambdoid craniosynostosis is the least commonly encountered presentation (1 in 300,000 births) [6], but has relevance as this presentation is the most likely to be mistaken for deformational plagiocephaly.

In understanding the aberrant head shapes associated with craniosynostosis, therapists should bear the following principles in mind [7]. In contrast to the more commonly encountered deformational presentations, where the abnormal head shape represents the primary problem, in craniosynostosis the abnormal cranial morphology is a merely symptom of the underlying problem. When synostosis occurs, growth will be restricted at the affected sutures and cranial plates, leading to compensatory growth elsewhere on the skull. Given the regularities observed in these compensatory growth patterns, the premature fusions in simple craniosynostosis can be diagnosed by a particular head shape [7]. The cranial morphologies associated with the various simple synostoses are listed in Table16.1.

These resultant head shapes are a product of three governing rules [8].

1. Compensatory growth will be greatest at those sutures adjacent to the fused suture.

TABLE 16.1
Cranial morphology of simple craniosynostoses

AFFECTED SUTURE	CRANIAL MORPHOLOGY
Metopic	Trigonocephaly
Unilateral Coronal	Frontal plagiocephaly
Bilateral Coronal	Frontal brachycephaly
Sagittal	Scaphocephaly
Unilateral Lambdoid	Occipital plagiocephaly

2. If the adjacent suture is more or less parallel to the fused suture, the compensatory growth will be symmetrical.

3. If the adjacent suture is more or less perpendicular to the fused suture, the majority of the compensatory growth occurs from the bone distal to the fused suture.

Applying these rules to each of the simple synostoses explains the resultant cranial morphologies (Figure 16.1). In cases of sagittal synostosis, compensatory growth occurs at the coronal and lambdoid sutures away from the parietal plates, creating the narrow, elongated head shape referred to as scaphocephaly [9, 10]. In cases of bilateral coronal synostosis, parallel compensatory growth occurs at the metopic and sagittal sutures, resulting in a tall, broad head shape with prominent frontal bones and reduced cranial length, described as frontal brachycephaly [9, 10]. In cases of unilateral coronal synostosis, growth of the ipsilateral frontal and parietal plates is restricted by the fusion while compensatory parallel growth occurs at the contralateral coronal suture into the contralateral frontal and parietal bones. Additional compensatory growth occurs into these plates at the metopic and sagittal sutures. The resultant head shape, described as synostotic frontal plagiocephaly, is characterized by the flattened frontal bone ipsilateral to the fusion and the frontal bossing contralateral to the fusion [9, 10]. In the case of metopic synostosis, the fusion precludes normal growth of the frontal bones, with parallel compensatory growth occurring bilaterally into the parietal bones and disproportionate growth at the coronal sutures into the parietal plates. The resultant trigonal cephalic head shape is characterized by bilateral parietal bossing and an extreme amount of frontal narrowing of the skull [9, 10]. In the rare cases of unilateral lambdoid synostosis, growth is restricted at the occiput ipsilateral to the fusion, with compensatory growth occurring at the contralateral lambdoid suture into the contralateral occiput and parietal plate [9, 10]. The resultant head shape, termed synostotic occipital plagiocephaly, is characterized by unilateral occipital flatness and can be confused with deformational plagiocephaly by the untrained eye [11].

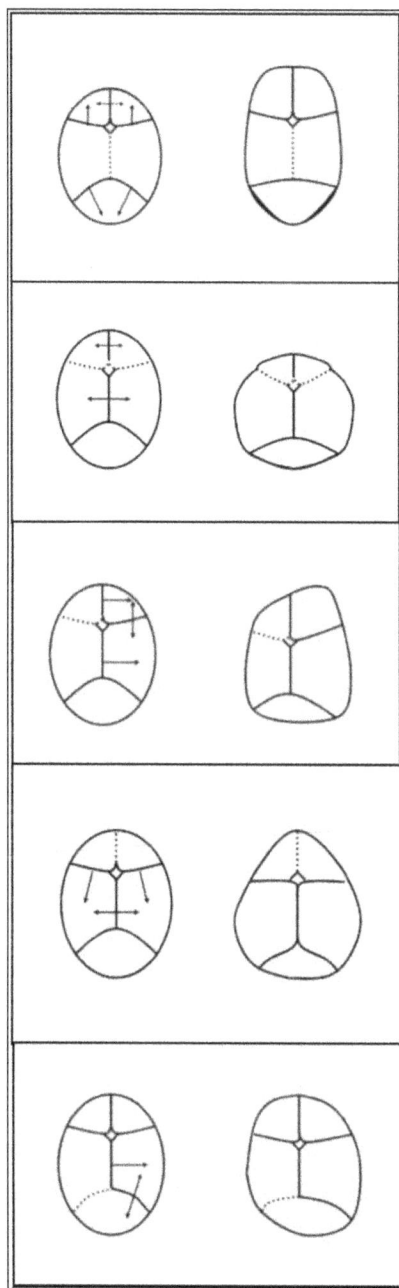

Figure 16.1. Common cranial morphologies associated with simple craniosynostoses. From top to bottom, sagittal, bilateral coronal, unilateral coronal, metopic and unilateral lambdoid.

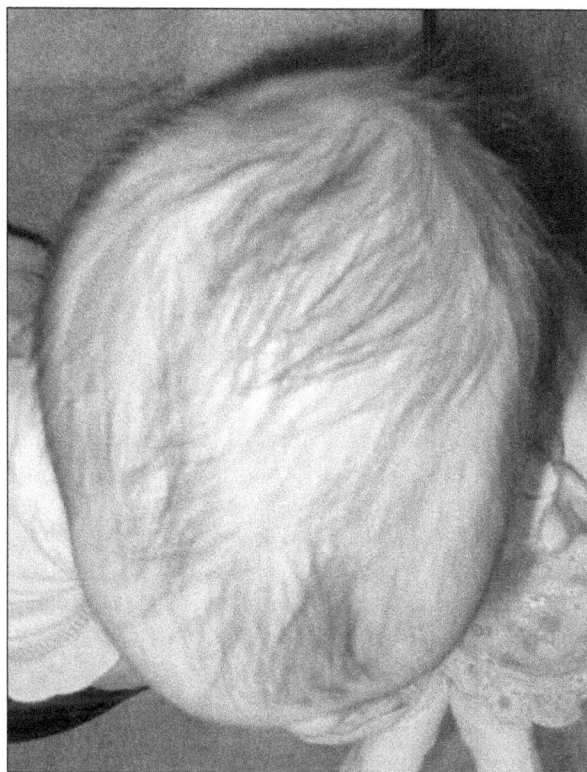

Figure 16.2. Topographic view of deformational plagiocephaly.

DEFORMATIONAL CRANIAL PRESENTATIONS

Nonsynostotic presentations in which the cranial sutures are open or "patent," include plagiocephaly, brachycephaly, and scaphocephaly. Deformational plagiocephaly is an asymmetrical presentation in which ipsilateral flatness of the occiput, forehead, or both is coupled with contralateral bossing [4].

Viewed superiorly, the resultant head shape generally resembles a parallelogram in which the bossing of the forehead is mirrored by a bossing of the contralateral occiput and the flatness of the forehead is mirrored by the flatness of the contralateral occiput [11] (Figure 16.2).

This presentation is the product of a rapidly growing infant cranium at a time when there is inadequate variation to its positioning, creating an environment in which the affected occiput is unable to grow because of the resultant gravitational forces acting upon it. These environmental forces create the characteristic shifting on the affected side that not only precludes occipital growth, but often causes an anterior translation of the ipsilateral ear relative to its counterpart, ipsilateral forehead bossing, and, in more extreme presentation, ipsilateral advancement of the facial zygoma.

While this presentation bears some resemblance to the synostotic plagiocephalies described earlier, differential diagnosis can generally be done observationally and confirmed by CAT scan or X-ray when craniosynostosis is suspected [12]. The principles of this differential diagnosis will be described later in the chapter.

Symmetrical deformational presentations include both brachycephaly and scaphocephaly. The former is more common and results when environmental forces are regularly applied symmetrically across the occiput during early infantile skull growth. The resultant symmetrical head shape is characterized by an exaggerated cranial width and a compressed cranial length. The normal contour of the occiput can be reduced or, in extreme

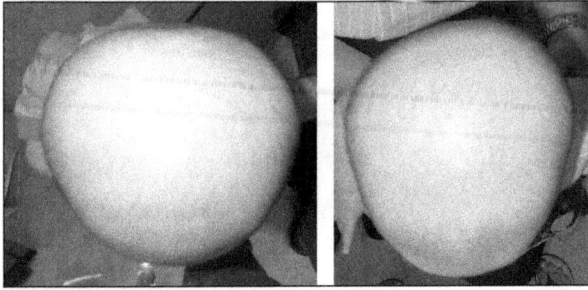

Figure 16.3. Topographical view of A. symmetrical brachycephaly and B. asymmetric brachycephaly/plagiocephaly

cases, absent entirely (Figure 16.3A). Frequently, these environmental forces occur with a bias to one side with a resultant head shape that is both asymmetric (plagiocephaly) and wide relative to its length (brachycephaly) (Figure 16.3B).

Less frequently, some infants that are positioned with their head turned fully to one side can develop a deformational scaphocephaly. This is more common in premature infants where the weak structure of the skull is unable to resist the gravitational forces associated with its own weight. Fortunately, such cases often resolve spontaneously within the first few months of life [13]. As with brachycephaly, these head shapes can present as both symmetric and asymmetric variants.

DIFFERENTIAL DIAGNOSES

While it is outside of a therapist's scope of practice to confirm a differential diagnosis of a craniosynostosis, therapists should be familiar with the guiding principles of differential diagnosis, allowing them to refer the family to the appropriate resources if synostosis is at all suspected.

An important consideration is found in the position of the ear relative to the occipital flatness [11]. In cases of

deformational plagiocephaly, this ear should be relatively advanced compared with its contralateral counterpart, consistent with the parallelogram presentation described earlier. When this is not the case, referral to a craniofacial specialist is warranted. This is summarized in the simple caution, "When the ear is near (to the flattened occiput or forehead), steer clear."

An additional sign of a synostotic occipital plagiocephaly due to unilateral lambdoid synostosis is an occipital bulge both distal and ipsilateral to the occipital flatness [11] (Figure 16.4). This bulge contributes to the appearance of a parallelogram shape that may be observed when the infant is viewed posteriorly [11]. Frontal flatness and bossing are observed inconsistently in this population, such that the cranial shape viewed superiorly may be seen as a trapezoid, a parallelogram, or an isolated occipital flatness.

Differential diagnosis of an anterior plagiocephaly is more visually apparent. As with synostotic occipital plagiocephaly, the position of the ipsilateral ear should be consistent with the parallelogram shape described earlier. That is, the ipsilateral ear should be relatively posterior to the flattened forehead in deformational cases. When the ear ipsilateral to the frontal flatness is relatively anterior to its contralateral counterpart, craniosynostosis can be reasonably suspected [14]. In addition, there are a number of characteristic facial asymmetries that are generally quite noticeable such that this presentation is generally observed and addressed by generalist primary care providers [14].

Particularly in recent years, the observed cranial morphologies associated with simple synostoses have not been immune to the deformational forces that occur in the rapidly growing infant. Thus, mixed presentations characterized by synostotic cranial morphologies overlaid with deformational asymmetries can be encountered. Importantly, cranial facial specialists must be engaged in any instance where the presence of a craniosynostosis might be reasonably suspected.

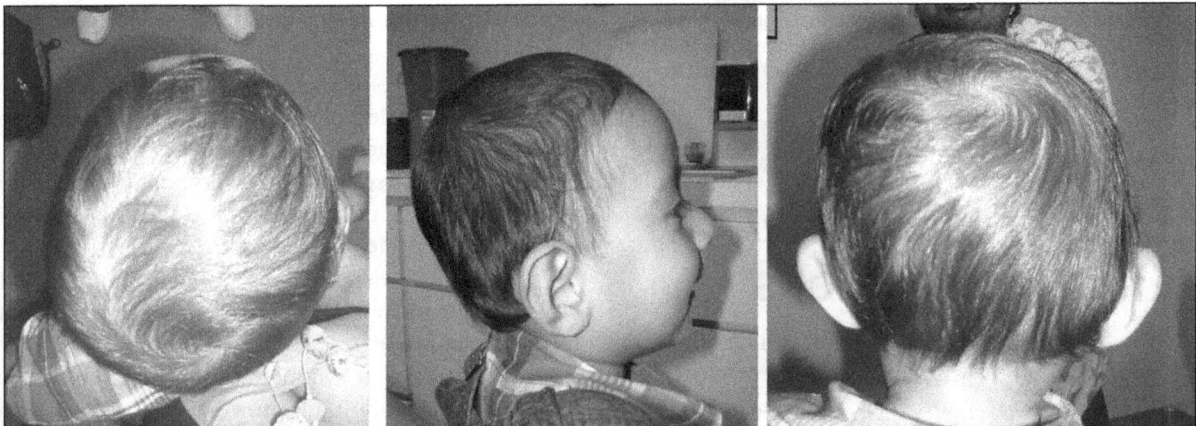

Figure 16.4. Topographic, side, and posterior view of right lambdoid synostosis

MANAGEMENT OF CRANIOSYNOSTOSIS

As stated earlier, the aberrant head shapes observed in craniosynostosis are best viewed as symptoms of an underlying problem. More specifically, the prematurely fused sutures must be surgically addressed before cranial morphology can be corrected, either intraoperatively, through guided post-operative remolding, or both. Historically, these cases were managed through challenging, extremely invasive calvarial vault remodeling surgeries [15, 16]. These procedures were characterized by substantial blood loss, 4–8-hour operative times, hospitalization periods ranging between 4 and 7 days, and mandatory blood transfusions [16]. Given the intensity of these procedures, they were delayed until approximately 8 months of age, when the infant was deemed strong enough to survive the procedures.

It was in association with these complex surgical approaches that several articles in the late 1980s described the use of skull molding caps as a post-operative treatment modality [6, 7, 17]. Provided by a treating therapist, these low temperature orthoses were used to guide postoperative cranial growth. Such guidance was desirable as intraoperative corrections were only partial and often incomplete. Additionally, left unmanaged, the skull might revert to either the original deformed shape or may develop a new abnormal form [17, 18]. As the use of cranial remolding orthoses became more frequent in the management of deformational plagiocephaly, this modality was also used to meet the objectives of skull molding caps, namely protecting the healing skull, guiding its postoperative growth to enhance correction, and preventing reversion to an apparent head shape [19, 20, 10].

In 2000, an alternate surgical management strategy for craniosynostosis was described by Jimenez and Barone [16]. Within this simplified endoscopic procedure, the fused suture and a reasonable margin of the adjacent cranial bone were surgically removed. A much less invasive procedure, operative times were reduced to less than 1 hour with substantially reduced blood loss. This permitted its use on much younger infants, allowing a longer window of postoperative cranial growth during which cranial morphology could be progressively corrected. Within this increasingly popular treatment model, endoscopic surgical procedures are performed as young as 3 months, followed immediately by a protracted course of cranial remolding orthoses to guide growth through over the subsequent months [21]. Today, such treatments are guideline-based and include improved diagnostics, expert consensus, and best evidence [22].

While the interaction of therapists with this population is generally unlikely and limited to screening potential instances of craniosynostosis, an awareness of general management strategies is ideal.

DEFORMATIONAL PLAGIOCEPHALY

The sharp increase in deformational plagiocephaly reported in the mid to late 1990s [23, 24, 25] has been justifiably linked with the introduction and adoption of the "Back to Sleep" campaign of the American Academy of Pediatrics [26]. While this public health initiative appears to have successfully reduced the prevalence of SIDS-related mortality [18, 27], an unintended consequence has been a dramatic increase in the observed prevalence of deformational plagiocephaly. However, assigning the increased prevalence of deformational plagiocephaly exclusively to this health initiative represents a gross oversimplification as the majority of children who adhere to this positioning strategy fail to develop deformational plagiocephaly and a number of additional characteristics have been associated with increased rates of deformational plagiocephaly. For example, the presentation is more common in first-born children, males, infants born prematurely, and among twins and triplets with the child who is delivered first being at the greatest risk [28, 29, 30].

Another strongly associated risk factor for deformational plagiocephaly is the presence of asymmetric strength and mobility of the neck, creating a preference to one side. The management of such asymmetries of the neck falls well within the therapist's scope of practice and will be described later in the chapter. Suffice it to say, some level of neck muscle imbalance has been reported in as many as 97% of all infants who are subsequently managed for their deformational plagiocephaly and has been identified as the most common associated finding in children with deformational plagiocephaly [31].

PREVALENCE

The prevalence rates of deformational plagiocephaly vary according to assessment ages and the severity thresholds for inclusion. At the time of Clarren et al.'s original description of deformational plagiocephaly and cranial remolding orthoses in 1979, a prevalence rate of 1 in 300 was cited [32]. However, modern prevalence rates are much higher. Mawji et al. recently reported an incidence of 47% among infants evaluated at their 2-month well-child visit [33, 34]. However, the majority of these cases were classified as "mild," with only 22% of the plagiocephalies defined as moderate to severe.

Hutchison et al. reported a comparable incidence of 16% at 6 weeks of age, but observed that, tracked longitudinally, incidence values change with age. Among their cohort, a peak incidence of roughly 20% was observed at 4 months with subsequent declines [35]. This longitudinal change in incidence was confirmed by van Vlimmeran, who found that, of the 23 infants observed with plagiocephaly at birth, 14 had reverted to normal by 7 weeks of age. However, of the 380 infants not initially diagnosed with plagiocephaly, 75 had developed the condition by 7 weeks of age [36].

Ultimately, prevalence rates in infant primary care centers have been reported at 15% [37] and 18% [38]. More recent sources indicate that since the "Back to Sleep" campaign and the very positive outcomes associated with it, the incidence of deformational plagiocephaly has increased 400–600% [39, 12, 40, 41]. Recent sources also indicate the incidence of anterior plagiocephaly to be 1/10,000 live births and that it occurs in 13–16% of children with craniosynostosis [42, 43, 39]. Deformational plagiocephaly prevalence is more recently estimated to be between 15 and 20% with reports as high as 47% [44, 45].

ASSESSING SEVERITY

Assessing the severity of deformational skull deformities is generally a combination of objective anthropometric measurement and subjective visual assessment. A number of cranial measurements should be obtained during the initial consultation and monitored throughout treatment. These consist of the cranial circumference, cranial length, cranial width, cephalic index (CI), occipital frontal transcranial diameters and the transcranial diagonal difference (TDD) [12], which are described in Table 16.2.

Cranial circumference is valuable as a longitudinal marker of cranial growth and can be used to assess the relative efficacy of an intervention (such as physical therapy or orthotic management). Cephalic index is a standardized measurement that is most useful in the assessment of a child with brachycephaly, where it should decrease with effective management. The transcranial diagonal difference is a measurement of cranial symmetry and is most useful in the assessment of a child with plagiocephaly. This number should also decrease with effective treatment.

While objective measurement remains the standard form of assessment, subjective visual assessments have also been advocated. Among these the most frequently advocated is the five-stage subjective classification of Argenta et al., based on such considerations as the presence or absence of posterior asymmetry, ear malposition, frontal asymmetry, and facial asymmetry [46].

A wide range of objective and subjective severity assessment strategies have been suggested. Looman and Kack Flannery proposed one set of standards [12] which combined the objective measurement standards of Hutchison et al. [35] with the visual observational criteria of Argenta et al. [46]. These were subsequently modified slightly through a Delphi consensus process by Lin et al. [47], resulting in the following descriptors:

- "Mild" plagiocephaly is defined as a TDD between 3 and 8 mm **AND** flatness that is restricted to the back of the head.
- "Moderate" plagiocephaly is defined as a TDD between 8 and 12 mm **AND** either ear malposition and/or forehead deformity.
- "Severe" plagiocephaly is defined as a TDD greater than 12 mm.

Looman and Kack Flannery also proposed a set of standards for brachycephaly [12] combining the objective measurement standards of Hutchison et al. [48] with the

TABLE 16.2
Anthropometric measurements used to track cranial deformations and abnormal ratios

ANTHROPOMETRIC MEASUREMENT	DESCRIPTION
Cranial circumference	Circumferential measurement taken at the equator of the skull obtaining the largest measurement in the horizontal plane.
Cranial length	Measured from the glabella (the most prominent midpoint between the eyebrows) and the opisthocranion (the most prominent point on the occiput).
Cranial width	Measured at the largest biparietal diameter proximal to the ears.
Cephalic index	Ratio of head width to head length multiplied by 100.
Long transcranial diameter	Measured from the apex of the bossed occiput to the to the apex of the contralateral bossed forehead.
Short transcranial diameter	Measured from the center of the affected (i.e., flattened) occiput to the center of the contralateral forehead.
Transcranial diagonal difference	Difference between the long transcranial diameter minus the short transcranial diameter.

visual observational criteria of Argenta et al. [46]. These were also subjected to Delphi consensus by Lin et al. [47], resulting in the following descriptors:

- "Mild" brachycephaly is defined as a CI between 82 and 90% **AND** no widening of the posterior skull.
- "Moderate" brachycephaly is defined as a CI between 90 and 100% **AND** widening of the posterior skull.
- "Severe" brachycephaly is defined as a CI greater than 100% **AND** a vertical head shape or temporal bossing.

CONGENITAL MUSCULAR TORTICOLLIS

While there are a number of overlapping risk factors for the development of deformational plagiocephaly, congenital muscular torticollis (CMT) is predominant among these. As deformational plagiocephaly is ultimately the result of disproportional loading of one side of the rapidly growing infantile cranium, it stands to reason that a comorbid muscle imbalance that precludes the ability of the infant or their caregivers to alternate head position during the first weeks and months of life will contribute to the child's overall risk.

Accordingly, torticollis is commonly observed in patients with deformational plagiocephaly and deformational plagiocephaly has been reported in up to 90% of children with CMT [49]. In younger infants with mild to moderate plagiocephaly, conservative management of the concomitant CMT through physical therapy and conscientious repositioning may adequately resolve the associated deformational plagiocephaly.

CMT is an idiopathic postural deformity evident shortly after birth, typically characterized by lateral flexion of the head to one side and cervical rotation to the opposite side due to unilateral shortening of the sternocleidomastoid muscle. CMT may be accompanied by other neurological or musculoskeletal conditions [50]. Clinical features include tilted and rotated head position, decreased range of motion, weakness on the opposite side of the involved SCM, tumor or tight band, and plagiocephaly [51].

The prevalence of CMT has ranged from 0.3% (15 of 5,079 live births) to 2.0% (43 of 2,190 live births) [52]. There has been an increase incidence of CMT and plagiocephaly since 1992 when the American Academy of Pediatrics recommended infants sleep in non-prone positions to reduce risk of SIDS in response to mounting evidence from Europe, New Zealand and Australia. In 1994 AAP initiated the "Back to Sleep" campaign [26, 53].

Etiology of CMT is unclear but there are a few possibilities, including: direct trauma, ischemic injury due to abnormal vascular patterns, heredity, and intrauterine compartment syndrome due to extreme head posturing in the birth canal [50].

There are three types of CMT: the sternomastoid tumor (SMT) group which is defined as a definite presence of a clinically palpable SCM (sternocleidomastoid) tumor; the muscular torticollis group (MT) with no palpable or visible tumor, but with clinical thickening or tightness of the sternomastoid muscle on the affected side; and the postural group (POST) in which all the clinical features of torticollis are present, but without tightness or tumor of the SCM [54, 55, 56].

Indications for treatment are children presenting with shortened/contracture of cervical musculature unilaterally with weakness on the uninvolved side, fibroses of the SCM or cervical muscles, mass, tumor or fibrosis in the cervical spine muscles or soft tissues, plagiocephaly, visual concerns, and intermittent torticollis positioning.

Contraindications to treatment include an unstable cervical spine as in Down syndrome, malignancy, vertebral anomaly, myelomeningocele or Arnold Chiari Malformation, compromised circulatory or respiratory systems, or clinical findings suggesting other pathology.

The objectives for treatment include the child being able to sustain a neutral or within 5° of neutral cervical spine in sitting and/or standing when age appropriate, symmetrical muscle function test, and full symmetrical passive range of motion for cervical rotation and lateral flexion. In addition, the child should have age-appropriate motor skills including symmetrical head and trunk righting responses, a cranial vault less than or equal to 4 mm, and parents competent to continue a home program including recognizing when return to therapy is appropriate [50, 51, 58, 57]. These objectives were derived from Kaplan's 2013 decision tree [50] by the Cincinnati Children's Hospital and Primary Children's Medical Center.

Evaluation or assessment of the child should start with a thorough history including pregnancy, birth, family history, medical/health concerns, current health and caregiver routine, and history of the torticollis/plagiocephaly. Physical screenings should canvas vision, skin appearance, hip stability, pain assessment, range of motion, and neurological presentation. Physical assessments include the infant's resting posture in supine, prone, sitting, and standing; spinal alignment; both active and passive cervical range of motion; muscular palpation; CMT classification (SMT, MT POST), motor development, and the presence of plagiocephaly based on anthropometric measurement [50, 56, 58].

Management includes repositioning, stretching tight muscles, improving active and passive range of motion (ROM), strengthening opposing cervical spine muscles, facilitating symmetrical motor skill acquisition, and cueing development of midline head orientation [50, 56, 58]. Parent education and home programming are an integral part of treatment as well. How to position the baby is addressed during first encounter with parents including positioning for feeding, passive rotation of head off of the flattened aspect of the cranium for sleeping, and carrying options to decrease plagiocephaly and promote strengthening and midline orientation of head. Decreased use of those devices that promote only supine positioning or semi reclined positioning like the car seats, bouncers, swings or other devices that promote upright positioning in a torticollis posture is encouraged. Ensuring parents understand how to position, stretch, and strengthen the cervical spine is imperative for a successful outcome [52, 53, 35, 59].

Treatment usually takes 3–4 months or an average of 9 visits to get resolution of CMT. The age at start of physical therapy plays into the success of conservative treatment. If therapy is started birth to 3 months, the CMT is resolved by 3–5 months. However, if it is started when the child is over 8 months it is not resolved until over 12 months of age. If conservative treatment is not successful in the first 4–6 weeks, additional therapy including kinesiotape®, TOT collar, and Botox injections can be implemented. Surgery would be the last option for treatment and an extreme measure for a very difficult torticollis [56].

CRANIAL REMOLDING ORTHOSES

Cranial remolding orthoses were first described by Clarren et al. in 1979 [32] in a preliminary report on 10 infants. This original publication described the foundational principles of cranial remolding therapy that remain in use today. Namely, an intimate impression of the child's head is obtained and used to create a positive model that is then modified through the addition of supplemental material in the flattened areas to obtain a symmetric shape while preserving an intimate fit over the bossed areas of the head [32].

While casting remained the method of choice for obtaining a positive model of an infant's head for many years, advances in technology have yielded several scanning-based approaches that allow for a digital capture of the child's head shape which can be modified in CAD-based computer programs [60, 61]. These files can then be carved as corrected 3-D models of the head and used to fabricate the cranial remolding orthosis. Given the ability of cranial remolding orthoses to directly influence the bony growth of the infant skull, the U.S. Food and Drug Administration (FDA) has declared them to be a class 2 device, such that their fabrication can only be performed in FDA-approved facilities.

Given the rapid cranial growth experienced by infants, cranial orthoses should be fit within 2 weeks of the initial data capture. Additional delays, particularly in younger infants, will compromise the fit and safety of the orthosis.

While some variations in helmet construction have been approved by the FDA, the most common helmet construction consists of internal closed cell foam lining reinforced by an external plastic shell (Figure 16.5). At fitting,

the orthotist verifies an intimate fit over the bossed areas of the skull and available growth room in the areas of undesirable flatness.

Given the heat retention initially experienced by infants with the use of remolding orthoses, a week-long period of acclimation is generally advised, through which wear times are progressively increased. Ultimately, a 23-hour daily wearing schedule is prescribed with removal of the helmet permitted for an hour every day. This daily break is permitted to allow cleaning of the helmet and bathing of the infant. Importantly, this period allows the family to ensure that any redness associated with helmet use dissipates within an hour's time, suggesting that the pressures and heat associated with the helmet are reasonable and appropriate. Regular follow-up is an integral part of helmet therapy, with appointments scheduled in approximately 2–4-week intervals, dependent on the child's age and growth rate.

Length of treatment can be quite variable, depending upon the severity of the cranial deformities and the age of the child at initiation of treatment, with younger children experiencing greater correction and completing treatment in less time [62]. Treatment times of 3–5 months are common.

Initiating Helmet Treatment

Just as different facilities and institutions may have individualized standards for determining the severity of deformational cranial deformities, there are a range of protocols for when to initiate helmet treatment. Such protocols are generally jointly based on the severity of the child's presentation and the age of the infant. Looman and Kack Flannery summarized a number of general management principles [12] that were refined by Lin et al. through a Delphi consensus model to create a treatment algorithm to determine when a cranial remolding orthosis is indicated [47].

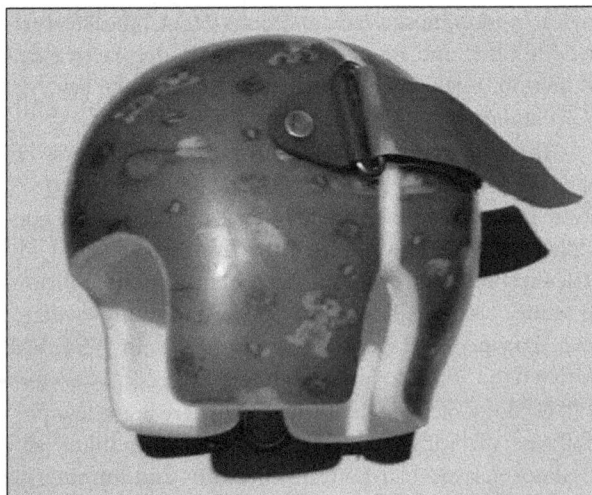

Figure 16.5. Cranial remolding orthosis with internal foam lining and external plastic shell.

Within this algorithm, children with more severe cranial deformities begin treatment at younger ages to take advantage of the rapid cranial growth experienced during this period. By contrast, children with less severe deformities can attempt longer courses of conservative management. Children presenting younger than 4 months of age are best managed through parental education on corrective repositioning and referral to a physical therapist in cases where torticollis is observed. Patients who present with severe deformational abnormalities at 4 months of age should begin helmet therapy, with mild and moderate deformities managed conservatively through repositioning and physical therapy. At 5 months of age, infants with moderate deformities are indicated for helmet therapy while infants with mild deformities are still managed conservatively. Infants who present with mild deformities at 6 months of age or older can pursue helmet therapy at the family's discretion.

As the efficacy of helmet therapy is dependent on cranial growth, optimal results are obtained during the first year of life. While some studies have documented continued benefits to helmet treatment in children older than 12 months [63], these improvements are very gradual and less than would have been experienced by earlier initiation of treatment.

Efficacy of Repositioning and Orthotics Treatment

A number of systematic reviews have been published on the efficacy of both conservative repositioning and cranial remolding orthoses [64, 65, 66, 67, 68]. In general, these reviews have observed that the body of literature in this area is comprised of retrospective, observational studies. Collectively, studies have demonstrated considerable evidence that cranial remolding orthoses reduce skull asymmetries more effectively than repositioning therapy [64]. These studies are not without limitation and areas of bias; however, such biases typically favor repositioning in that those observation cohorts representing orthotic remolding are comprised of older infants, infants with more severe cranial deformities and infants who have failed to attain adequate correction from conservative repositioning strategies [64].

One randomized controlled trial yielded findings highly contradictory to the remainder of the published literature [69]. Its methods and data interpretation have been highly criticized, causing the American Academy of Pediatrics to assert, "In summary, we find significant weaknesses in the methodology employed by van Wijk et al. that necessarily call into question any conclusions about the lack of effectiveness of helmets" [70].

More representative to clinical experience and prior publications are the observations of Eberle et al. [71] and Steinberg et al. [72]. Eberle et al. retrospectively reported on 4,248 patients managed over a 5-year period. Within a conservative treatment group of 3,186 infants managed with repositioning, 75% achieved complete correction, defined as a cranial diagonal difference of less than 6 mm. The remaining 25% were moved to a second treatment group managed with a remolding orthosis. Of these 1,062 infants, 95% achieved full correction as defined above, over an average treatment duration of 5 months [71].

Near the same time, authors from Children's Memorial Hospital in Chicago released their collective observations from a 7-year time period [72]. A conservative treatment group, comprised of 3,381 infants, was managed through prescribed repositioning and in the majority of cases, physical therapy. Of these, 77% obtained complete correction (defined by this clinic as a transcranial diagonal difference of less than 5 mm). Of those who failed to attain complete correction, the majority transitioned to a helmet treatment group, with a minority failing to obtain complete correction and declining further treatment. The helmet group was comprised of 997 infants who were initially prescribed a helmet and the 534 infants who were added to the group after conservative treatments failed, yielding a total population of 1,531 infants. Complete correction by the standards reported above was obtained by 94% of those infants initially managed with a remolding helmet, and by 96% of those infants who transitioned after failed conservative management attempts. Collectively, 4,062 of the 4,378 infants in the retrospective analysis attained successful correction of their cranial deformations through a combination of active repositioning, physical therapy and orthotic remolding. The authors' conclusions were direct: "Conservative treatment and helmet therapy were found to be effective for correcting positional cranial deformation in 92.8 percent of infants."

DEVELOPMENTAL DELAY

While the literature to date has not suggested a causal relationship between deformational skull deformities and developmental delays, a correlation has been observed [73, 74]. Robinson and Proctor [66] have suggested that the presence of deformational plagiocephaly may indicate to primary care providers that there is an increased possibility of developmental delay and that additional screening is necessary.

SUMMARY

With the recently increased prevalence of deformational skull deformities and their strong association with congenital muscular torticollis, it is increasingly important for physical therapists to understand the range of abnormal cranial presentations that may be encountered and their underlying etiologies. Deformational and synostotic cranial morphologies must be understood and recognized to ensure appropriate medical care. Deformational plagiocephaly is the most commonly encountered form of aberrant infantile head shapes with a prevalence that varies according to the ages of the examined children. Severity assessments often represent a combination of objective measurement and subjective appearance considerations. These severity ratings can, in turn, aid clinical decision making with regard to the initiation of treatment. For the physical therapist, the presence of deformational plagiocephaly is frequently associated with congenital muscular torticollis. This comorbid condition also requires targeted intervention. The management of deformational plagiocephaly in the infant population is conservative in its nature, ranging from parent education, targeted stretching and strengthening programs and the use of cranial remolding orthoses.

References

[1] Cohen MM, MacLean RE. Anatomic, genetic, nosologic, diagnostic, and psychosocial considerations. In: Cohen M, MacLean R. eds. *Craniosynostosis: Diagnosis, Evaluation, and Management*, 2000. 2nd edition, pp. 119–143. Oxford University Press, New York.

[2] Filisetti M, Cattarelli D, Bonomi S. Positional plagiocephaly from structure to function: Clinical experience of the service of pediatric osteopathy in Italy. *Early Hum Dev*. 2020;146:105028.

[3] Ballardini E, Sisti M, Basaglia N, et al. Prevalence and characteristics of positional plagiocephaly in healthy full-term infants at 8–12 weeks of life. *Eur J Pediatr*. 2018 Oct;177(10):1547–1554.

[4] Kabbani H, Raghuveer TS. Craniosynostosis. *Am Fam Phys*. 2004;69(12):2863–2870.

[5] Boulet SL, Rasmussen SA, Honein MA. A population-based study of craniosynostosis in metropolitan Atlanta, 1989–2003. *Am J Med Genet A*. 2008;146A(8):984–991.

[6] Ham CK, Meyer SW. Skull molding caps: an adjunct to craniosynostosis surgery. *Plast Reconstruct Surg*. 1987;80:737–741.

[7] Ham CK. Skull molding caps: external splinting to correct cranial vault deformities. In: Persing JA, Edgerton MT, eds. *Scientific Foundations to Surgical Treatment of Craniosynostosis*, 1989. Williams & Wilkins, Baltimore, MD. 1989, pp. 270–274.

[8] Jane JA Jr, Lin KY, Jane JA Sr. Sagittal synostosis. *Neurosurg Focus*. 2000 Sept 15;9(3):e3.

[9] Delashaw JP, Persing JA, Broaddus WC, Jane JA. Cranial vault growth in craniosynostosis. *J Neurosurg*. 1989;70:159–165.

[10] Stevens PM, Hollier LH, Stal S. Post-operative use of remoulding orthoses following cranial vault remodelling: a case series. 2007;31(4):327–341.

[11] Huang MH, Gruss JS, Clarren SK, et al. The differential diagnosis of posterior plagiocephaly: true lambdoid synostosis versus positional molding. *Plast Reconstr Surg*. 1996;98:765–774.

[12] Looman WS, Kack Flannery AB. Evidence-based care of the child with deformational plagiocephaly, part 1: assessment and diagnosis. *J Pediatr Health Care*. 2012;26(4):242–250.

[13] Huang MH, Mouradian WE, Cohen SR, Gruss JS. The differential diagnosis of abnormal head shapes: separating craniosynostosis from positional deformities and normal variants. *Cleft Palate Craniofac J*. 1998 May;35(3):204–211.

[14] Bruneteau RJ, Mulliken JB. Frontal plagiocephaly: synostotic, compensational or deformational. *Plast Reconstr Surg*. 1992;89:21–31.

[15] Jane JA, Persing JA. Neurosurgical treatment of craniosynostosis. In: Cohen M, MacLean R. eds. *Craniosynostosis: Diagnosis, Evaluation, and Management*, 2000. 2nd edition, pp. 209–227. Oxford University Press, New York.

[16] Jimenez DF, Barone CM. Endoscopy-assisted wide-vertex craniectomy, "barrel-stave" osteotomies, and postoperative helmet molding therapy in the early management of sagittal suture craniosynostosis. *Neurosurg Focus*. 2000;9(3):1–6.

[17] Persing JA, Nichter LS, Jane JA, Edgerton MT Jr. External cranial vault molding after craniofacial surgery. *Ann Plast Surg*. 1986;1:274–283.

[18] Persing J, James H, Swanson J, Kattwinkel K & American Academy of Pediatrics Committee on Practice and Ambulatory Medicine, Section on Plastic Surgery and Section on Neurological Surgery. Prevention and management of positional skull deformities in infants. *Pediatrics*. 2003;112(1 Pt 1):199–202.

[19] Seymour-Dempsey K, Baumgartner JE, Teichgraeber JF, et al. Molding helmet therapy in the management of sagittal synostosis. *J Craniofac Surg*. 2002;13:631–635.

[20] Higuera S, Hollier LH, Stevens PM, Stal S. A preliminary investigation of postoperative molding to improve the result of cranial vault remodeling. *J Prosthet Orthot*. 2005;17:125–128.

[21] Jimenez DF, Barone CM, Cartwright CC, Baker L. Early management of craniosynostosis using endoscopic-assisted strip craniectomies and cranial orthotic molding therapy. *Pediatrics*. 2002;110:97–104.

[22] Mathijssen IMJ. Updated guideline on treatment and management of craniosynostosis. *J Craniofac Surg*. 2021 Jan–Feb;32(1): 371–450.

[23] Kane AA, Mitchell LE, Craven KP, Marsh JL. Observations on a recent increase in plagiocephaly without synostosis. *Pediatrics*. 1996;97:877–885.

[24] Turk AE, McCarthy JG, Thorne CH, Wisoff JH. The "Back to Sleep Campaign" and deformational plagiocephaly: is there cause for concern? *J Craniofac Surg*. 1996;7(1):13–18.

[25] Argenta LC, David LR, Wilson JA, Bell WO. An increase in infant cranial deformity with supine sleeping position. *J Craniofac Surg*. 1996;7(1):5–12.

[26] AAP Task Force on Infant Positioning and SIDS. Positioning and SIDS. *Pediatrics*. 1992;89:1120–1126.

[27] Willinger M, Hoffman HJ, Hartford RB. Infant sleep position and risk for sudden infant death syndrome: report of meeting held January 13 and 14, 1994, National Institutes of Health, Bethesda, MD. *Pediatrics*. 1994 May;93(5):814–819.

[28] Bialocerkowski AE, Vladusic SL, Ng CW. Prevalence, risk factors, and natural history of positional plagiocephaly: a systematic review. *Dev Med Child Neurol*. 2008;50(8):577–586.

[29] Oh AK, Hoy EA, Rogers GF. Predictors of severity in deformational plagiocephaly. *J Craniofac Surg*. 2009;20:685–689.

[30] McKinney CM., Cunningham ML, Holt VL, et al. A case-control study of infant, maternal, and perinatal characteristics associated with deformational plagiocephaly. *Paediatr Perinat Epidemiol*. 2009;23(4):332–345.

[31] Rogers GF, Oh AK, Mulliken JB. The role of congenital muscular torticollis in the development of deformational plagiocephaly. *Plast Reconstr Surg*. 2009;123(2):643–652.

[32] Clarren SK, Smith DW, Janson JW. Helmet treatment for plagiocephaly and congenital muscular torticollis. *J Pediatrics*. 1979;94:43–46.

[33] Mawji A, Vollman AR, Hatfield J, et al. The incidence of positional plagiocephaly: a cohort study. *Pediatrics*. 2013;132:298–304.

[34] Unnithan AKA, De Jesus O. Plagiocephaly. StatPearls [Internet]. Accessed August 30, 2024. https://www.ncbi.nlm.nih.gov/books/NBK564334/.

[35] Hutchison BL, Hutchinson LAD, Thompson JMD, Mitchell EA. Plagiocephaly and brachycephaly in the first two years of life: a prospective cohort study. *Pediatrics*. 2004;114(4):970–980

[36] van Vlimmeren LA, van der Graaf Y, Boere-Boonekamp MM, et al. Risk factors for deformational plagiocephaly at birth and at 7 weeks of age: a prospective cohort study. *Pediatrics*. 2007;119(2).

[37] Littlefield TR, Saba NM, Kelly KM. On the current incidence of deformational plagiocephaly: an estimation based on prospective registration at a single center. *Semin Pediatr Neurol*. 2004;11(4):301–304.

[38] Glasgow TS, Siddiqi F, Hoff CC, Young PC. Deformational plagiocephaly: development of an objective measurement and determination of its prevalence in primary care. *J Craniofac Surg*. 2007;18(1):85–92.

[39] Borad V, Cordes EJ, Liljeberg KM, et al. Isolated lambdoid craniosynostosis. *J Craniofac Surg*. 2019 Nov–Dec;30(8):2390–2392.

[40] Hauck FR, Tanabe KO. Beyond "Back to Sleep": ways to further reduce the risk of sudden infant death syndrome. *Pediatr Ann*. 2017 Aug 01;46(8):e284–e290.

[41] Marshall JM, Shahzad F. Safe sleep, plagiocephaly, and brachycephaly: assessment, risks, treatment, and when to refer. *Pediatr Ann*. 2020 Oct 1;49(10):e440–e447.

[42] Di Rocco C, Paternoster G, Caldarelli M, et al. Anterior plagiocephaly: epidemiology, clinical findings, diagnosis, and classification. A review. *Childs Nerv Syst*. 2012 Sep;28(9):1413–1422.

[43] Rhodes JL, Tye GW, Fearon JA. Craniosynostosis of the lambdoid suture. *Semin Plast Surg*. 2014 Aug;28(3):138–143.

[44] Renz-Polster H, De Bock F. Deformational plagiocephaly: the case for an evolutionary mismatch. *Evol Med Public Health*. 2018;2018(1):180–185.

[45] Mawji A, Vollman AR, Fung T, et al. Risk factors for positional plagiocephaly and appropriate time frames for prevention messaging. *Paediatr Child Health*. 2014 Oct;19(8):423–427.

[46] Argenta L, David L, Thompson J. Clinical classification of positional plagiocephaly. *J Craniofac Surg*. 2004;15(3):368–372.

[47] Lin RS, Stevens PM, Wininger M, Castiglione CL. Orthotic management of deformational plagiocephaly: consensus clinical standards of care. *Cleft Palate Craniofac J*. 2016 Jul;53(4):394–403.

[48] Hutchison BL, Stewart AW, De Chalain TB, Mitchel EA. A randomized controlled trial of positioning treatments in infants with positional head shape deformities. *Acta Paediatr*. 2010;99(10):1556–1560.

[49] Nilesh K, Mukherji S. Congenital muscular torticollis. *Ann Maxillofac Surg*. 2013 Jul-Dec;3(2):198–200.

[50] Kaplan S, Coulter C, Fetters, L. Physical therapy management of congenital muscular torticollis: an evidence-based clinical practice guideline. *Pediatr Phys Ther*. 2013 Winter;25(4):348–394.

[51] Cooperman DR. The differential diagnosis of torticollis in children. *Phys Occup Ther Pediatr*. 1997;17:1–12.

[52] Cheng JC, Wong MW, Tang SP, et al. Clinical determinants of the outcome of manual stretching in the treatment of congenital muscular torticollis in infants. A prospective study of eight hundred and twenty one cases. *J Bone Joint Surg Am*. 2001;83(5):679–687.

[53] American Academy of Pediatrics Task Force on Infant Sleep Position and Sudden Infant Death Syndrome. The changing concept of sudden infant death syndrome: diagnostic coding shifts, controversies regarding the sleeping environment, and new variables to consider in reducing risk. *Pediatrics*. 2005;116(5):1245–1255.

[54] Cheng JC, Tang SP, Chen TM, et al. The clinical presentation and outcome of treatment of congenital muscular torticollis in infants—a study of 1,086 cases. *J Pediatr Surg*. 2000 July;35(7):1091–1096.

[55] Macdonald D. Sternomastoid tumor and muscular torticollis. *J Bone Joint Surg*. 1969 Aug;51(3):432–443.

[56] Karmel-Ross K, Lepp M. Assessment and treatment of children with congenital muscular torticollis. *Phys Occup Ther Pediatr*. 1997;17(2):21–67.

[57] Ohman A, Nilsson S, Beckung E. Stretching treatment for infants with congenital muscular torticollis: physiotherapist or parents? A randomized pilot study. *PM R*. 2010 Dec;2:1073–1079.

[58] Ohman AM, Nilsson S, Beckung ERE, et al. Validity and reliability of the muscle function scale, aimed to assess the lateral flexors of the neck in infants. *Physiother Theory Pract*. 2009;25(2):129–137.

[59] Hutchison BL, Stewart AW, Mitchell EA. Deformational plagiocephaly: a follow-up of head shape, parental concern, and neurodevelopment at ages 3 and 4 years. *Arch Dis Child*. 2011;96:85–90.

[60] Da Silveira AC, Daw JL, Kusnoto B, et al. Craniofacial applications of three-dimensional laser surface scanning. *J Craniofac Surg*. 2003;14(4):449–456.

[61] Lam S, Pan IW, Strickland BA, et al. Factors influencing outcomes of the treatment of positional plagiocephaly in infants: a 7-year experience. *J Neurosurg Pediatr*. 2017;19(3):273–281.

[62] Freudlsperger C, Steinmacher S, Saure D, et al. Impact of severity and therapy onset in helmet therapy in positional plagiocephaly. *J Craniomaxillofac Surg*. 2016;44:110–115.

[63] Littlefield TR, Pomatto JK, Kelly KM. Dynamic orthotic cranioplasty: treatment of the older infant. Report of four cases. *Neurosurg Focus*. 2000;15(9):e5

[64] Xia JJ, Kennedy KA, Teichgraeber JF, et al. Nonsurgical treatment of deformational plagiocephaly: a systematic review. *Arch Pediatr Adolesc Med*. 2008;162(8):719–727.

[65] McGarry A, Dixon MT, Greig RJ, et al. Head shape measurement standards and cranial orthoses in the treatment of infants with deformational plagiocephaly. *Dev Med Child Neurol*. 2008;50(8):568–576.

[66] Robinson S, Proctor M. Diagnosis and management of deformational plagiocephaly. *J Neurosurg Pediatr*. 2009;3(4):284–295.

[67] Naidoo SD, Skolnick GB, Patel KB, et al. Long-term outcomes in treatment of deformational plagiocephaly and brachycephaly using helmet therapy and repositioning: a longitudinal cohort study. *Childs Nerv Syst*. 2015 Sep;31(9):1547–1552.

[68] Paquereau, J. Non-surgical management of posterior positional plagiocephaly: orthotics versus repositioning. *Ann Phys Rehabil Med*. 2013 Apr;56(3):231–249.

[69] van Wijk RM, van Vlimmeren LA, Groothuis-Oudshoorn CGM, et al. Helmet therapy in infants with positional skull deformation: randomized controlled trial. *BMJ*. 2014;348:g2741.

[70] Steinberg JP et al. American Academy of Pediatrics Executive Committee—Plastic Surgery Section. Rapid response to *BMJ* 2014;348:g2741. Accessed April 8, 2025. https://www.bmj.com/content/348/bmj.g2741/rapid-responses

[71] Eberle NA, Stelnicki EJ, Boland B. Efficacy of conservative and cranial orthotic therapy in over 4000 patients treated for positional plagiocephaly over a five-year period. *Plast Reconstr Surg*. 2015;136(4S):5–6.

[72] Steinberg JP, Rawlani R, Humphries LS, et al. Effectiveness of conservative therapy and helmet therapy for positional cranial deformation. *Plast Reconstr Surg*. 2015;135(3):833–842.

[73] Fowler EA, Becker DB, Pilgram TK, et al. Neurologic findings in infants with deformational plagiocephaly. *J Child Neurol*. 2008;23(7):742–747.

[74] Speltz ML, Collett BR, Stott-Miller M, et al. Case-control study of neurodevelopment in deformational plagiocephaly. *Pediatrics*. 2010;125(3):e537–e542.

CHAPTER 17

Orthoses for the Upper Extremity

Brigid Driscoll and Bonnie Leshuk

OBJECTIVES

Following completion of this material, the reader will be able to:

1. Identify appropriate upper extremity orthotic needs for patients with a variety of diagnoses that range from neuromuscular to sports-related injuries.
2. Formulate an appropriate therapeutic plan for the patient who could benefit from utilization of an orthosis for the upper extremity(ies).
3. Identify specific adaptations for orthotic interventions based on injuries, individual patient needs, and age.

INTRODUCTION

This chapter provides an overview of upper extremity orthotic intervention that ranges from multiple diagnoses to a large variety of upper limb devices. Typically, orthotic devices are named for the body part with which they are used. However, some orthoses are named using an eponym naming convention after a key designer or given nicknames. It is helpful to be familiar with all the commonly used upper extremity orthoses. When fitting an orthosis there should be a well-defined purpose for the device with the main goal of functional gains that allow patients to return to daily activities of life. This is achieved through a team approach that includes the patient, caregivers, therapists, orthotists, and physicians. Enabling the patient to be the center of the decision-making process

through adequate education empowers them to assist in choosing an appropriate device and increases orthotic compliance. Simplicity of design, cosmesis, device weight, dynamic versus static movement, adjustability for growth, comfort, ease of donning, and affordability are all factors to consider when recommending an orthotic device for a patient. Educating the patient and/or caregiver is critical for sufficient understanding of upper extremity orthotic use and device rationale. Most upper extremity orthoses require patient and family training during therapy sessions that translate to a home program. Consistent education from therapists and orthotists will produce optimal results and provide realistic expectations. Careful assessment of the recommended device is necessary to ensure it does not compromise a patient's compensatory movements or overall function. It is common to have a progression of upper

DOI: 10.4324/9781003526025-19

extremity orthoses based on a patient's progress through the rehabilitation process.

CEREBROVASCULAR ACCIDENT/TRAUMATIC BRAIN INJURY

Upper extremity hemiplegia is common post cerebrovascular accident (CVA) and traumatic brain injury (TBI). Considerable impairments are endured by patients with brain injuries, including contractures, loss of functional activities, loss of motor control, abnormal muscle tone, pain, and cognitive or behavioral involvement. Frequently, the upper extremities are more severely affected compared to the lower limbs in CVA patients. The coordination and control of detailed movements of the upper extremity are also more difficult to relearn after a CVA [1]. Over 50% of patients with upper extremity impairment post CVA fail to regain functional arm use [2]. Physical and occupational therapy and orthotic devices appropriate for the patient's respective progress through the stages (i.e., acute, subacute, chronic) of CVA and TBI rehabilitation are needed. Purposes of these devices include increasing function through maintenance of or increasing range of motion, reducing abnormal tone or supporting the limb.

Shoulder subluxation, loss of motion, and pain are common in hemiplegic patients. Shoulder pain can affect up to 70% of CVA patients [1]. The upper extremity typically begins in a flaccid state. Overall general shoulder muscle weakness is still present even when spasticity begins to emerge [3]. Shoulder slings can be used with flaccid upper extremities for support and protection during ambulation. The use of lap boards, arm troughs on assistive devices, and dynamic shoulder orthosis are other forms of shoulder support. The goal is to prevent inferior shoulder subluxation due to limited motor activity and the pull of gravity on the affected limb [4, 1]. It is important with the use of any of these devices that the patient removes them periodically for shoulder and elbow range of motion and for active movement if possible.

Flexor spasticity often presents in the flaccid limb. Coupled with compensatory movement patterns, this can foster the development of shoulder adduction and elbow flexion contractures. This can lead to skin breakdown, increased difficulty with functional tasks and nerve injuries. Compression neuropathies of the ulnar nerve are seen in 10% of patients with brain injuries [3]. Serial casting of elbow flexion contractures is an effective form of treatment. Weekly cast changes at 5–7 days with progressive increased elbow extension as range increases towards full extension are recommended. Casts should be set at the first angle of catch when moving a joint through its

range (also known as the R1 measurement). This will avoid stretching or forcing range of motion at the elbow, especially with spasticity present, because it will cause pain and skin breakdown. Once full extension is obtained, the final cast can be bivalved and relined to maintain the corrected range of motion. An alternative device could be a bi-valve thermoplastic orthosis molded in full elbow extension. Stockinette as a protective liner is used with both devices to preserve skin integrity. The cast or orthosis should be removed multiple times daily for cleaning and skin care, along with range of motion exercises. Dynamic elbow orthoses can also be used to increase range of motion. Devices consist of an arm and forearm cuff attached by medial and lateral elbow joints. Ultraflex joints (Ultraflex Systems Inc., Pottstown, PA) are commonly used. The joint is aligned at the center of the anatomical elbow joint and set in the measured available range of the elbow and most typically produces a low load extension force [3]. This type of device is for a selective group of brain injury patients with the ability to express if too much tension is being applied and the ability to monitor skin integrity. If the patient is not capable of providing this feedback, an attentive caregiver must be present to ensure the device is properly used and monitored.

Compensatory patterns and movements are developed early post brain injury. Therapy is initiated once the patient is medically stable to begin intervention for motor relearning and avoidance of poor pattern development while increasing functional independence [5]. Upper extremity orthotic management traditionally immobilized the limb to provide support to the extremity, maintain range of motion or reduce spasticity, but failed to improve function. Additionally, electrical stimulation of weakened wrist and finger extension muscles has been used to improve strength and function of the extensors. However, it is unclear how long the correction is maintained once the stimulation stops [1, 6]. There is an increased trend in the development of functional electrical stimulation (FES) orthoses. A variety of dynamic orthoses has been developed to focus on completion of functional tasks. Some are used as training devices at rehabilitation facilities, whereas others are wearable exoskeleton type dynamic devices to assist in carrying out activities of daily living (ADLs) [5, 7, 8]. The MyoPro Motion (Myomo Inc., Boston, MA) is a myoelectric device designed to support the weak extremity while controlling movement [9]. The design of the brace includes molded arm and forearm sections connected by a myoelectric elbow joint and includes a manually articulated wrist system. The device is activated by self-initiated movement of the paretic arm, and then a sensor in the brace detects the movement and amplifies the weak muscle signal in order to move the arm [10]. As with most orthotic devices, therapy intervention is needed to train individuals to use the new dynamic movement orthosis properly and efficiently. Clinicians need to be selective when recommending this type of device based on patient's abilities and expectations [8]. Dynamic movement orthoses allow tasks to be completed on a repetitive basis for motor relearning and have been found to be effective at increasing motor skills and improving functional abilities [5].

Hand and wrist splints are commonly used orthoses post brain injury. Brace designs vary based on whether the upper extremity is paralyzed or if partial paresis is present. The purpose is also to prevent contractures, reduce tone, and support the extremity. Forearm spasticity can lead to wrist and forearm flexion deformities, making it difficult to complete functional tasks, cause skin breakdown, and develop fixed deformities. Casts, custom thermoplastic devices, soft foam or thermoplastic over the counter devices, and more dynamic wrist hand orthoses can be used to encourage extension.

Serial casting of the wrist and fingers can also be performed. The technique is similar to the elbow extension cast described earlier. Here, the cast is made on the forearm and extends into the palm of the hand to gradually increase wrist extension. The casts are changed on a weekly basis with each new cast being set in the newly achieved available range of motion. It is important to cast at the length of the muscle and not to force unavailable range to avoid skin breakdown and lack of tolerance to casting. Casting typically focuses on increasing wrist extension due to the high incidence of flexion deformities. Once full range of motion is achieved, the cast can be bivalved and relined for maintenance of range, with the ability to remove the device throughout the day for active or passive range of motion exercises. A bivalved custom thermoplastic device can also be made. If the contracture is more flexible, use of a dynamic wrist extension orthosis, such as an Ultraflex (or JAS device (Joint Active Systems, Inc., Effingham, IL)) can be used for gradual increases in range of motion.

Resting hand splints can also be used to support wrist extension of approximately 10–30° and may extend the full length of the fingers to promote extension. If adduction and flexion of the thumb is present, the thumb may be incorporated and held in extension, opposition, and abduction. Clinicians must choose between a dorsal or volar device (Figure 17.1). Factors to consider include ease of donning the device and the severity of the deformity. If significant flexor spasticity is present, a dorsal splint may be more effective to extend the wrist and fingers. This is because bracing on the volar side may elicit a sensory response encouraging increased flexion into the hand splint and increased spasticity [10]. If ROM is adequate and severe deformities are not present, use of off-the-shelf wrist orthoses are often effective and appropriate. With more severe range limitations, the wrist hand orthosis (WHO) would require custom fabrication. These are commonly made with low temperature plastics such

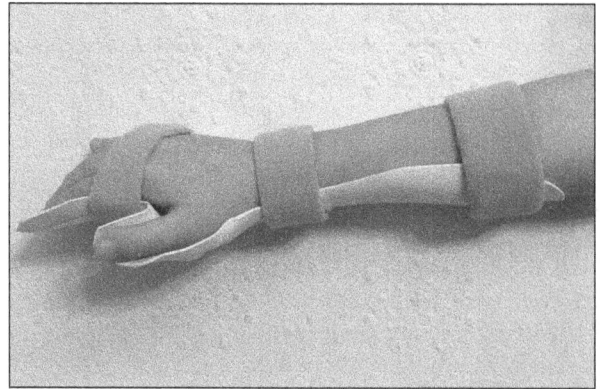

Figure 17.1. Example of a resting hand splint used to support 10–30° of wrist extension.

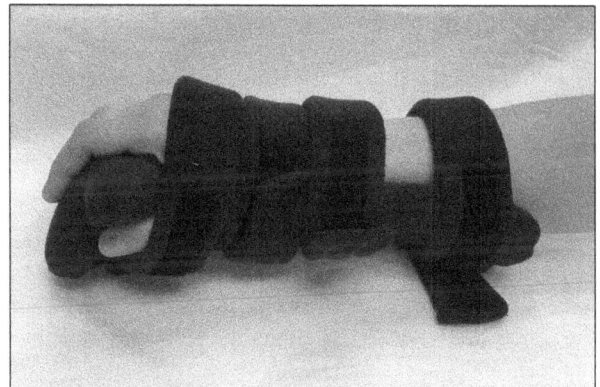

Figure 17.2. Prefabricated soft splint providing an open wrist and hand space to facilitate increased joint range, skin integrity, and proper hygiene.

as polyform or EZ-form to accommodate contractures and deformities. Some patients do not tolerate the thermoplastic WHOs well due to severe spasticity and deformities. Soft splints (Figure 17.2) are available to open the wrist and hand space with increased comfort to encourage increased range of motion to protect skin integrity and to allow proper hygiene.

When finger extension is compromised by flexor spasticity, dynamic wrist hand finger splints are an option to encourage grasp. They consist of a thermoplastic forearm section with outriggers and rubber bands which position the hand for grasping objects by opening the fingers and abducting the thumb. This style of brace is bulky and can challenge compliance [3]. Therefore, it is important to assess how functional this device will be for a patient considering motivation, goals of the patient, and ease with ADLs.

Recovery post stroke is a combination of spontaneous recovery and complex brain reorganization. These concepts are slowly becoming better understood through more accurate diagnostic tools known as brain mapping technology such as functional MRIs or transcranial magnetic stimulation. Neuroplasticity, which is the ability of the nervous system to reorganize, has been proven to occur in the brain post CVA or TBI [11]. Intense amounts of repetitive movement of specific motor tasks appear to stimulate neuroplasticity in the brain [12]. The term "learned nonuse" is used when referring to patients with hemiplegia post brain injury. This is when compensatory movements are adopted, and the unaffected limb takes over to complete functional daily tasks. To improve function in the impaired upper extremity, it has been shown that constraint-induced movement therapy (CIMT) is effective in improving function for chronic brain injury patients in the hemiparetic limb through intensive repetitive motor learning tasks. When learned nonuse persists, individuals are unable to rehabilitate. Thus, it is not surprising that over 50% of patients still present with significant hemiparesis [2, 11, 13]. CIMT was designed to overcome learned nonuse by constraining the uninvolved limb with devices such as slings with a resting hand splint or a sling with a mitt over the hand. The constraint device is used 90% of awake time. Intense functional therapy is then instituted up to 6 hours per day focusing on repetitive motor tasks to improve overall function and use of the involved upper extremity in activities of daily living [11, 13, 14].

There are many orthotic options for managing patients with brain injuries. The important factors to consider are the patient's ability to functionally use them, caregiver support, the patient's motivation level, orthotic goals, and optimal fit based on anatomical alignment and underlying tone.

Spinal Cord Injury

Patients with quadriplegia have a unique challenge as they may require an extensive and expensive amount of technology, orthotics, and durable medical equipment. Greater than half the orthotic devices prescribed may not be used 1–2 years post hospital discharge. This emphasizes the importance of recommending only the most functional devices with patient-centered input [15].

MyoPro Motion-G orthosis (Myomo, Inc., Cambridge, MA) is an option to replace the wrist-driven flexor hinge orthoses for C5 and C6 level SCIs. It may also be used with the following diagnoses: brachial plexus injury, stroke, multiple sclerosis, TBI, amyotrophic lateral sclerosis, and cerebral palsy. The device uses surface EMG to power the motors of the elbow joint and three jaw chuck finger grasp. The number of electrodes will determine if the grasp is voluntary with automatic release (1 electrode) or sustained (2 electrodes). Typically, the electrodes would be positioned for moving the elbow and fingers. The wrist and forearm require manual positioning. MyoPro is appropriate for ambulatory patients with intact cognition, a stable

shoulder (one finger or less subluxation allowable) and a viable EMG signal in the proximal and distal upper extremity. It is not for use in cases with hypertonicity or when Botox injections have been used. Full hand and finger passive range of motion (PROM) is necessary as well as wrist ROM to neutral or greater extension [9]. Because the device uses sensors to amplify the weak muscle signal via software rather than electrical stimulation, it is better tolerated on the skin and can produce more power than alternatives. The goal of this device is to provide the user with a stabilizing assist for bilateral activities and to improve lifting ability of the elbow and three jaw chuck prehension for ADLs. Functional uses of this device may include increasing safety by allowing the user to hold an object with the device while using the unaffected/opposite arm to hold onto a railing or open a door, decreasing postural compensations and increasing energy conservation by increasing the affected arm's power, increasing function by allowing tasks such as pouring or carrying a laundry basket to be completed bimanually. It typically takes 4–6 sessions to become adept at using this device.

The Rehabilitation Institute of Chicago (RIC) tenodesis splint provides improved functional prehension strength by using the hand's natural tenodesis wrist extension force translated into finger prehension. This type of dynamic, hinged orthosis is appropriate for a C6–C7 spinal cord injury. Patients may not need these splints for all-day wear, but rather for a specific functional skill such as removing laundry from a machine or driving.

Static orthotic devices for the wrist and hand include short and long opponens type WHOs with extension stops. Again, these devices may be used for specific tasks during the day. They may also serve as a base for stabilizing adaptive equipment for self-care, work, or sports. Night-time resting hand splints or wrist hand finger orthoses (WHFOs) are necessary to prevent contractures that would interfere with dressing and hygiene as well as to preserve the tenodesis function of the wrist and hand.

Fractures

Orthotic management is indicated for specific upper extremity fractures. Sarmiento et al. introduced functional brace therapy in 1967, initially used for tibial fractures, and in 1977, presented an orthosis for humeral shaft fractures [16–18]. The concept of functional bracing is based on circumferential compression of the soft tissues surrounding the fracture site. This provides external stabilization with improved fracture alignment and control of limb length while healing occurs. Through use of functional bracing the joints adjacent to the fracture are free, which allows early range of motion and functional mobility. Early movement of the limb facilitates muscle contractions surrounding the fracture which stimulates blood flow and osteogenesis while promoting rapid healing [16, 17].

Midshaft humeral fractures are successfully treated with an anterior and posterior prefabricated shell that accommodates the arm musculature (Figure 17.3). The majority of humeral fractures are treated with this method. Acceptable alignment and healing is observed in over 90% of cases [16–20]. Typical treatment for a humeral fracture begins with a coaptation splint and sling to provide proper stabilization and pain control while allowing reduction of swelling. Once the majority of swelling is resolved, usually between 10 and 14 days [17], a functional brace is likely implemented. As stated earlier, this allows early movement of the limb and prevents loss of motion and inflammation at the elbow and shoulder.

Proper brace fit is essential for successful healing and treatment. The medial aspect of the shell should rest 2.5 cm beneath the axilla and extend 1 cm proximal to the medial epicondyle. The lateral shell placement is just distal to the

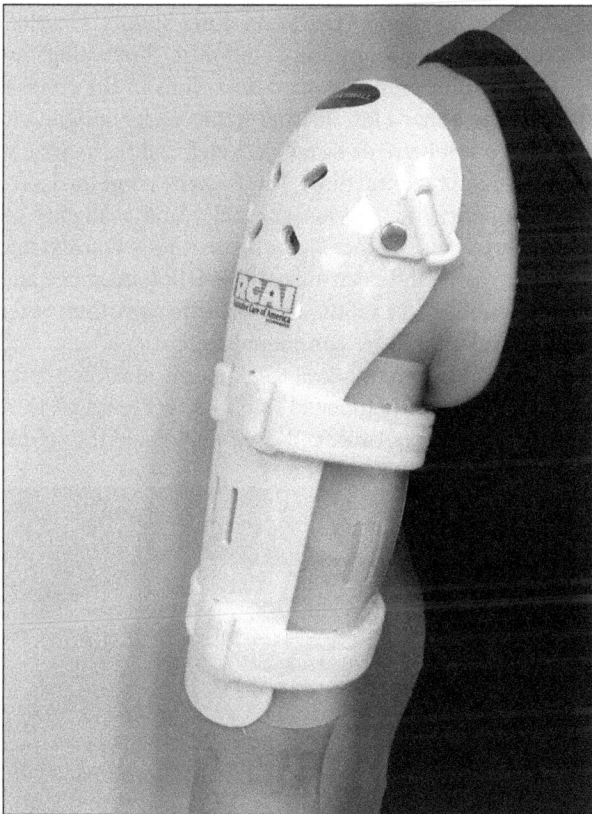

Figure 17.3. Anterior and posterior prefabricated shell to accommodate arm musculature in the presence of a midshaft humeral fracture.

lateral aspect of the acromion process while extending to just proximal the lateral epicondyle [17]. Velcro® straps attach the anterior and posterior shell and allow adjustability to accommodate changes in swelling while maintaining proper circumferential pressure for bone healing. Stockinette is worn between the brace and skin to prevent irritation or breakdown.

The device is worn until fracture healing is radiographically confirmed which may take approximately 10 weeks [18–21]. Acceptable parameters for healing and fracture reduction are 30° of varus angulation, 20° of anterior bowing, and up to 15° of internal rotation. Beyond these ranges, clinical loss of function and cosmetic deformities are noted [17]. Not all humeral fractures can be functionally braced for fracture management. Functional brace management is not indicated for open fractures, fractures with extensive soft tissue damage due to the risk of infection, individuals who have suffered multiple traumas, and certain fracture patterns [17]. There is also risk of radial nerve injury, an average of 11–12%, due to its contact with the humerus. Recovery of the nerve with observation alone is noted in over 90% of cases [17, 19, 21].

Ulnar fractures are also documented to produce bone union with functional bracing. The key to successful fracture management is proper indication of use. Isolated ulnar shaft fractures of the middle to distal third of the long bone may likely result in proper bone union and positive functional results. The success of functional bracing may be based on forearm stability from the integrity of the interosseous membrane. Stable ulnar shaft fractures are defined as having an intact interosseous membrane and displacement of the ulnar fragment that is less than half the width of the shaft in the anteroposterior and lateral radiographic planes [22].

The course of treatment is quite similar to that of the humeral functional bracing. Long arm casts are applied at the time of injury in a neutral position for stability while controlling pain and reducing swelling. On an average of 5 days, the cast is removed, and use of a prefabricated brace is initiated [22, 23]. The brace consists of an anterior and posterior shell that wraps circumferentially around the forearm with Velcro® closures that can be adjusted for changes in swelling. The shell has an interior liner with a figure 8 contour promoting a total contact fit preventing rotation within the device [23]. A stockinette liner is used over the skin for protection and to prevent irritation. Functional activities and use of the affected extremity, along with therapy intervention should commence with brace use. Bone union is commonly achieved in approximately 7–8 weeks [22, 23].

Good functional return and bone union are both indicators of successful fracture management. Use of functional bracing has proven to be effective in managing certain types of upper extremity fractures and allows avoidance of risks associated with surgery while maintaining lower costs.

ARTHRITIS

While early orthotic intervention is helpful, medications may decrease inflammation and improve range of motion to make a considerable impact on the recommended orthotic intervention. The goal of the orthosis for an arthritis patient is to prevent and reduce contractures, decrease pain and inflammation, and protect the involved joints during daily living activities.

For patients requiring long-term joint stabilization who also have soft tissue changes due to swelling, custom orthoses may be better tolerated. An orthosis fabricated from low temperature material allows for repeated heating and remolding to accommodate changes in shape and range of motion due to inflammation. High temperature fabricated orthoses have a durability benefit but are less adjustable.

A simple prefabricated or custom low temperature elbow or wrist hand finger orthosis can provide the necessary stretch, support, and pain relief for night use. If only the fingers are involved, a low temperature plastic "gutter" type splint provides sagittal and coronal plane control. Some patients may better tolerate soft neoprene finger sleeves if the goal is contracture prevention isolated to the fingers. While there are dynamic torsion joint devices available for night use, it is important to remember the weight of the device may have more of an impact on the patient with arthritis. Arthritis patients may benefit from lighter weight spring wire and foam hand and finger products. Neoprene type elbow orthoses which have Velcro® openings are generally easier to don than pull-type sleeves. Dynamic orthotic devices with outriggers are typically used for post-operative joint replacements. They may interfere with ADLs and may not provide optimal alignment during sleep.

Daytime orthoses need to provide stability without impeding function. There are many prefabricated wrist hand orthoses on the market but some require customization. For example, a typical wrist hand orthosis equipped with a metal reinforcement (i.e. stay) may require removal and re-contouring to the patient's functional wrist position and anatomy and to increase comfort. Acceptance and tolerance for the orthosis may be further improved by replacing the metal stay with low temperature plastic molded to the patient. This offers support without rigid immobilization. Newer 3D printed products, such as the ActivArmor (ActivArmor, Port St. Lucie, FL) wrist hand and finger orthosis, can be worn during activities that require getting hands wet. Such technologies allow for increased joint support and compliance during activities of daily living.

The 3D-printed orthoses can be designed for some edema fluctuation but have limited adjustability.

Arthritic metacarpophalangeal (MCP) joints may be addressed with versions of wrist hand orthoses that include the thumb or in carpometacarpal (CMC)/MCP specific devices. The Push ortho thumb brace CMC (Push Braces, Maastricht-Airport, The Netherlands) provides stability and pain relief for CMC instability by supporting abduction. Ulnar deviation or drift at the MCPs is typically seen in patients with rheumatoid arthritis. It is important to prevent and control ulnar deviation of the fingers at the MCP joints. This may be achieved with a combination of a WHFO and daytime hand orthoses (HO) or wrist hand orthoses (WHO).

In general, when finger contractures are less than 20–25°, metal ring splints or prefabricated plastic splints are beneficial. Dynamic spring foam and wire type finger splints can be used for contractures up to 45° of flexion. Serial casting of the joint is needed for contractures greater than 45°. Serial casting the proximal interphalangeal (PIP) joints is an effective method to reduce PIP joint flexion contractures in patients with rheumatoid arthritis or juvenile idiopathic arthritis. Individual PIP joint casting may result in less stiffness in non-contracted joints, but children and smaller adult hands may not accommodate the bulkier plaster cast material on multiple involved fingers [24]

Metal ring splints (i.e., Silver Ring Splints, Charlottesville, VA) are a long-term solution to fluctuating finger contractures and alignment deviations in the coronal plane. Using a sizing kit, the ring splint can be designed to address Boutonniere or Swan Neck deformities as well as individual joint contractures. These can be combined with lateral supports to provide coronal plane realignment. Once fabricated, the metal can be bent to accommodate subtle increases and decreases of PIP/DIP joint range and inflammation. These splints are more expensive than other options and should be considered for patients who will require them long term. Oval 8 splints are a low-cost, prefabricated alternative to metal ring splints (Figure 17.4). A sizing kit is also available, and combinations of the splints

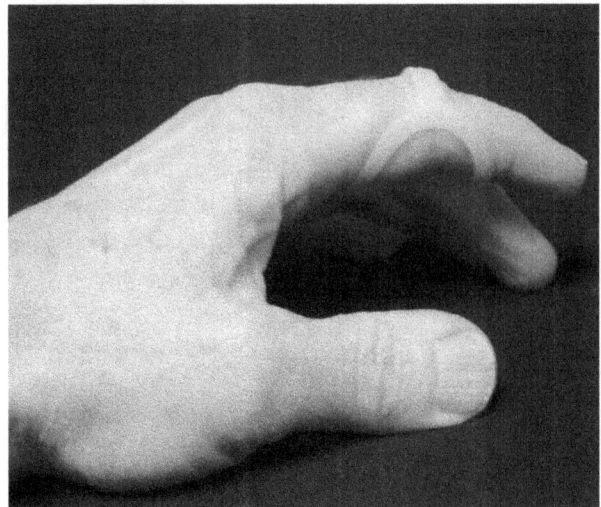

Figure 17.4. Oval 8 splint used in the case of a Boutonniere deformity.

being used in the sagittal and coronal planes can simulate the effect of metal ring splint lateral supports. Minor adjustments can be made to the plastic with a heat gun.

BURNS

Burn patients present unique challenges. For instance, involved tissue can contract rapidly. Additionally, the burn may involve surfaces in multiple planes which may limit use of traditional straps to secure the orthosis. Clam shell type orthoses can help distribute pressure over a broader area. The design of hand orthoses for burn victims needs to be well planned due to potential multi-joint involvement. For example, individual slotted straps or finger troughs may help expand the palmar area. These patients often use static or static-progressive devices. They are typically worn for a length of 6–18 months. Often, they are used in combination with pressure garments for scar control. It is important to consider this when choosing a volar or dorsal based orthotic device to avoid uncomfortable pressure and potential skin irritation from zippers.

Two plastic materials that particularly benefit burn patients are high temperature Silon-STS and low temperature Silon-LTS. Both are silicone lined, likely eliminating the need for separate silicone pads that may slip out of place. Low temperature has the advantage of being reheated if additional range of motion is expected or for smaller joints. High temperature materials tend to be stronger which allows for stable attachment of metal bars/joints. This strength may be needed for larger joints, active children and adults.

Axillary burns require a prefabricated or custom shoulder elbow wrist hand orthosis (SEWHO). Low temperature elbow orthoses are helpful as they can be reheated to accommodate volume changes in dressings. In the rehabilitation phase, static-progressive or dynamic elbow orthosis may be needed. If the hand is not involved, it may need to be included regardless to help keep the orthosis in the correct position and prevent compression of the wrist anatomy. The hand may also need to be included to preserve supination, which is more challenging to restore and

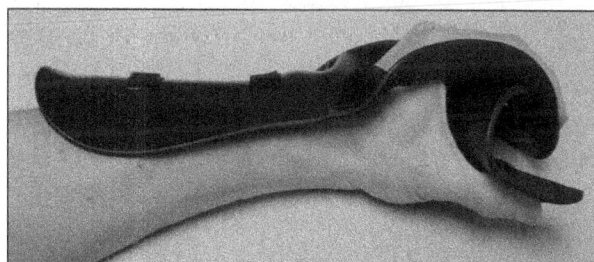

Figure 17.5. Non-circumferential orthosis applied to the extensor surface of the forearm in the case of a volar burn to the hand at risk for developing an intrinsic minus (claw hand) deformity. The goal in this case is to position the hand in an intrinsic plus or "safe" position of 15–30° wrist extension, 70–80° MCP flexion, full IP joint extension, and thumb abduction.

cannot be compensated for like pronation by internally rotating at the shoulder.

A volar burn to the hand is at risk for developing an intrinsic minus or "claw hand" deformity. It needs to be positioned in an intrinsic plus or "safe" position of 15–30° wrist extension, 70–80° MCP flexion, full IP joint extension and thumb abduction [3]. (See Figure 17.5.)

CHRONIC PAIN

The causes of chronic pain are numerous: orthopedic (post fracture, arthritic development), neurologic, tendonitis, and syndrome-related. Because pain has a personal and cultural component, pain can be challenging and complex. Patients and caregivers need to play an active role in choosing whether or not to add an orthotic device to their treatment plan. Some patients may require limiting movement due to joint instability and overuse, others may require mobility assist due to joint stiffness. It is wise to systematically evaluate each involved joint to determine which movements require a stop, limit or assist and in which anatomical plane (sagittal, coronal, transverse). A rule of thumb when recommending a dynamic corrective orthosis to treat soft tissue contractures is that the contracture must be less than a year old in adults, but can be of indefinite duration in children [25]. Since fatigue is a concern for chronic pain patients, consideration of device weight over benefit of support is very important.

A common diagnosis with a chronic pain component is Ehlers Danlos Syndrome, a connective tissue disorder resulting in hypermobility of the joints. Due to the ligament hyperlaxity, patients with the diagnosis of Ehlers Danlos commonly present with shoulder instability, elbow hyperextension, and finger and thumb hyperextension. These patients may benefit from orthoses similar to those recommended for arthritis patients. Compared with patients with traumatic shoulder instability, their shoulders are more likely to experience recurrent subluxation and dislocation [26]. The goal of shoulder orthoses is to increase proprioceptive feedback, increase shoulder stability, reduce pain, improve postural alignment, and increase active range of motion of the shoulder. Shoulder stabilization orthosis options include the custom DMO™ (DM Orthotics, Redruth, United Kingdom) or prefabricated devices such as Bauerfeind's OmoTrain® (Bauerfeind, Atlanta, GA). Ehlers Danlos and other elbow instabilities may benefit from a prefabricated elbow anti-hyperextension orthosis such as Breg's HEX elbow (Breg Inc., Carlsbad, CA) with hinges and extension stops and anterior elbow strapping which can limit movement. Hypermobile wrists and fingers may be addressed with custom or prefabricated WHOs and Oval 8 type finger orthoses.

One barrier to patient compliance for a WHO returning to work or during daily living activities is the ability to use the device in a wet or dirty environment. As mentioned in the arthritis section, 3D-printed orthoses can be a solution to this problem. ActivArmor is one example of a waterproof 3D-printed exoskeleton device made from a body scan. Use of an optical 3D scanner to produce a customized orthosis is a more recent development in the field but is making access to scanners increasing production efficiency and cost effectiveness is in its early stages [27, 28].

SPORTS

Preventative Orthoses

Upper extremity orthotics designed for sports activities can prevent injury or allow patients to return to sports post injury. Preventative orthoses (protective equipment) provide support to braced anatomical joints to limit motion and distribute external forces over a larger surface area [3]. Protective equipment is typically made of a thin thermoplastic outer shell that is as lightweight as possible to allow distribution of pressure. The shells contain linings made of soft low-density materials to absorb as much energy as possible [3, 29, 30]. In order for protective equipment to be effective, it is essential that the device fits properly.

Shoulder pads for athletes primarily involved in American football, hockey, and lacrosse are common protective equipment. The exact design varies from sport to sport, and also based on a specific position. Shoulder pads are intended to protect the chest, shoulder girdle, and upper back. Football shoulder pads consist of an outer plastic shell for high impact and a foam liner for shock absorption. Proper fitting shoulder pads should encompass the shoulder while covering the deltoid area. Straps should be securely donned to minimize movement of pads [3].

Elbow sleeves, typically prefabricated, made of neoprene or more breathable materials such as BioSkin (BioSkin, Ashland, OR) can be used for soft tissue compression and therapeutic warmth. The sleeve can control swelling or prevent pain; in addition it can protect the skin during sports activities where sliding occurs against turf or grass. Modifications can be made to elbow sleeves for additional protection. In instances where protection of the olecranon process is needed, a plastic shell can be fabricated and placed over the olecranon to protect against elbow fractures in sports such as inline skating. Dense foam padding along the forearm can also be used to prevent injuries where potential stick impact can occur [3].

Wrist guards have been noted to prevent injuries in snowboarding, inline skating, and skateboarding [29, 30]. Fractures of the distal radius, carpal fractures, and ligament tears are some of the most common injuries associated with athletes involved in these sports [30]. Wrist guards are typically made of a nylon glove that is against the athlete's skin with a volar and dorsal plate extending from the proximal aspect of the wrist to the metacarpophalangeal

joint. The plastic plates prevent excessive wrist extension and should limit the range to 30° [30]. Velcro® straps at the wrist and hand provide a total contact fit and prevent device migration. Studies show that wrist guards protect the wrist by load sharing and absorbing energy [29, 30]. It is also noted that additional soft padding can be effective in force reduction, while a thin outer shell is necessary to spread the load over a greater surface area to reduce peak pressures [29].

Orthoses Post Injury

When an athlete is injured, the goal is to return to the previous level of function. This requires proper healing, strengthening, and educating the athlete on realistic expectations for return to activities. It is important to determine when to push aggressively through the rehabilitation process and when to slow the process down to allow healing and strengthening. A team approach is needed when managing patients returning to sports post injury. The team includes the athlete, physician, therapists, coaches, trainers, orthotists, and team officials. Once the athlete has successfully completed the rehabilitation process, they need to be properly braced for joint protection and injury prevention. The use of taping, custom splints, off-the-shelf braces, soft casts, or hard casts are all options that may be used as protective bracing [31]. The key is to use sound judgment during goal setting, risk factor analysis, and assessment, and to assure the athlete is medically ready to return to activity.

Acromioclavicular (AC) joint injuries are common shoulder injuries in sports. The AC joint acts as a strut for the scapula to rest against the thorax. It stabilizes the scapula while allowing translation of the joint with shoulder elevation and rotation to attain full abduction [32]. This joint is easily sprained and susceptible to trauma from falls. Rehabilitation is aimed at regaining proper scapulohumeral movement through soft tissue release, modalities, stretching, strengthening, and proprioceptive re-training. Taping of the joint is known to be a positive adjunct to the rehab process. The mechanical effects of taping re-locate the joint in order to stabilize it with proper length–tension relationships for normal musculoskeletal alignment and motor patterns [32]. Taping also provides proprioceptive feedback to the joint [32, 33]. AC taping method is applied at the coracoid process and attaches over the shoulder in a posterior direction toward the mid-section of the thoracic cage [32]. Use of a donut pad over the AC joint can be used for additional protection. If more protection is needed, a plastic dome shell can be placed over the joint. This can be prefabricated or custom made from low temperature thermoplastics. In sports where additional shoulder padding is used, such as football or lacrosse, it is important to ensure the AC padding or shell rests properly over the joint with the addition of the protective shoulder pads [3].

The glenohumeral joint allows significant joint mobility to function, thus making the joint very unstable and the most frequently dislocated joint in the body [35]. In order to return to activities post dislocation it is necessary to complete a regimented rehabilitation program for dynamic shoulder stability. Rehabilitation consists of specific strengthening exercises with a focus on scapular stabilization, dynamic stability activities, neuromuscular training, and proprioceptive exercises [35]. Once functional range of motion is regained, strength is symmetrical, and dynamic stability is achieved, athletes can and often return to sports with supportive bracing [34, 35] and at times with taping of the shoulder [32]. Supportive bracing and taping are used for control of shoulder external rotation and abduction. One technique is the Rigney Strap, which is applied with the shoulder abducted to 90°and in full internal rotation. Taping begins from the posterior and inferior aspect of the humerus bringing the rigid tape anteriorly across the superior aspect of the glenohumeral joint and attaching at the mid thorax. Multiple layers are applied, limiting range of motion and the likelihood of dislocation [32]. Shoulder stability braces such as the DonJoy brace (Enovis/, DJO GLOBALLewisville, TX) or Duke Wyre brace are often required for return to play in contact sports such as football or hockey [35, 34] The Sully brace (DJO GLOBAL, Vista, CA) (Figure 17.6) could be used for athletes who overhead throw, such as basketball players, allowing greater shoulder range of motion while still providing stability [34].

Common elbow injuries in athletes are inflammation such as lateral epicondylitis, muscle contusions, and elbow dislocations. Lateral epicondylitis is managed with taping, bracing, and therapeutic exercises. Bracing of the wrist extensors proximally near their origin on the lateral epicondyle is effective in compressing the tendons and reducing pain. Simple single strap counterforce braces

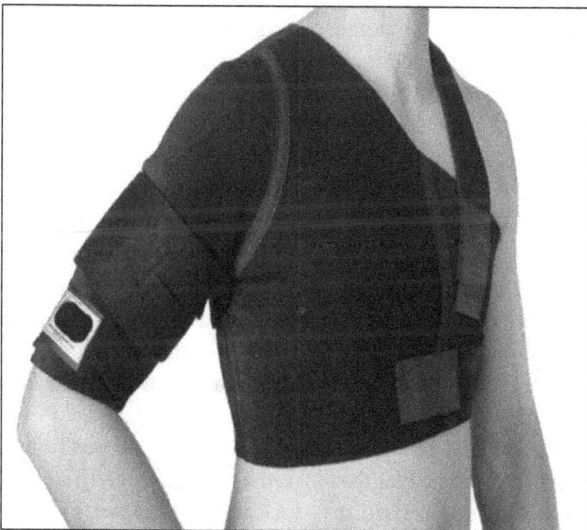

Figure 17.6. A shoulder stability brace. Shoulder stability braces such as this one are often required for return to play in contact sports such as football or hockey.

wrap around the proximal forearm just distal to the elbow, essentially adding to the proximal origin of the involved muscles and redirecting the magnitude and vector of force application [36]. Dislocation injuries may require greater stability and range of motion limitations. Hinged elbow braces can be utilized with adjustable range of motion depending on the extent of injury and necessary range limitations. Braces with bilateral hinges can help control varus or valgus elbow stress [3].

Wrist and hand injuries can be managed with protective equipment allowing injured athletes to safely return to play. Taping, custom-made splints, and over-the-counter splints are decided upon based on specific sport demands, healing, rehab status, and recommendations of the therapist or trainer directly involved with the patient [31]. Gymnasts and football players use taping or neoprene wraps to avoid wrist hyperextension [3, 31]. "Buddy taping" is utilized for protecting reduced phalangeal dislocations and subluxations, soft tissue injuries, and healing phalangeal fractures. Taping should stabilize the joint while allowing necessary range of motion for the athlete's needs. The intact finger acts as a splint for the adjacent injured finger with application over the mid-phalangeal level and not over the joints. Taping of the MCP and carpometacarpal joint of the thumb is also effective for stability while allowing functional thumb range of motion [31]. Thermoplastics can be used for injuries, such as mallet fingers, a simple spring extension assist splint, which is attached with tape for sports activities [37]. Thermoplastic rigid splints can be used over tape of the wrist and hand, but they need to be approved by team officials for safety of use during play.

Adaptive Sports Equipment

Protective equipment used when returning to sport has been presented thus far; however, adapting actual sporting equipment can also be appropriate. It is important to research individual sports to best understand their respective athletic demands. Listen to athletes to learn about the position they play and how they maneuver their upper extremity during sporting activities. Additionally, be aware what is within regulation with respect to orthotic intervention for return to sport activities [37]. Regulatory sporting agencies include the National Collegiate Athletic Association, www.NCAA.org, the National Federation of State High School Associations, www.NFHS.org, others. When preparing an athlete for return to sport post rehabilitation, it is important to assess the condition of their sporting equipment, their interaction with it, as well as how they maneuver the upper extremity during sporting use. Equipment adaptations and orthotic fabrication can occur based on this evaluation. An example would be for a thumb ulnar collateral ligament (UCL) injury, gamekeeper's thumb, for a hockey player. A hand-based low temperature splint can be fabricated to immobilize

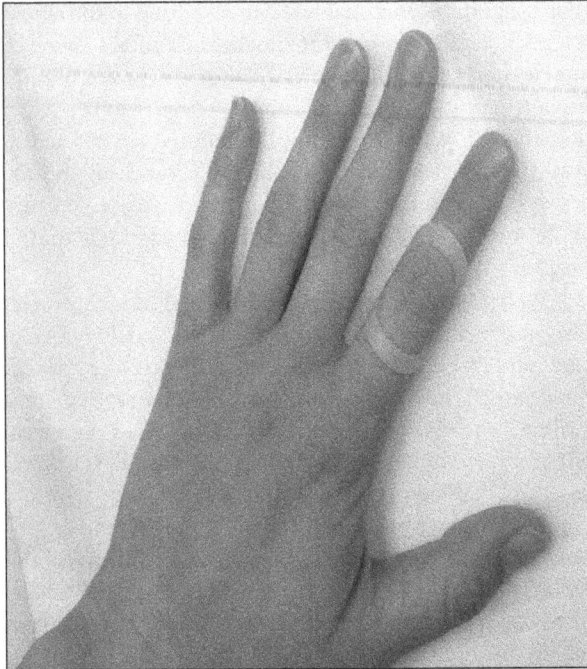

Figure 17.7. Simple over-the-counter thermoplastic PIP extension restriction splint.

the thumb while making sure it fits into the hockey glove [38]. Another example could be for a cyclist with ulnar nerve compression within Guyon's canal. Modifications can be made to handlebars to decrease pressure or excessive extension of the wrist. In addition, fabrication of an ulnar-based custom thermoplastic splint with a gel liner can be used to reduce pressure. Again, this should be fabricated to accommodate padded cycling gloves. Simple over-the-counter thermoplastic PIP extension restriction splints (Figure 17.7) can be used during ball sports, such as basketball, to prevent finger hyperextension in healing injuries [39]. There are numerous adaptations that can be made for athletes returning to sports. The point is to individualize each athlete's orthotic and sporting needs.

BRACHIAL PLEXUS INJURY

The brachial plexus involves the nerves of C5–C8 and T1. Lesions to the brachial plexus can result from a variety of causes such as traction during birth or motor vehicle accident, direct trauma from a bullet wound or radiation, or compression. Because the brachial plexus is tethered by the clavicle and scalene muscles, forceful neck motion to the side frequently produces a traction injury to the upper brachial plexus (C5–C6) [40]. Traction to the brachial plexus may also occur because of arm movement; as the arm is brought up and over the head, traction will occur within the lower brachial plexus (C8–T1) [41]. Compression injuries to the brachial plexus occur between the clavicle above and the first rib below.

Damage to these nerves during birth is referred to as an obstetric brachial plexus injury (OBPI). The infant will present with decreased upper extremity muscle and sensory function. The lesions are often due to traction during labor and occurrence is 2 in 1,000 births [41]. Prognosis is based on severity of the traction injury: neuropraxia to axontomesis will have complete to near complete recovery; neurotomesis and root avulsion will have permanent loss of arm function. While the majority of lesions resolve, 20–30% will have residual deficits [41]. The most common OBPI involves the C5–C6 nerve roots and is frequently referred to as Erb's palsy. In this type of lesion the upper extremity is typically resting in adduction, internal rotation, and elbow extension. If C7 is also involved, the wrist and fingers rest in flexion.

The goal for upper extremity orthosis for brachial plexus injuries is to prevent deformity and support the maximal range of motion for self-care, assist in positioning the limb, and promote the hand's transverse and longitudinal arches. Depending on the location of the BPI and age of patient, different orthoses may be utilized.

The most extensive device, a shoulder elbow wrist hand orthosis (SEWHO), has adjustable shoulder, elbow, and forearm positions. Commercially available SEWHO devices include the pediatric "High Five" and the adult MyoPro which was previously discussed in the spinal cord injury section. The High Five device can be used pre-operatively to provide stretch or post-operatively to protect the surgical release/transfer for an OBPI. A gentle, low-load force over a prolonged period is most effective [42]. It is critical to not be too aggressive and attenuate the nerve. A custom device is necessary when the soft tissue contours are outside the normal anatomy, in the presence of soft tissue contractures or if the patient is too small to fit the parameters of a prefabricated device.

During the day, the flail BPI shoulder should be protected with a sling to prevent attenuation of the joint capsule and protect the insensate arm. While there are many options for routine daily sling use, patients who wish to participate in high caliber sports and work may require a custom sling to secure and protect the arm. The United Brachial Plexus Network (www.ubpn.org) provides a resource for the custom sling.

If the shoulder is able to attain a functional position and the range of motion restrictions are in the elbow, forearm and wrist, an elbow wrist hand orthosis (EWHO) evaluation is needed. Elbow motion serves to position the hand in space. The functional arc of elbow motion during activities of daily living are considered to be 100° for both flexion–extension (30° to 130°) and pronation–supination (50° in either direction) [43]. Supination/pronation range of motion must be assessed with the elbow flexed at 90° to avoid shoulder compensations. This is also the position to provide optimal length–tension relationships. Therefore, the orthosis will require a locking mechanism for flexion as close to this position as possible. The patient who has restrictions in extension and supination may need to initially focus on extension as a priority to provide protection during falls. Supination may be addressed more aggressively later in treatment by alternating nights of extension with supination, locking the device in 90°of flexion for static progressive supination.

A commercially available device such as the JAS Orthosis uses multiple static progressive splinting sessions (typically 30 minutes, three times a day) during the day to restore range of motion. These prefabricated, customized devices usually require the patient to be stationary. Ultraflex uses a dynamic spring tension joint (unidirectional or bidirectional) for increasing elbow flexion and extension via night-time use [44, 45]. For pediatrics or adults with soft tissue contours outside of the norm, a custom forearm rotation elbow orthosis (FREO) will help achieve functional elbow and forearm range of motion. The FREO combines an Ultraflex dynamic tension joint at the elbow with a static progressive configuration (interlocking forearm cuffs with Velcro® hook and loop) at the forearm [46]. (See Figure 17.8.) General guidelines for contracture management with dynamic orthosis is anytime in children, less than one year in adults.

Dynamic movement orthoses (DMO) full- and short-length gloves can help improve resting position and functional day use [47]. The DMO fabricated from a Lycra® base material, can be designed with reinforcement panels to promote forearm supination and wrist extension. It is critical that the patient have adequate passive range of motion present to achieve the functional goal position. The DMO is not intended to improve passive range of motion; its goal is to facilitate functional position through the elasticity of the panels. When designing the device, it is important to consider multiple layers and pre-stretching of the material to facilitate an optimal functional position of supination and wrist extension. Recall that DMO fabric is susceptible to catching and tearing, thus the device may require further protection with leather-type biking gloves depending on the patient's activity. The additional glove layer may decrease sensation to an already impaired hand. Open finger tips are usually recommended by the manufacturer. Patients returning to work may not be able to use

some orthotic devices if there is a safety risk while using heavy machinery or due to hygiene requirements.

Functional day use WHOs are commonly used. Many prefabricated versions and customized, latex-free alternatives are available through companies such as Benik (Benik Corp., Silverdale, WA) and McKie (McKie Splints, Duluth, MN). They can retain heat/moisture so enzyme cleaners are available, but they tend to be tolerated well due to their soft interface and cosmetic appearance. It is important to evaluate the device to ensure that the thumb and wrist are secured in neutral alignment and deviations are not simply obscured by the material. One way to customize a prefabricated orthosis is by removing standard metal stays and contouring them to the patient. Also, flaring the metal edges at the distal and proximal ends, away from the patient's tissue, avoids facilitating a flexion response (Figure 17.9). For patients requiring less support, the metal

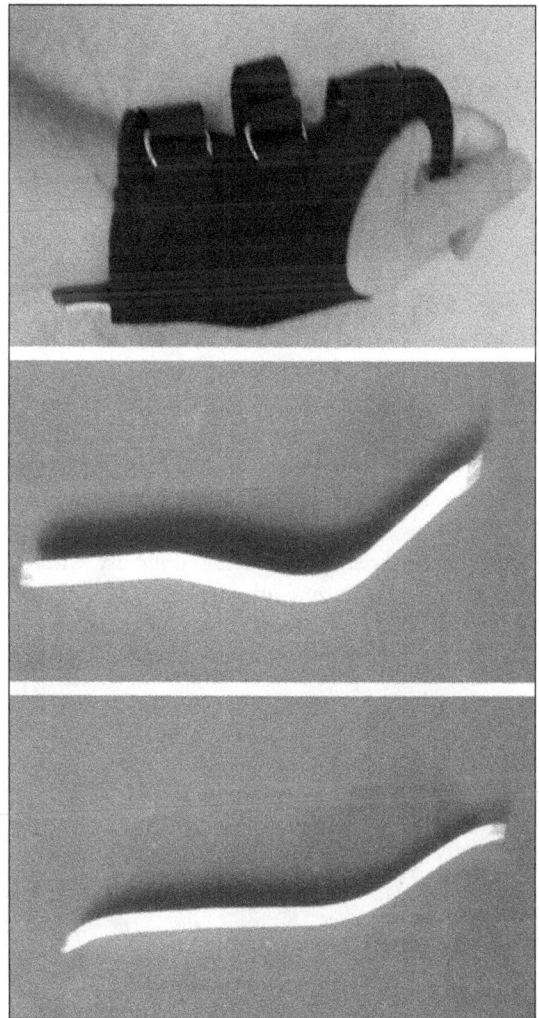

Figure 17.9. A functional day use wrist hand orthosis (WHO) with the thumb and wrist secured in neutral alignment. Metal stays can be customized to the patient via contouring, flaring metal edges at the distal and proximal ends, or by replacing them with low temperature molded stays that can be heated in a microwave and shaped to fit. A. Fully assembled. B and C. Demonstrations of the customizability of the orthotic structure, specifically in the sagittal plane.

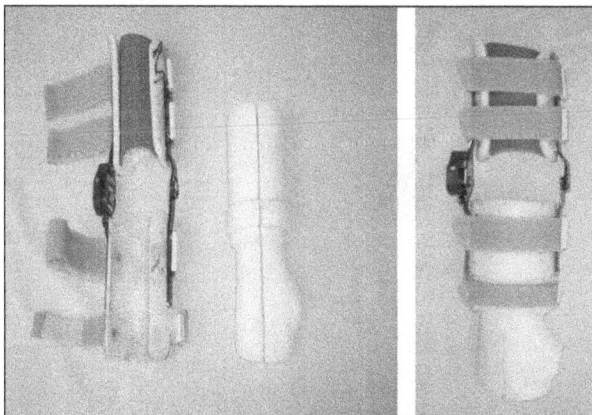

Figure 17.8. A forearm rotation elbow orthosis (FREO) combining an Ultraflex dynamic tension joint at the elbow with a static progressive configuration (interlocking forearm cuffs with Velcro® hook and loop) at the forearm. A. Disassembled. B. Fully assembled.

stay can be replaced with a low temperature molded stay to allow some active movement and resistance. Further support can be provided by ordering single to multiple layers of THK (thin, high-temperature plastic covered in Velcro®-sensitive material) to reinforce areas such as the thumb and ulnar border. The THK-reinforced orthosis can be heated in a microwave oven and molded directly on the patient to support the corrected position.

For the patient requiring support or facilitation of wrist extension who does not have significant radial or ulnar deviation, a MacKinnon splint [48] will provide washable support with minimal palmar coverage. Patients who require more support will benefit from a dorsal-based plastic WHO which can provide improved alignment in the coronal and sagittal planes while supporting wrist and palmar arches. The benefits of a dorsal design with minimal palmar coverage maximizes sensory input and is especially helpful for young children's participation in sensory play (painting, shaving cream, etc.). If needed, a universal cuff can be attached at the palmar support to assist in holding utensils, paint brushes, markers, and other tools. A focus rigidity casting univalve WHO can be helpful to improve prehension for infants and small children who need circumferential support whereas objects may slip out of a traditional WHO (Figure 17.10).

CEREBRAL PALSY

Cerebral palsy (CP) is a non-progressive lesion of the brain but the manifestations of the disease are not static. Joint contractures may progress, limb malalignment and disuse can occur with growth, fluctuations in tone may occur, and musculoskeletal compensations may be noted during activities of daily function. Up to 60% of individuals with CP experience significant difficulty with hand skills [49]. Many children with CP have spasticity which increases the tone in their upper extremities and compromises functional hand skills. When spasticity persists or increases, contractures of the upper extremity can develop, making activities of daily living even more challenging. Abnormal posturing can occur in the hand and arm causing wrist flexion, thumb adduction, forearm pronation, and more proximal compensations such as elbow flexion. These patterns make it difficult to manipulate the hand and wrist for fine motor activities [50, 51]. Flexion contractures of the upper extremity develop, and extensor muscles may weaken. Two types of therapy intervention are supported by research as effective forms of treatment: CIMT, which was discussed earlier in the CVA/TBI section, and intensive bimanual therapy [49, 51]. Bimanual therapy teaches children with hemiplegia to use both hands together to complete everyday tasks. It is an intensive program that incorporates repetitive practice of two-handed activities. In addition to therapy for strengthening and improved motor control, orthotic intervention is also indicated for individuals with CP.

Orthotic management of the upper extremity for CP can be divided into two groups: "non-functional" and "functional" hand splints. Non-functional hand splints are typically made of low temperature thermoplastics or casting materials. The purpose of these splints is to prevent contracture or increase muscle length. Resting hand splints can be made dorsal or volar, or as a combination of the two in a bivalved design. In treating the spastic upper extremity in CP, thermoplastic such as polyform or aquaform is molded to encourage extension of the wrist and fingers with the thumb abducted and in the opposed position. Due to the movement limitation and potential for disuse atrophy from this type of splint, they are primarily used at night to increase muscle length. It can be challenging to keep hand splints in place, specifically with the pediatric patient particularly regarding material weight, thickness, and strapping techniques. Use of thinner thermoplastic

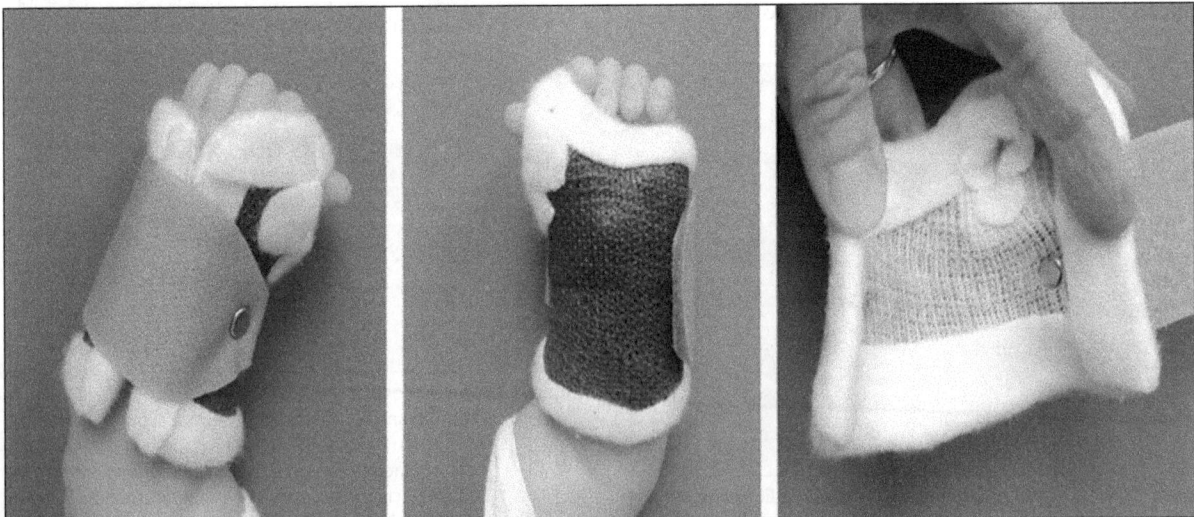

Figure 17.10. A universal cuff attached to a palmar support can assist in holding utensils etc. Shown is an infant's focus rigidity casting univalve WHO: A. dorsal view; B. volar view; C. interior surface.

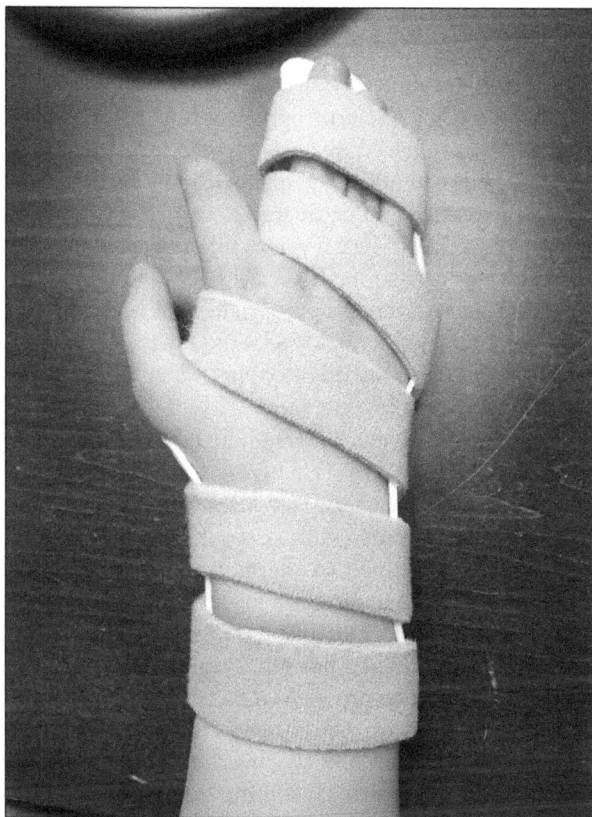

Figure 17.11. Spiral strapping technique for securing a hand splint in a child with cerebral palsy.

allows for improved molding and contouring of the child's anatomy, especially in the web space of the thumb and fingers. Maintaining a total contact fit with respect to orthotic trimlines and the use of strapping that is snug can minimize bridging away from the skin and minimize device migration. Use of slot straps can prevent migration of the device. Rivets can be used to secure the straps on the splint and avoids the potential of a choking hazard. Other strapping techniques such as diagonal application or spiral strapping (Figure 17.11) can provide a more secure closure and avoid unwanted splint removal. Use of excessive padding or linings in thermoplastic splints should be avoided to prevent bacterial build-up and skin irritation. Use of appropriate, minimal padding optimizes daily cleaning of thermoplastic splints using a damp cloth with soap and water or alcohol for hygiene and to protect skin integrity. Orthotic management of more proximal tightness at the elbow can be addressed with custom elbow extension splints or with off the shelf devices. Increasing elbow ROM can be achieved with devices such as an ultraflex system or a JAS brace (Effingham, IL) where low-load prolonged stretch can be applied to the joint.

Functional hand splints are used to improve biomechanical alignment and to provide support to the hand and wrist for successful completion of functional tasks. When choosing the design for functional hand splints, one needs to consider avoiding excessive palmar and volar coverage as this can impair sensory feedback [49, 51]. The primary

goal of functional hand splint such as the McKie splint (McKie Splints, Duluth, MN) or Joe Cool splint (The Joe Cool Company, South Jordan, UT) is to improve thumb position into abduction and opposition for grasp [52]. The addition of a supinator strap may encourage supination for tasks such as picking up a cup or holding a pencil. Wrist extension orthoses are indicated when a more functional wrist and hand position are needed. Flexion of the wrist and adduction of the thumb is the typical spastic pattern noted. Use of a neoprene-type wrist extension and thumb abduction splint, such as the Benik (Benik Corporation, Silverdale, WA), places the arm in a functional position for increased distal control of the thumb and fingers for activities such as grasp and release. When choosing a neoprene device, it is important that the material is not so thick that it blocks movement and function. This style of bracing can improve the spontaneous use of an involved extremity during bi-manual tasks in children with hemiplegic CP [53]. Addition of a supinator strap can also be used with the wrist hand orthosis.

As in patients with CVA and TBI, use of electrical stimulation with orthotic devices can be effective in reducing tone and improving upper extremity function. Dynamic bracing of the hand, wrist, and elbow is fabricated and used two to three times a day with electrical stimulation of the antagonist muscle groups, extensors. Retention of improved hand function upon cessation of therapy intervention is only for a limited amount of time [55, 54].

Compliance with upper extremity orthotics needs to be considered. Compliance for upper limb orthosis is less than 50% in children with hemiplegia [51]. When treating individuals with CP, most often you are dealing with the pediatric population and their family and caregivers. Orthotic compliance can be challenging. Multiple factors require discussion such as determining patient and family goals, history of previous orthotic failures and successes, orthotic expectations and more. Education regarding design and functions of each orthotic option will help the clinician, patient, and family to determine the most appropriate orthoses for the individual. Empowering patients and families in the decision-making process will improve compliance and effectiveness of the device in achieving functional goals [56].

ARTHROGRYPOSIS

Arthrogryposis Multiplex Congenita (AMC) is an orthopedic condition in which patients present with multiple congenital contractures. While the contracture pathology is usually non-progressive, the contractures need to be addressed as the lack of muscle balance and the patient's movement patterns will allow the contractures to progress, thus decreasing upper extremity function. Primary deformities created by nerve and muscle damage during the early fetal stage tend to recur after correction and will require long-term orthotic use. Positional deformities which occur later during the fetal stage due to lack of movement usually will improve with therapy and freedom of movement. Commonly seen contractures are internal rotation of the shoulder, extension of the elbow, pronation or supination of the forearm, wrist and finger flexion.

Common goals for the patient who present with elbow extension and wrist flexion contractures include a neutral functioning wrist and 90° of elbow flexion. This position promotes functional hand to face and mouth patterns and desk access from a seated position. Once this goal is achieved, night-time use of an orthosis is most effective for preventing recurrence as sleep accounts for one-third to half of a child's daily schedule. This minimizes interference to play or tactile input [57].

Daytime orthotic use requires consideration relative to functional goals. Arthrogryposis presents a challenge in upper extremity orthotic intervention as each patient's presentation of functional use and their ability to adapt is unique. Often devices are rejected due to the patient's ability to adapt to their muscle function and be more efficient and comfortable without any orthosis. Intervention should address alignment issues and minimize long-term wear and tear on joints.

A typical pattern seen with arthrogryposis is to weight bear on a flexed wrist with the dorsal hand or MCPs. Often this is seen to assist in transitioning in and out of standing. This flexed wrist pattern can impair grasp. WHOs, either dorsal- or volar-based, position the wrist in neutral to extension for transfers and provide a functional position to stabilize the wrist for hand function. The addition of individual finger tubes with extension assist straps on the WHO may further improve function by bringing the fingers away from the palm, which can provide fingertip access to buttons. It also increases the functional hand

opening needed for tasks such as doorknob access. This allows the patient use of the lever and mass of their arm to open a door or cabinet (Figure 17.12).

Serial casting for arthrogryposis can be successful, particularly if followed by goal-oriented, consistent daily and/or nightly orthotic use to maintain gains realized from casting. A plaster and/or fiberglass cast that is changed every 1–2 weeks or with a removable univalve polyester fiberglass tape casting method called Focus Rigidity Casting (FRC) is a clinically appropriate therapeutic option. Over the course of several weeks the range of motion is gradually increased, usually stopping when the range has plateaued after two cast changes.

Plaster casting can be removed by soaking and by means of bandage scissors whereas fiberglass and plaster casts require a cast saw for safe removal. Casts may be bivalved and secured with straps if there is a need for regular skin inspection. An alternative to the bivalve cast is a univalve cast that ensures a more intimate fit and less chance of migration. FRC may be used for serial casting the upper extremity and has other applications including fracture and wound care management. The univalve cast is ideal for families whose concerns are about compliance to skin precautions such as keeping the cast clean and dry or their ability to return for routine cast change appointments. For families that travel considerable distances to the casting clinic, the univalve cast provides some flexibility. The polyester casting tape is flexible with no sharp fiberglass edges and can be donned and doffed through a single opening. Additional layers of the polyester casting material are applied to areas requiring reinforcement while minimal layers are used in the circumferential wrap. This, for example, allows the clinician to create a cast design to stop ulnar deviation and flexion at the wrist, as well as flexion or extension at the elbow. The univalve type requires edge finishing with adhesive liner at the opening and straps.

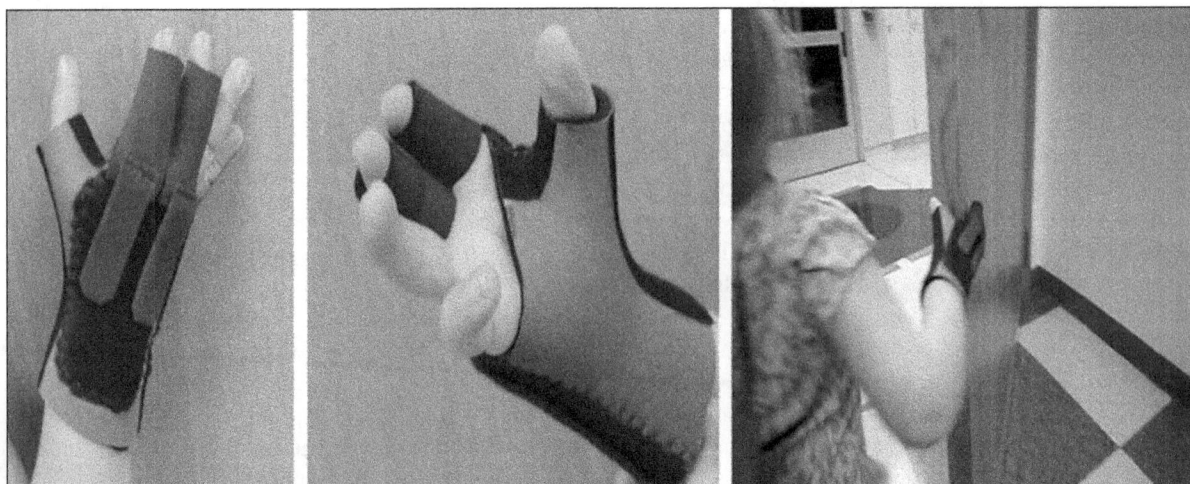

Figure 17.12. Additional individual finger tubes with extension assist straps on a WHO used to improve prehension by bringing the fingers away from the palm A. Dorsal view showing extensor straps; B. palmar view; and C. demonstration of functional utilization.

PEDIATRIC CONSIDERATIONS AND TIPS

For pediatric patients under the age of three or older children with developmental delays, it is important to confirm that there are no small straps, pads, or parts that may come loose and become a choking hazard. Additionally, orthoses for children under the age of three may need to be hand-/wrist-based in order to be secured in place well. Spiral wrapping a long strap distal to proximal will eliminate the need for small straps. Another method is to use CoFlex® wrap (Andover Healthcare Inc. [DBA Ovik Health], Salisbury, MA) to secure an orthosis (Figure 17.13). Coflex® wrap adheres to itself without leaving adhesive residue. It is important to use a large enough piece to prevent it from becoming a choking hazard. Secure it at the thumb by cutting a hole in the material to create an anchor site. Finally, it is important to wrap from distal to proximal and to instruct the caregiver in checking correct tension through capillary refill.

It can be challenging to attain measurements or tracings for a low temperature orthosis on small or distractible children. Placing the child's hand on a copier machine to get an accurate tracing of the hand may be helpful. For the child who is in pain or anxious about the process, tracing or measuring the non-involved hand can be helpful if there is not a size discrepancy.

GENERAL CONSIDERATIONS AND TIPS

Scheduling a follow-up visit within the first couple of weeks following the initial fitting can help facilitate orthotic compliance and appropriate device use. If the orthosis is to be used long term, additional follow-ups on a quarterly basis can help monitor device fit and function. It is important to confirm that there is adequate relief at bony prominences to avoid contact with any plastic or metal. Straps should be total contact with the skin and not bridging the borders of the orthosis. Reducing trim lines or the addition of a pad can achieve a total contact fit. The correct pull of straps needs to be at 90° in order

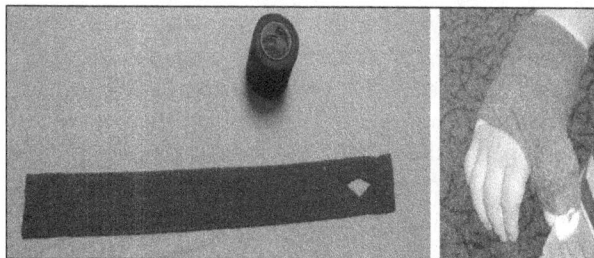

Figure 17.13. Self-adherent Coflex® wrap used to secure a thumb spica orthosis.

to maximize correction and avoid shear forces that can irritate the skin. Slotted straps can improve the angle of pull and also minimize straps from being lost or pulled off. Finally, it is recommended to verify correct anatomical alignment in all planes while wearing the orthotic device.

SUMMARY

This chapter presented pathologies and impairments that can benefit from orthotic and rehabilitative management of the upper extremity(ies). It should be emphasized that outcomes tend to be improved when a multidisciplinary team, utilizing evidence-based practice, is engaged in patient management. The chapter culminates with two case studies described below.

CASE STUDY: ELBOW CONTRACTURE MANAGEMENT

History

Patient is a 13-year-old male with primary diagnosis of left elbow osteochondronal fragment and elbow soft tissue contracture. He was initially immobilized in a splint due to a fall on his outstretched arm/hand while skateboarding. His pain was resolved, and he returned to his normal activities. One month after the initial injury he fell again on his elbow while skateboarding. He was immobilized but due to persistent pain and swelling had an MRI performed. The patient also had eight sessions of physical therapy without improvement. He presented in clinic for a second opinion about 4 months after the initial injury.

Presentation

	RIGHT	LEFT
ELBOW EXTENSION	0°	−35°
ELBOW FLEXION	140°	132°
FOREARM SUPINATION	90°	75°
FOREARM PRONATION	85°	85°

The patient complained of a small amount of pain but primarily was bothered by the lack of movement and strength. He also participated in speed skating, requiring protective extension and arm strength.

The second MRI indicated a minimally displaced osteochondral fragment. Non-surgical and surgical options were discussed with the family and a non-surgical treatment plan of aggressive physical therapy and orthotic management was chosen.

Intervention

The treatment options included static progressive low temperature orthosis remolded to the patient's range of motion gains from therapy and home program every 1–2 weeks, serial casting, and a dynamic orthosis.

The goal of the orthosis was to increase both flexion and extension range of motion for decreased pain and improved functional reach of the upper extremity. The functional arc of elbow range of motion for ADLs is 100° for both flexion and extension, less than 45° pronation and supination. The loss of supination is more disabling; pronation can be compensated with shoulder abduction. A lesser range of motion loss may be considered nonfunctional if it significantly impairs lifestyle [43].

The orthopedic physician prescribed a dynamic, torsion style, left elbow orthosis to initially address limitation in elbow extension and later augment flexion. Due to the patient's thin build and age, a custom orthosis was necessary to obtain optimal positioning of the left upper extremity impression and measurements were taken.

The patient was fit with left Ultraflex elbow orthosis with a bi-directional tension joint set-up for addressing increasing elbow extension (elbow flexion to be addressed once full elbow extension is achieved). The elbow orthosis consisted of plastic posterior shells, free motion medial joint, tension Ultraflex lateral joint, a foam anterior humeral cuff, and four anterior straps. At the initial fitting, the dynamic joint tension was set at '1/2' to begin treatment; tension set at '1' caused discomfort at the posterior, distal humeral cuff during trial wearing period.

His mother expressed concern regarding frequency of appointments for tension adjustments on the mechanical elbow joint with her work traveling schedule and patient's school schedule. The patient's mother was provided with instructions on how to adjust the joint in 1/2 increments, joint precautions, and importance of increasing length of time wearing orthosis rather than tension. The mother was also instructed that tension should not be increased over a 3 or 4 during the course of treatment and that before increasing the tension by a 1/2 increment, he must be able to tolerate a week of full nightly use without discomfort in the morning.

After a trial of conservative range of motion therapy and orthotic intervention for approximately 3 months, his range of motion gains plateaued and the patient could not tolerate increasing the tension on the dynamic extension joint. At his orthopedist follow-up visit, the decision was made to remove the bone fragment. After surgery the patient continued with orthotic use and resumed physical therapy.

At 2 months post-op the patient was pain-free and pleased with his elbow range of motion (–25° extension and 125° flexion). The physician instructed the patient to continue his home program and orthotic use. At 5 months post-op the patient was able to resume all activities with his range of motion (–25° extension and 135° flexion).

Case study question: When would a dynamic elbow orthosis such as the Ultraflex elbow extension orthosis not be recommended as a treatment intervention?

Answer: *When the contracture has been present for greater than one year.*

CASE STUDY: BILATERAL UPPER EXTREMITY MANAGEMENT FOR PEDIATRIC PATIENT WITH CEREBRAL PALSY

History

The patient is a 7-year-old female with primary diagnosis of CP with left hemiplegia, developmental delay and Williams syndrome. Children with Williams syndrome typically present with low muscle tone and joint laxity but are at risk for joint contractures later in childhood (www.williams-syndrome.org).

Presentation

	RESTING POSTURE	PASSIVE RANGE OF MOTION
Elbow	35° flexion	0–145°
Forearm	80° pronation	80–45°
Wrist	20–60° flexion with 10–20° ulnar deviation	Within Normal Limits (WNL)
Digits 2–5	45° flexion	WNL
Thumb	0° adduction	WNL

Her mother reports the patient tends not to use her left upper extremity without cueing. Functionally, she can raise her arms to push a stroller by resting her hands on the handle with her forearms pronated but has difficulty with functional grasp of the handle due to thumb adduction bilaterally. Her mother reports previously using a right neoprene-style WHO with a volar stay but notices that she is still able to flex and ulnar deviate her wrist. The patient did complain of some pain with end range stretch in supination. Her occupational therapist and physical therapist provided input for the orthoses. Her mother was involved, and the patient was cooperative and motivated to participate.

Her goals include decreasing upper extremity pain, increasing range of motion for improved grasp and reach, and improving left upper extremity use as a functional assist.

Intervention

The patient was fit with the following.

1. A left, elbow wrist hand orthosis with joints, supination with full hand included for night time stretching.
2. A right Benik-type neoprene wrist hand finger orthosis, with a volar THK panel wrapped around the ulnar side.
3. A Bilateral Benik type neoprene wrist hand orthosis with THK volar/ulnar panel for use during the day.

All the Benik devices were heated (THK panels) and molded to patient in 15°–20° wrist extension and neutral in the coronal plane, thumbs in functional abduction position.

The family was familiar with the WHFO and WHO devices. The patient demonstrated improved alignment of the wrist and thumb at rest. Functionally she demonstrated a stronger and more efficient grasp with her thumb abduction. Time was taken to have the mother practice donning the two-piece interlocking EWHO for supination. The patient tolerated an extended stretch in 15°–20° supination without complaints of discomfort. The family was pleased with the devices and was given the expectation that some adjustments and follow-up visits may be needed to optimize function as the patient begins routine wear and to monitor her progress with supination.

Case study question: What is the optimal position to obtain assessment and stretch into supination?

Answer: *90° elbow flexion with stabilization.*

REFERENCES

[1] Aoyagi Y, Tsubahara A. Therapeutic orthosis and electrical stimulation for upper extremity hemiplegia after stroke: a review of effectiveness based on evidence. *Top Stroke Rehabil.* 2004;11(3):9–15.

[2] Tyson SF, Kent RM. The effect of upper limb orthotics after stroke: a systematic review. *NeuroRehabilitation.* 2011;28(1):29–36.

[3] Hsu JD, Michael JW, Fisk JR, eds. *AAOS Atlas of Orthoses and Assistive Devices,* 2008. 4th edition. Mosby Elsevier, Philadelphia, PA.

[4] Ada L, Foongchomcheay A, Canning CG, Cochrane Stroke Group. Supportive devices for preventing and treating subluxation of the shoulder after stroke. In: The Cochrane Collaboration, ed. *Cochrane Database of Systematic Reviews,* 2005. John Wiley & Sons, Chichester, UK. Accessed October 4, 2016. http://doi.wiley.com/10.1002/14651858.CD003863.pub2.

[5] Cappato de Araújo R, Rocha D, Pitangui A, Pinotti M. The influence of dynamic orthosis training on upper extremity function after stroke: a pilot study. *J Healthc Eng.* 2014;5(1):55–66.

[6] Höhler C, Hermsdörfer J, Jahn K, Krewer C. The assistive potential of functional electrical stimulation to support object manipulation in functional upper extremity movements after stroke: a randomized cross-over study. *J Cent Nerv Syst Dis.* 2024 May 6;16.

[7] Cempini M, Giovacchini F, Vitiello N, et al. NEUROExos: a powered elbow orthosis for post-stroke early neurorehabilitation. *Proc Int Conf IEEE Eng Med Biol Soc EMBC.* 2013:342–345.

[8] Long C. Advances in myoelectric bracing. *O&P Alm.* 2016 June;65:28.

[9] Myomo–myoelectric orthosis arm brace upper limb c brace MyoPro. Accessed October 14, 2016. http://myomo.com/.

[10] Lannin N., Horsley S, Herbert R, et al. Splinting the hand in the functional position after brain impairment: a randomized, controlled trial. *Arch Phys Med Rehabil.* 2003;84(2):297–302.

[11] Schaechter JD. Motor rehabilitation and brain plasticity after hemiparetic stroke. *Prog Neurobiol.* 2004;73:61–72.

[12] Cadman P. Neuroplasticity: achieve the best outcomes with neurological patients. *Phys Ther Prod.* 2015;26:14–17.

[13] Kunkel A, Kopp B, Müller G, et al. Constraint-induced movement therapy for motor recovery in chronic stroke patients. *Arch Phys Med Rehabil.* 1999;80:624–628.

[14] Page SJ, Sisto S, Levine P, McGrath RE. Efficacy of modified constraint-induced movement therapy in chronic stroke: a single-blinded randomized controlled trial. *Arch Phys Med Rehabil.* 2004;85:14–18.

[15] Garber SL, Gregorio TL. Upper extremity assistive devices: assessment of use by spinal cord-injured patients with quadriplegia. *Am J Occup Ther.* 1990;44(2):126–131.

[16] Sarmiento A, Latta L. The evolution of functional bracing of fractures. *J Bone Jt Surg Br.* 2006;88(2):141–148.

[17] Walker M, Palumbo B, Badman B, et al. Humeral shaft fractures: a review. *J Shoulder Elbow Surg.* 2011;20(5):833–844.

[18] Koch PP, Gross DFL, Gerber C. The results of functional (Sarmiento) bracing of humeral shaft fractures. *J Shoulder Elbow Surg.* 2002;11(2):143–150.

[19] Ekholm R, Tidermark J, Törnkvist H, et al. Outcome after closed functional treatment of humeral shaft fractures. *J Orthop Trauma.* 2006;20(9):591–596.

[20] S. Rutgers M, Ring D. Treatment of diaphyseal fractures of the humerus using a functional brace. *J Orthop Trauma.* 2006;20(9):597–601.

[21] Papasoulis E, Drosos GI, Ververidis AN, Verettas D-A. Functional bracing of humeral shaft fractures. A review of clinical studies. *Injury.* 2010;41(7):e21–e27.

[22] Ostermann PA, Ekkernkamp A, Henry SL, Muhr G. Bracing of stable shaft fractures of the ulna. *J Orthop Trauma.* 1994;8(3):245–248.

[23] Gebuhr P, Hölmich P, Orsnes T, et al. Isolated ulnar shaft fractures. Comparison of treatment by a functional brace and long-arm cast. *J Bone Joint Surg Br.* 1992;74(5):757–759.

[24] Uğurlu Ü, Özdoğan H. Effects of serial casting in the treatment of flexion contractures of proximal interphalangeal joints in patients with rheumatoid arthritis and juvenile idiopathic arthritis: a retrospective study. *J Hand Ther.* 2016;29(1):41–50.

[25] Nandi S, Maschke S, Evans PJ, Lawton JN. The stiff elbow. *HAND.* 2009;4(4):368–379.

[26] Shirley ED, DeMaio M, Bodurtha J. Ehlers-Danlos syndrome in orthopaedics: etiology, diagnosis, and treatment implications. *Sports Health.* 2012;4(5):394–403.

[27] Baronio G, Harran S, Signoroni A. A critical analysis of a hand orthosis reverse engineering and 3D printing process. *Appl Bionics Biomech.* 2016;2016:1–7.

[28] Silva R, Silva B, Fernandez C, et al. A review on 3D scanners studies for producing customized orthoses. *Sensors.* 2024 Feb 20;24(5):1373.

[29] Maurel ML, Fitzgerald LG, Miles AW, Giddins GEB. Biomechanical study of the efficacy of a new design of wrist guard. *Clin Biomech.* 2013;28(5):509–513.

[30] Staebler MP, Moore DC, Akelman E, et al. The effect of wrist guards on bone strain in the distal forearm. *Am J Sports Med.* 1999;27(4):500–506.

[31] Almekinders LC, Tao MA, Zarzour R. Playing hurt: hand and wrist injuries and protected return to sport. *Sports Med Arthrosc Rev.* 2014;22(1):66–70.

[32] Kneeshaw D. Shoulder taping in the clinical setting. *J Bodyw Mov Ther.* 2002 January;6(1):2–8.

[33] Chu JC, Kane EJ, Arnold BL, Gansneder BM. The effect of a neoprene shoulder stabilizer on active joint-reposition sense in subjects with stable and unstable shoulders. *J Athl Train.* 2002;37(2):141–145.

[34] Buss DD, Lynch GP, Meyer CP, et al. Nonoperative management for in-season athletes with anterior shoulder instability. *Am J Sports Med.* 2004;32(6):1430–1433.

[35] Wilk KE, Macrina LC, Reinold MM. Non-operative rehabilitation for traumatic and atraumatic glenohumeral instability. *N Am J Sports Phys Ther.* 2006;1(1):16–30.

[36] Bisset LM, Collins NJ, Offord SS. Immediate effects of 2 types of braces on pain and grip strength in people with lateral epicondylalgia: a randomized controlled trial. *J Orthop Sports Phys Ther.* 2014;44(2):120–128.

[37] Russell CR. Therapy challenges for athletes: splinting options. *Clin Sports Med.* 2015;34(1):181–191.

[38] Jacobs MA, Austin NM. *Orthotic Intervention for the Hand and Upper Extremity Splinting Principles and Process,* 2014. 2nd edition. Lippincott Williams & Wilkins, Philadelphia, PA.

[39] Jacobs MA, Austin NM. *Splinting the Hand and Upper Extremity Principles and Process,* 2003. Lippincott Williams & Wilkins, 2003, Philadelphia, PA.

[40] Michael JW, Nunley JA. Special considerations: brachial plexus injuries: surgical advances and orthotic/prosthetic management. In: Bowker HK, Michael JW, eds. *Atlas of Limb Prosthetics: Surgical, Prosthetic, and Rehabilitation Principles,* 2002. American Academy of Orthopedic Surgeons (AAOS), Rosemont, IL, Originally published 1992.

[41] Malessy MJA, Pondaag W. Obstetric brachial plexus injuries. *Neurosurg Clin N Am.* 2009;20(1):1–14.

[42] Nuismer BA, Ekes AM, Holm MB. The use of low-load prolonged stretch devices in rehabilitation programs in the Pacific northwest. *Am J Occup Ther.* 1997;51(7):538–543.

[43] Morrey BF, Askew LJ, Chao EY. A biomechanical study of normal functional elbow motion. *J Bone Jt Surg Am.* 1981;63(6):872–877.

[44] Stevens P, DiBello T. The use of dynamic orthoses in reducing knee flexion contractures in a pediatric patient with myelomeningocele. *Acad TODAY.* 2006 October:A10–A11.

[45] Light KE, Nuzik S, Personius W, Barstrom A. Low-load prolonged stretch vs. high-load brief stretch in treating knee contractures. *Phys Ther.* 1984;64(3):330–333.

[46] Yasukawa A, Cassar M. Children with elbow extension and forearm rotation limitation: functional outcomes using the forearm rotation elbow orthosis. *JPO.* 2009;21(3):160–166.

[47] Scott-Tatum L. Lycra-based splinting, can it really help? Second Skin, 2003. Accessed October 14, 2016 https://www.secondskin.com.au/files/c71bf8f0-3b6e-11e7-9907-57fd0036ed80/Can%20Lycra%20Based%20Splinting%20Help%2018_10_2006.pdf.

[48] Flegle JH, Leibowitz JM. Improvement in grasp skill in children with hemiplegia with the MacKinnon splint. *Res Dev Disabil.* 1988;9(2):145–151.

[49] Jackman M, Novak I, Lannin N. Effectiveness of hand splints in children with cerebral palsy: a systematic review with meta-analysis. *Dev Med Child Neurol.* 2014;56(2):138–147.

[50] Barroso PN, Vecchio SD, Xavier YR, et al. Improvement of hand function in children with cerebral palsy via an orthosis that provides wrist extension and thumb abduction. *Clin Biomech.* 2011;26(9):937–943.

[51] Basu AP, Pearse J, Kelly S, et al. Early intervention to improve hand function in hemiplegic cerebral palsy. *Front Neurol.* 2015 Jan 6;5:281.

[52] Teplicky R, Law M, Russell D. The effectiveness of casts, orthoses, and splints for children with neurological disorders. *Infants Young Child.* 2002;15(1):42–50.

[53] Louwers A, Meester-Delver A, Folmer K, et al. Immediate effect of a wrist and thumb brace on bimanual activities in children with hemiplegic cerebral palsy: bracing and bimanual activities in cp. *Dev Med Child Neurol.* 2011;53(4):321–326.

[54] Ozer K, Chesher SP, Scheker LR. Neuromuscular electrical stimulation and dynamic bracing for the management of upper-extremity spasticity in children with cerebral palsy. *Dev Med Child Neurol.* 2006;48(7):559–563.

[55] Scheker LR, Chesher SP, Ramirez S. Neuromuscular electrical stimulation and dynamic bracing as a treatment for upper-extremity spasticity in children with cerebral palsy. *J Hand Surg Br.* 1999;24(2):226–232.

[56] Russo RN, Atkins R, Haan E, Crotty M. Upper limb orthoses and assistive technology utilization in children with hemiplegic cerebral palsy recruited from a population register. *Dev Neurorehabil.* 2009;12(2):92–99.

[57] Flowers KR, LaStayo P. Effect of total end range time on improving passive range of motion. *J Hand Ther.* 1994;7(3):150–157.

A special thank you to Erin Claussen, MPO, orthotics resident, for her assistance in writing this chapter.

BASIC LOWER EXTREMITY PROSTHETIC CHECKOUT

Below are basic and essential items the PT should consider evaluating when conducting a basic lower extremity prosthesis checkout. The PT may wish to include additional items depending on patient needs and goals.

1) Prescription

2) Gait evaluation

3) Sitting inspection

4) Doff prosthesis

5) Sock ply? Half socks?

6) Liner? Type of liner? Pin position?

7) Skin inspection
   ** Redness is WNL (within normal limits) if it dissipates within a few minutes; persistent redness for several hours is not OK and may indicate beginning skin breakdown

8) Breakdown?

9) Previous adjustments to interface?

10) Inspect prosthesis (visual/palpation)

11) Is the patient able to don/doff shoe onto prosthetic foot? (appropriate foot size)

12) Don prosthesis

INDEX

Note: Page numbers in *italics* refer to figures and those in **bold** to tables.

For Product Safety Concerns and Information please contact our EU
representative GPSR@taylorandfrancis.com
Taylor & Francis Verlag GmbH, Kaufingerstraße 24, 80331 München, Germany

www.ingramcontent.com/pod-product-compliance
Lightning Source LLC
Chambersburg PA
CBHW081056220326
41598CB00038B/7124